The 30-Day Blood Pressure Cure

The Drug-Free, Step-by-Step Plan to Reverse Your Hypertension and Drop Your Blood Pressure into the Safety Zone

Roy Heilbron, MD, and Jim Healthy

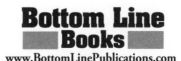

Bottom Line Books
www.BottomLinePublications.com

Bottom Line Books® Edition 2014
Published by arrangement with Jim Healthy Publications, Inc.
ISBN 0-88723-702-9

10 9 8 7 6 5 4 3 2 1

This book is based on the research and observations of the author. The information contained in this book should by no means be considered a substitute for the advice of the reader's personal physician or other medical professional, who should always be consulted before beginning any health program.

The information in this book has been carefully researched, and all efforts have been made to ensure accuracy as of the date published. Readers, particularly those with existing health problems and those who take prescription medications, are cautioned to consult with a health professional about specific recommendations for supplements and the appropriate dosages. The author and the publisher expressly disclaim responsibility for any adverse effects arising from the use or application of the information contained in this book.

Bottom Line Books® is a registered trademark of Boardroom® Inc.
281 Tresser Blvd., Stamford, CT 06901
www.BottomLinePublications.com

Bottom Line Books® publishes the opinions of expert authorities in many fields. The use of this book is not a substitute for health or other professional services. Please consult a competent professional for answers to your specific questions.

Offers, prices, addresses, telephone numbers and Web sites listed in this book are accurate at the time of publication, but they are subject to frequent change.

Bottom Line Books® is an imprint of Boardroom® Inc., publisher of print periodicals, e-letters and books. We are dedicated to bringing you the best information from the most knowledgeable sources in the world. Our goal is to help you gain greater wealth, better health, more wisdom, extra time and increased happiness.

Printed in the United States of America

TABLE OF CONTENTS

PHASE THREE

Appendices

Endnotes

THE NONDRUG SOLUTION FOR HIGH BLOOD PRESSURE

Blood pressure is a term that describes the force of blood pushing against the walls of the arteries as the heart pumps blood. The higher your blood pressure, the harder your heart pumps. *High blood pressure,* also known as hypertension, is a condition in which the force of blood in arteries is chronically elevated. If this pressure remains high over time, it can wreak havoc throughout the body.

WHAT CAN BE DONE ABOUT HYPERTENSION?

Is there a true solution for high blood pressure? Indeed there is. A nondrug solution *does* exist even though doctors stubbornly insist that drugs are the best way to deal with this serious health threat.

That's the good news. Better news: There is nothing new or high-tech about it. The solution involves simple lifestyle changes that can be adopted in merely 30 days.

There is no doubt that high blood pressure has reached epidemic rates in the US and other Western cultures. More than 60% of the US adult population has abnormal blood pressure, including hypertension and pre-hypertension. More than 50% of Americans over age 60 are diagnosed with hypertension. Of those patients currently taking antihypertension drugs—many on multiple medications—a considerable number *don't* have their blood pressure under control. Yet doctors remain stumped and mind-boggled by it, professing that 90% of all high blood pressure is "idiopathic," meaning it has "no known cause." Of the factors they attribute to high blood pressure, excessive salt consumption and uncontrolled stress lead their list.

HIGH BLOOD PRESSURE IS A DISEASE OF CIVILIZATION

We have reliable records that high blood pressure did not exist in primitive cultures before the appearance of European settlers. Nor does it exist today in those indigenous tribes where modern civilization hasn't fully intruded.

So then, is rampant high blood pressure the consequence of the high-sodium foods and high-stress lifestyle that are hallmarks of modern, civilized culture? Doctors would have us believe so—but please don't accept either notion because both are unsubstantiated. As you'll see in this book, neither of these causes plays a major role (if any at all) in this widespread problem.

In light of these facts, it's fair to say that the modern medical approach to treating hypertension is failing. A major reason for this is that doctors are almost entirely invested in pharmaceutical solutions. It's no big surprise why. Blood pressure medications alone are worth $17 billion a year to the pharmaceutical industry; and drugmakers, being the profit-oriented business people that they are, would eagerly ignore or try to discredit any option that might discourage drug use. Yet, as you'll see in this book, diet and lifestyle modifications can produce dramatic improvements in blood pressure for those patients who are willing to make them.

WHY WE WROTE THIS BOOK

For the majority of our careers, we have committed ourselves to providing the public with information about a more balanced approach to health and healing. As helpful as drugs and surgeries can sometimes be, they are almost always fraught with risks. Our mission is to help everyone achieve a level of optimal health that makes risky medical interventions unnecessary. And for those instances when a health problem does manifest itself, we are dedicated to providing patients and readers, alike, with safe, effective and well-documented non-pharmaceutical healing alternatives to help people improve their own health in noncritical situations.

YOUR DOCTOR SHOULD BE YOUR PARTNER

The trick to good self-care, of course, is in the timing. Generally speaking, a medical emergency is no time to employ a natural remedy. While conventional medicine certainly has its shortcomings, its great strength lies in its ability to intervene successfully at the eleventh hour. If you are in an emergency situation (say, if your blood pressure is 200/140 or higher), please follow your doctor's recommendations without hesitation. Not to do so is foolish and potentially deadly.

Whether your current blood pressure is critical or not, we urge you to read this book carefully and thoroughly—and to discuss its contents with your physician. Under his or her watchful eye, you're invited to try some of the suggested remedies described in these pages and to monitor your results by taking your blood pressure at home several times during the day. This way, you and your doctor can note the positive effects that our suggestions may elicit, and under his direction have your medication dose lowered or entirely eliminated.

Please don't accept anything in this book on blind faith. Like a good scientist, approach these ideas with a healthy skepticism and an objective desire to discover the truth. Observe your body's response carefully—and then draw your own conclusions.

Of course, you should *never* stop your medication or change your dose without your doctor's knowledge and consent. But if you're seeing consistent reductions in your blood pressure by following the tips in this book, your doctor should be delighted by your improvements and eager to lower your dose or take you off of antihypertensive drugs entirely.

HOW TO USE THIS BOOK

We've divided this book into two parts. Part One presents you with a basic understanding of hypertension—what causes it, what exacerbates it, and what helps reverse it. You'll discover the most recent clinical findings by researchers and see how to apply that knowledge to your own life.

In Part Two, which begins on page 175, we have created a step-by-step plan to begin to reverse your hypertension and significantly improve your overall health in just 30 days.

PART ONE

REVERSE YOUR HYPERTENSION NOW

CHAPTER ONE

GOT HIGH BLOOD PRESSURE?
YOU ARE NOT ALONE

So, you've just visited the doctor, perhaps for your regular checkup, and the nurse strapped a compression cuff on your arm to check your blood pressure. In pops the doctor to listen to your heart with his stethoscope and then the verdict: "You have hypertension." Next thing you know he hands you a prescription for a drug (or two), tells you to cut back on your sodium, lose some weight, get some exercise, and then sends you on your way.

If you've picked up this book, chances are you've been searching for a better way to treat your condition than Big Medicine's approach. The good news: *"You just found it!"*

The truth, which most people are not hearing, is that there are *plenty* of effective ways to improve and reverse hypertension—and not one involves drugs. The dietary advice, healing foods, herbs, supplements, and lifestyle changes you'll discover in the chapters ahead have proven highly successful for tens of thousands of hypertension patients, so you can be confident that they'll work for you, too.

And these are not radical, superhuman changes that turn your life upside down. On the contrary, we've made this really easy because small changes can work wonders when it comes to healing your hypertension. Here's a sneak peek: Add a little olive oil to your diet, start eating more berries and yogurt, and skip the bread and baked goods. How hard is that?

HYPERTENSION IS EPIDEMIC THESE DAYS

This may come as a shock, but nearly 60% of adults in the US have hypertension—or may be on the verge of developing it—according to research published in the *Archives of Internal Medicine.* [1]

This conclusion comes from national health data collected for the Centers for Disease Control and Prevention (CDC), which found that more than half of all adults surveyed (58.2%) had blood pressure readings that placed them into the categories of either "hypertensive" or "pre-hypertensive." Nearly 36 million of those adults—more than half—have *uncontrolled* high blood pressure, even though many of these people have insurance coverage and easy access to healthcare. [2]

According to the survey, hypertension and pre-hypertension occur most commonly among non-Hispanic blacks (63%), especially men (69%); among all adults surveyed age 60+ (88%); those with less than a high school education (65%); and those with body-mass indexes over 30, indicating obesity. If you fit into any of these groups, this book should be of great interest and help to you.

"The prevalence of either pre-hypertension or hypertension among both men and women who were not overweight was 47%. But among overweight individuals, it increased to almost 60%, and among those who were obese, the prevalence was 76%," said the study's lead author. "This is of great concern…recent national survey data show that approximately two-thirds of American adults are overweight or obese."

Most troubling of all: Research reveals that awareness and appropriate management of high blood pressure is very poor. One-third of all hypertensives aren't even aware of their condition. And among those who do know they have it, more than half don't have it under control.[3] Mexican-Americans have the lowest awareness of their hypertension and are least likely to have it under control. Only 58% were ever told by their doctors that they had the condition. [4]

HYPERTENSION IS SPREADING AMONG THE YOUNG

Once a condition associated with aging, hypertension is now showing up in young adults. A study funded by the US National Institutes of Health (NIH) found that nearly 20% of young people aged 24 to 32 now have high blood pressure, even though many of them don't even realize they have this potentially life-threatening condition. [5]

This represents a five-fold increase in the incidence of hypertension in our younger population since the last time such a survey was conducted of the same age group. Health officials are understandably concerned. "With high blood pressure happening at this younger age, the chances that we will see heart (problems) developing earlier is likely," said Dr. Suzanne Steinbaum, a preventive cardiologist at Lenox Hill Hospital in New York City.

WHY HEALING YOUR HYPERTENSION NOW IS CRITICAL

As you'll see, heart problems and high blood pressure are intimately linked. Cardiovascular disease (CVD) is America's leading cause of death and disability, claiming more victims than any other illness. One million people die of CVD each year—that's one fatality every 33 seconds. More than 50,000 of these deaths are from heart attack, many occurring in the prime of life. A stunning 50% of first-time attacks are fatal. And in the majority of cases, a heart attack is the first sign that there is a problem. It is estimated that 20% to 40% of middle-aged people currently have early or advanced CVD due to atherosclerosis (hardening of the arteries); most have neither symptoms nor knowledge of their condition.

Here's what's most important: Having hypertension increases your risk of dying from cardiovascular-related disease, such as heart attack and stroke, by 300% or more. Because it usually causes no symptoms, uncontrolled hypertension can damage your arteries, heart, and brain. It can also cause death before the situation is ever diagnosed. [6]

We believe it's a mistake to think of hypertension as a "medical condition," per se (although this is exactly how conventional medicine characterizes it). Instead, it is more accurate—and far more helpful—to view hypertension as a *symptom* or warning sign that things are not right with your cardiovascular system. Like the little red warning light on your car's dashboard that signals engine problems, hypertension is alerting you and your physician to problems "under the hood." By turning this warning light off (which is, in effect, what anti-hypertensive drugs do), you and your doctor may believe the problem is solved. In reality, the underlying dysfunction can continue to develop until serious health trouble strikes.

In the pages ahead, we will examine some of the cardiovascular problems that hypertension usually signals, as well as the simple lifestyle solutions that can help correct them.

HYPERTENSION RARELY EXISTS BY ITSELF

Doctors do their patients a great disservice by failing to see hypertension as a possible clue to undisclosed cardiovascular danger. That's because hypertension rarely presents itself as a lone condition. More frequently, it is accompanied by a cluster of co-symptoms, including:

- Elevated triglycerides (a type of blood fat).

- Low HDL ("good") cholesterol.

- Accumulated abdominal fat.

- Chronically high blood sugar level.

- Chronically high insulin level.

This cluster of symptoms was identified by Gerald M. Reaven, MD, in the 1970s and is now referred to as "metabolic syndrome."

Metabolic syndrome is the most reliable predictor of impending heart attack or stroke that we currently have, although most doctors continue to overlook it. A review of more than 70 recent studies involving one million patients found that people with metabolic syndrome are two to four times more likely to have a heart attack or stroke compared with the general population.[7] It also significantly increases the risk of Type 2 diabetes. [8]

Not only is metabolic syndrome extremely dangerous, but it is becoming quite common, now affecting an estimated 25% of the US population.[9] If you have hypertension and your physician hasn't tested you for metabolic syndrome yet, we strongly encourage you to make an appointment right away.

IS THERE A CURE FOR HYPERTENSION?

Most physicians will tell you there is no "cure" for hypertension, though not everyone agrees. At best, they say, you can get hypertension under control with a combined strategy of:

- Medication

- Careful monitoring of your blood pressure

- Proper diet

- Sodium restriction

- Weight loss

- Regular physical activity

- Stress reduction

This approach, they advise, can significantly lower your risk of a life-threatening heart attack or stroke.

Unfortunately, current medical treatment leaves little room for any therapy other than pharmaceutical drugs—even though lifestyle approaches have been shown to reduce blood pressure far more effectively than drugs, while dramatically reducing the risks of a CVD event or other serious complications. [10]

This means that the vast majority of hypertensive patients are not receiving the best treatment we have for this condition. And this really concerns us.

MEDICAL POLITICS IS LARGELY TO BLAME

Although lifestyle measures have proven themselves more successful than drug therapy, very few hypertensive patients are receiving a proper education about them from their doctors. This is largely due to the refusal of most health insurance providers to reimburse physicians for any time they spend on "patient education." The result is that physicians don't go into much detail about lifestyle modifications for hypertension, which leaves a lot of patients in the dark.

Most doctors are too busy to bother, anyway. Their workload is so heavy these days that the average patient visit lasts between seven and 12 minutes. That's hardly enough time for adequate instructions, questions or explanations.

On the other side of the issue, doctors are quick to prescribe hypertension drugs because they can be sued and lose their licenses if they stray from standard treatment protocols (in other words, medications). Should you have any health difficulties after a physician tells you about a hypertension-healing diet or helpful supplement, he can be accused of malpractice and brought into court and/or brought before a license review board. Drug therapy, therefore, is a safe strategy for doctors, even if it's not necessarily the most effective treatment for blood pressure patients.

WHY MORE PATIENTS ARE CHOOSING THE HOLISTIC ROUTE

Treating blood pressure with drugs has several drawbacks, not the least of which is that they're fairly ineffective. (Remember: More than half of all people with hypertension don't have their blood pressure under control. [11]) This is undoubtedly why more hypertension patients are seeking physicians who are familiar with nondrug treatment plans and advice.

Another factor: The numerous side effects of blood pressure drugs can actually harm your body while you're trying to heal it. When you choose to combat hypertension with diet, physical activity, nutritional supplements, and smart lifestyle changes, you'll be helping your body to heal itself—without risking any side effects. And this natural approach will have a positive effect on your entire health, not just your blood pressure. This is what *holistic* healing is really all about.

According to the *Encarta Dictionary,* "Holistic healing" means "...considering all factors when treating illness: taking into account all of somebody's physical, mental, and social conditions in the treatment of illness." In other words, we are going to look at your body, your health, and your life as a *whole,* because each aspect has its own unique effect on your blood pressure.

To your doctor, your hypertension may just be a couple of numbers. He/she is not necessarily considering the many causes behind your high blood pressure. Maybe your boss makes a sport of breathing down your neck. Or you have not taken a walk outside since you had kids. Or you're addicted to eating donuts in the morning and drinking a six-pack before bed.

The holistic approach wants to know about all of these factors—the details of how you got out of balance and what it will take to help you find health again. No pill can possibly achieve this.

Although we wish it weren't the case, modern medicine often reminds us of the John Godfrey Saxe poem about six blind men who encountered an elephant and tried to describe it without being able to see. One felt its tail and declared that the elephant was like a rope. Another felt its ear and said, "No, an elephant is like a fan." Another felt its leg and said, "You are wrong. An elephant is like a tree." Each of the men was mistaken because they missed the whole of what an elephant is.

The goal of holistic medicine is to see (and heal) "the whole elephant" in treating your hypertensive condition—so it doesn't trample your health and quality of life.

As part of our educational, self-help approach to healing hypertension, we challenge some of mainstream medicine's biggest sacred cows, such as the supposed importance of reducing your sodium consumption. As you'll read a little later, dietary sodium isn't the bogeyman that conventional health authorities make it out to be.

We also believe that the relatively new clinical category of "pre-hypertension" needs to be viewed with some healthy skepticism. Both of us feel that too many doctors have a quick trigger-finger when it comes to prescribing antihypertensive drugs—and this is almost certainly due to Big Pharma's intrusive influence over physicians, the medical community and Big Medicine.

It really upsets us that the health and quality of life of trusting patients often take a backseat to profits. And we can tell you from clinical experience—and from the thousands of people who visit Jim's popular website www.jimhealthy.com—that the combination of healing foods and supplements, plus regular physical activity, can definitely improve (if not completely reverse) most cases of high blood pressure without drugs. So let's get started!

CHAPTER TWO

WHAT IS HYPERTENSION?

Having a diagnosis of hypertension is very common in the US these days. As we've already shared, some sources say the incidence is as high as 60% of the adult population. Yet, despite its widespread prevalence, hypertension is not to be taken lightly. More than 40 million people wind up in the hospital each year because of it. Doctors call it the "silent killer" because you can have it without ever experiencing any symptoms—until it's too late.

We're not trying to scare you, but getting (and keeping) your high blood pressure, and its root causes, under control is one of the most important things you can do to save and lengthen your life. That's because, next to cigarette smoking, hypertension is the leading cause of heart disease, heart attack, stroke, and kidney failure.

We believe knowledge is power, especially when it comes to your health. So, in order to heal your hypertension, it's important to first understand how it develops.

WHY DOCTORS MEASURE BLOOD PRESSURE

Blood pressure is the measurement of the force that blood flow exerts on the walls of arteries. Under normal circumstances, your arteries are flexible, like a new garden hose. When your heart pumps harder, as it does when you're exercising or under physical exertion or emotional stress, healthy arteries expand to accommodate the extra pressure. This is called *dilation*.

As you age, arteries can become more narrow, rigid and inflexible. This narrowing increases the pressure inside arteries and veins, forcing the blood to flow more forcefully. This higher pressure damages artery walls and strains your heart, thus increasing the risk of heart attack, stroke, peripheral artery disease (clogged arteries, most often in your legs), and congestive heart failure (a weakened heart muscle that can't pump blood efficiently).

Many lifestyle factors contribute to this narrowing of the arteries, including:

- Cigarette smoking.

- Being overweight.

- Insufficient physical activity.

- Diabetes or pre-diabetes.

- Inflammation.

- Chronic stress.

- Poor diet.

We'll discuss each of these risk factors in more detail in a moment.

IS YOUR BLOOD PRESSURE NORMAL OR ABNORMAL?

Blood pressure is measured in millimeters of mercury (mmHg) and is expressed in two numbers as a fraction, such as 120/80. The top number (systolic pressure) measures the pressure of the blood flow when your heart is contracting. The bottom number (diastolic pressure) identifies the arterial pressure when the heart is relaxing.

"Hypertension" occurs when the pressure inside the blood vessels is too high and considered to be a health danger.

The American Heart Association (AHA) ranks blood pressure into five categories: [12]

- "Normal" is less than 120/80.

- A relatively new category called "pre-hypertension" is characterized by readings in the range of 120–139/80–89. (We'll explain later—many other health authorities strongly believe this category is unnecessary.)

- Hypertension stage 1 is 140–159/90–99.

- Stage 2 is 160 or higher/100 or higher.

- A hypertension crisis occurs when systolic is higher than 180, and diastolic higher than 110.

Levels	Numbers
Normal	Less than 120/80
Pre-Hypertension	120-139/80-89
Hypertension Stage 1	140-159/90-99
Hypertension Stage 2	160 or higher/100 or higher
Hypertension Crisis	Higher than 180/110

When your numbers start to rise, so does the concern for your health because high blood pressure is related to strokes, heart attack, heart failure, and kidney failure.

A large case-controlled study called Interstroke concluded that hypertension leads the list of the top 10 risk factors associated with 90% of all strokes.[13] New research also shows that hypertension may contribute to a scarring of brain tissue that is linked to the development of Alzheimer's disease.[14]

THE TYPES OF HYPERTENSION

Hypertension is classified as either "primary" (also referred to as "essential") hypertension or "secondary" (or "inessential") hypertension.

Primary (or essential) hypertension is the most prevalent type, affecting 90% to 95% of all hypertensive patients. Although no direct cause has been identified by doctors, many factors are suspect, including:

- Sedentary lifestyle.

- Smoking.

- Stress.

- Abdominal fat accumulation.

- Potassium deficiency (hypokalemia).

- Obesity (more than 85% of cases occur in those with a body mass index greater than 25).

- Salt (sodium) sensitivity.

- Excess alcohol consumption.

- Vitamin D deficiency.

- Air pollution.

- Heavy metal toxicity including lead, mercury, arsenic, and cadmium.

Each of these factors is thought to increase the risk of developing hypertension.

Untreated, essential hypertension is a risk factor for stroke, myocardial infarction (MI, or heart attack), congestive heart failure, and arterial aneurysm (weakened, expanded section of artery that can rupture). It also is a leading cause of chronic kidney failure. Even a moderate elevation of arterial blood pressure leads to shortened life expectancy.

The risk of hypertension also increases with aging, inherited genetic mutations and having a family history of hypertension. Elevated levels of renin, a hormone secreted by the kidneys, is another risk factor. Insulin resistance, a component of metabolic syndrome, is also believed to contribute to hypertension.

Secondary (or inessential) hypertension is caused by an identifiable underlying secondary cause and affects only 5% of hypertensive patients. It has many different causes, including endocrine disease, kidney disease, and tumors. Another common cause is Cushing's syndrome, a

13

condition in which the adrenal glands overproduce the hormone cortisol. Secondary hypertension also can be a side effect of many medications, such as erythropoietin, corticosteroids, cough/cold and asthma medications, migraine medications, and estrogens.*

OTHER TERMS YOUR DOCTOR MAY USE

Persistent hypertension is another way of saying "chronic hypertension."

Accelerated hypertension is associated with headache, drowsiness, confusion, vision disorders, nausea, and vomiting. These symptoms are collectively called hypertensive encephalopathy, which is caused by severe small blood vessel congestion and brain swelling. These symptoms are reversible if blood pressure is lowered.

Pulmonary hypertension is high blood pressure in the arteries leading to your lungs. It is a serious condition. If you have it, the blood vessels that carry oxygen from your heart to your lungs become hard and narrow. As a result, your heart must work harder to pump blood. Over time, the heart muscle weakens and can no longer do its job, leading to heart failure. Although pulmonary hypertension isn't curable, treatments are available that can help lessen symptoms and improve the patient's quality of life.[15]

Gestational hypertension (or pregnancy-induced hypertension) is defined as the development of new arterial hypertension (blood pressure exceeding 140/90) in a pregnant woman after 20 weeks gestation, but without the presence of protein in the urine. When gestational hypertension is present with protein in the urine, the condition is called preeclampsia.

WHEN DRUGS ARE NECESSARY

Most physicians, including many who practice holistic medicine, believe that anyone with a pressure reading of 160/100 or higher should immediately go on medications to stabilize it. In such cases, a blood pressure drug can be a lifesaver. However, once blood pressure is normalized, natural therapies can be very effective at keeping it at a healthy level. Using natural therapies to maintain a healthy blood pressure will allow your doctor to gradually withdraw the drugs as your condition improves.

It's absolutely vital that you work with a physician who is familiar with and in favor of natural therapies. The average doctor is taught that once a patient has been diagnosed with high blood pressure, that person must remain on hypertensive medications for the rest of his life. This is not a good situation. You want to do everything in your power to avoid this. Many of these drugs have nasty side effects (you'll read all about them in the next chapter) and can drain your body of essential nutrients. In fact, use of hypertension drugs can actually shorten your life.

*http://www.nlm.nih.gov/medlineplus/ency/article/000155.htm

TOP OR BOTTOM: WHICH NUMBER IS MORE IMPORTANT?

Until the 1980s, doctors believed that the bottom number of a reading (diastolic blood pressure, or DBP) was more important than the top reading (systolic blood pressure, or SBP). Accordingly, most treatment goals were aimed at lowering DBP. Since then, there has been a radical change in thinking, based on studies showing that an elevated top number (SBP) is a more significant risk factor, especially with respect to stroke risk.

For this reason, the term "isolated systolic hypertension" (ISH) now refers to patients with an elevated SBP (when the top number is persistently higher than 140 mmHg) and a normal—or even lower—DBP (the bottom number). This condition is the most common type of hypertension in the elderly, and it is the most prevalent type of untreated hypertension among persons over 60 years of age. (SBP tends to rise with advancing age, whereas DBP usually levels off and then tends to decrease in the elderly.) [16]

Isolated systolic hypertension, therefore, is defined as a systolic pressure (top number) that is above 140 mmHg with a diastolic pressure (bottom number) that remains at or below 90. This usually indicates the presence of hardened arteries.[17]

PULSE PRESSURE: A NEW WAY TO GAUGE YOUR HEALTH

The standard blood pressure reading isn't the only way to gauge the health of your cardiovascular system. Some doctors are beginning to recognize the diagnostic value of pulse pressure, which is the difference that remains when the diastolic (bottom) number is subtracted from the systolic (top) number. For example, if your blood pressure reading is 120/80, your pulse pressure is 40 (120 minus 80), which is considered normal and healthy.

An elevation of the systolic pressure without an elevation of the diastolic pressure, as in isolated systolic hypertension, increases the pulse pressure. Many forward-thinking physicians now believe elevated pulse pressure is an even better predictor of potential stroke and cardiovascular events[18] in elderly hypertensives.

Generally speaking, a pulse pressure greater than 40 is considered abnormal and may indicate trouble ahead, particularly heart attack or stroke. Pulse pressure lower than 40 may signal weak heart function.

Once considered harmless, a high pulse pressure is now an important indicator of health problems and potential organ damage. Elevated pulse pressure may be caused by calcification of the aorta, the body's largest artery. Isolated systolic hypertension is associated with two to four times greater risk for heart enlargement or dying from a heart attack or stroke.

8 WAYS HIGH BLOOD PRESSURE
SECRETLY AGES YOUR BODY AND BRAIN

- Your doctor worries about your high blood pressure because it can suddenly kill or cripple you through a stroke or heart attack.

- But high blood pressure is even more insidious. It speeds up the aging of your body and brain—making you chronically fatigued, sexually impaired, and feeble-minded by stealing your "youth." Here's how...

- **Brain damage.** High blood pressure decreases the normal blood flow to the brain. This can cause recurring mini-strokes (called transient ischemic attack or TIA)...forgetfulness...memory loss...loss of balance and frequent falls...dementia and cognitive impairment.

- **Enlarged heart.** High blood pressure forces your heart to work harder, which leaves you breathless, tired, and chronically fatigued. By working harder, the heart becomes enlarged—a risk factor for heart attack, heart failure, and cardiac arrest.

- **Failing eyesight.** High blood pressure damages the tiny blood vessels of the eyes, causing retinopathy (disease of the retina). It can cause blurred vision or even total blindness.

- **Erectile dysfunction.** Hardened arteries impair blood flow to sexual organs, causing underperformance, frustration, and depression.

- **Hardened arteries.** High blood pressure damages delicate artery linings, triggering calcified plaque buildup. Because hardened arteries can't expand, they force your heart to work harder—which leads to early heart failure.

- **Kidney failure.** Properly functioning kidneys are essential to your good health because they purify your blood. Excess blood pressure scars these filtration cells, which can lead to kidney failure, sepsis (whole body inflammation and self-poisoning), and frequent infections.

- **Aneurysms.** Excess blood pressure can weaken portions of your blood vessels, forming bubbles that can burst suddenly. When this happens it can be a very serious matter. If it occurs in the brain, death may result before medical attention can be found.

- **Physical disability.** More than 80% of all strokes cause permanent disability, making you unable to talk, walk, or care for yourself—and leaving you dependent upon others for life's most basic tasks.

It's all so sad and unnecessary—because this sneaky destruction of your brain and body can *easily* be prevented (and even reversed) simply by keeping your blood pressure in the safety zone.

CHAPTER THREE

DIRTY LITTLE SECRETS ABOUT HYPERTENSION DRUGS

Mild to moderate hypertension represents the vast majority of hypertension cases. Yet even though it responds well to lifestyle modifications, such as maintaining a more healthful diet, increasing physical activity, and reducing stress, most physicians today automatically choose to treat it with drugs—and in many cases, *multiple* drugs.

According to the Center for Disease Control and Prevention, while the percentage of patients with hypertension has remained steady for the last decade, the prevalence of patients receiving drug treatment for this condition has increased.[19]

This means the chances are very good that you're currently on drug therapy for your blood pressure, or soon will be. And because the best result that drugs can accomplish is to artificially force down your numbers, it's likely that you'll be on one or more of these drugs for the rest of your life—unless you make some important lifestyle changes.

As you'll understand after reading this chapter, this isn't the outcome you want. There are numerous problems related to taking anti-hypertensive drugs, even in the short-term. You definitely do *not* want to be on these drugs for the long term if you can avoid it.

PROBLEMS WITH HYPERTENSION DRUGS

Hypertension can have a variety of mechanical, physical, and biochemical causes, yet current treatment guidelines make no real distinction between the different types of hypertension, notes Curt D. Furberg, MD, PhD, professor emeritus of Public Health Sciences at Wake Forest School of Medicine. In a paper tellingly entitled "Treatment of Hypertension: A Failing Report Card," published in a recent issue of the *American Journal of Hypertension*, Dr. Furberg points out the shortcomings associated with current drug treatment for hypertension:

"The mantra [is] 'choose any of the large number of antihypertensive agents representing 10 different drug classes with different mechanisms of action, and if the first choice doesn't work, add a second, a third or a fourth drug type. This approach leads to an over-utilization of drugs per patient and has been associated with poor outcomes.'" [20]

The type of hypertension a person has can make a big difference in choosing an approach to treatment. One size does not fit all. For example, in a recent meta-analysis of four randomized control trials comprised of nearly 9,000 patients, Diana Diao, MD (University of British Columbia, Vancouver) and her colleagues demonstrated that using prescription drugs for mild hypertension (140/90 to 159/99 mmHg) had no demonstrable benefit in preventing stroke, coronary heart disease, cardiovascular events, or death from any cause for up to five years following treatment.

On the other hand, these drugs all produce side effects in many of the people who take them. Many participants withdrew from the four studies because of adverse drug effects, so can we in any way conclude that the benefits outweigh the risks here? Not likely.[21,22]

DRAWBACKS OF HYPERTENSION DRUGS

Uncontrolled hypertension is quite dangerous because it increases your risk for heart attack, stroke, and premature death. But blood pressure drugs carry their own dangers and may actually *shorten* your lifespan, according to a University of Florida study published in the *Journal of the American Medical Association*.

The study was performed on individuals with both Type 2 diabetes and coronary artery disease (CAD). Each person in the study received one or more blood pressure medication (calcium antagonist, beta-blocker, ACE inhibitor, and diuretic) in whatever combination was required to achieve a systolic blood pressure less than 130 mmHg (the standard hypertension guideline for diabetics).

Much to their surprise, the researchers discovered that tighter control of blood pressure in these patients did not produce better outcomes compared with the group whose systolic blood pressure was held between 130 and 140. This second group actually displayed a slightly lower risk of death than the group whose systolic was maintained at the recommended level—under 130 mm Hg.

Tight Control Group	12.7% risk for death
Usual Control Group	12.6% risk for death
Uncontrolled Group	19.8% risk for death

The authors write: *"In this observational study, we have shown for the first time, to our knowledge, that decreasing systolic BP to lower than 130 mmHg in patients with diabetes and CAD was not associated with further reduction in morbidity beyond that associated with systolic BP lower than 140 mmHg, and, in fact, was associated with an increase in risk of all-cause mortality. Moreover, the increased mortality risk persisted over the long term."*

THE MANY SIDE EFFECTS OF BLOOD PRESSURE DRUGS

Allow us to translate the medical lingo here. "Poor outcomes" mean a lousy quality of life due to the side effects of these drugs. This can include:

- Chronic headaches.

- Dizziness.

- Shortness of breath.

- Nagging cough.

- Fatigue.

- Constipation.

- Frequent urination.

- Weight gain.

- Insomnia.

- Depression.

- Erectile dysfunction.

And these aren't the worst that can happen. More serious complications include:

- Gout.

- Elevated blood sugar (and even diabetes).

- Congestive heart failure.

- Shortened longevity.

- Sudden death.

Some of the side effects that blood pressure drugs produce are a direct result of the action they encourage. Beta-blockers, for example, weaken the strength of the heartbeat to decrease blood pressure. In doing so, they can weaken it too much and cause heart failure.

Other side effects occur because of indirect consequences. For instance, diuretics (or any blood pressure drug containing hydrochlorothiazide) reduce the volume of fluid in the blood by encouraging frequent urination. But this also flushes away valuable vitamins, nutrients, and minerals such as potassium, which has an important role in regulating sodium and magnesium (as you'll see in Chapter Seven).

Magnesium is absolutely necessary for healthy heart function, blood sugar control, and muscle relaxation. A magnesium deficiency can result in poor cardiovascular function, thicker blood and, ironically, higher blood pressure.

Suzy Cohen, RPh, a retired pharmacist and author of *The 24-Hour Pharmacist* (HarperCollins, 2007), calls antihypertensive drugs "vitamin and mineral muggers" because they rob your body of the nutrients it needs for proper functioning and optimal health.

One way to protect yourself is to make sure you're taking in more of the vitamins and minerals than are being "mugged" by these drugs. You can also replenish potassium by consuming more bananas, oranges, figs, bran, apricots, grapes, squash, beans, baked potatoes with skins, watermelon, and spinach.

Foods rich in magnesium include dark chocolate (yum!), halibut, nuts, oatmeal and oat bran, pumpkin seeds, and artichokes. Some people find it helps them sleep better, remain calmer during the day, and regulates their bowels. (Too much magnesium produces a runny stool, but given the choice, it certainly beats constipation!)

Another reputable magnesium product is Magnesium Infusion (www.activationproducts.com/store/magnesium-infusion) or Norm Shealy MD's Magnesium Lotion at www.norm-shealy.com. These do not go in your mouth; instead, you rub them on your skin. Your body absorbs only the amount it needs—and there are no loose stools to deal with. Since it is applied topically, you're able to get your magnesium level up to peak very quickly, even from a very low starting point.

Beta-blockers, another large class of blood pressure drugs, are known to decrease protective HDL cholesterol levels and increase triglycerides. Furthermore, for those with borderline or mild hypertension, reduction in blood pressure by medications alone has not been found to decrease the rate of coronary heart disease. This is contrary to what your doctor may tell you, since one of the primary goals in controlling hypertension is to reduce your risk of a heart attack or stroke.[23]

Beta-blockers are high on our list of drugs to avoid for a lot of reasons. They contribute to fatigue. They slow down your metabolism. They can even trigger asthma attacks. And as if all that wasn't enough, one new study shows that they're practically useless, too. These medications (which include *atenolol*, Lopressor, and *metoprolol*) are designed to lower blood pressure. But after following 45,000 patients in NYU Langone Medical Center's data registry for 44 months, researchers discovered that the drugs *don't* ward off heart attacks or stroke.

Among patients with coronary artery disease (CAD), 12.9% died of a heart attack or stroke despite being on beta-blockers. Those who didn't take the blood pressure meds died at a rate of 13.6%, not even one full percentage point of difference.

Of the patients taking beta-blockers due to CAD risk factors (like diabetes or high blood pressure), 14.2% suffered a negative outcome—as opposed to 12% among those not on the drugs. That's still only a 2.2% difference. We would not risk a bad hair day on a "success" rate like that—never mind our energy levels or waistlines.

Researchers did find a slight benefit among patients who had suffered a heart attack within the past year. [24] But even so, it's clear that the majority of heart disease patients have no good reason to take beta blockers.

So why are doctors still prescribing them?

One nutrient mugging that may occur with beta blockers is the depletion of coenzyme Q10 (CoQ10). The main job of this naturally occurring substance is to help convert your food into *adenosine-5'-triphosphate* or more simply ATP, which is the life force that animates us. The highest concentrations of CoQ10 are found in muscle cells, particularly the heart muscle. A randomized double-blind study published in the *European Heart Journal* (September, 2007) found that CoQ10 supplementation (100 mg three times daily) improved blood flow to the heart by relaxing blood vessels in patients with coronary artery disease. [25] Recent research also supports this heart-healthy benefit in diabetics.

SHOULD YOU TAKE BLOOD PRESSURE DRUGS?

This is a serious conversation you should have with your physician (if you haven't yet) because, as with all drugs, there is a trade-off in taking blood pressure meds. Too few doctors take the time to explain the side effects and long-term consequences of these drugs. It's neither fair nor ethical to allow a patient to discover this downside after the fact.

Not all physicians are gung ho on blood pressure drugs. "The issue of whether hypertension needs to be treated has also vexed researchers for many years," says Thomas Cowan, MD, author of *The Fourfold Path to Healing*. "If the pressure of the blood inside the arteries is too high, leading to kidney damage and stroke, it's obvious that we should try to lower blood pressure. But several studies now show that while it is clear that having normal blood pressure is better for your long-term health than elevated blood pressure, lowering pressure with medicines does not demonstrably improve the outcome."

Here's Dr. Cowan again: "Many of the drugs in use to treat hypertension have unfortunate side effects. Diuretics cause the loss of valuable electrolytes (minerals), thereby predisposing the patient to cardiac arrhythmia. Beta-blockers alter lipid levels and can worsen the tendency toward Type 2 diabetes, which can lead to the same adverse outcome as elevated blood pressure. Similar problems have been found with calcium channel blockers, and even with the new ACE inhibitors."

WHAT DOCTORS USUALLY DON'T TELL YOU

Most patients don't know all of the problems with taking the pharmacological approach to hypertension. Here are some of the most important:

Drugs don't always do the trick. From 30% to 50% of patients taking antihypertensive medications don't have their blood pressure under control, despite taking drugs. Clearly, these drugs don't work for everyone.

Hypertension drugs can produce nasty side effects. Blood pressure medications can be so troublesome that airline pilots were once prohibited to fly while on them. These reactions are so bad that 50% of patients who start taking them soon stop because of the side effects.

Hypertension drugs can sometimes *raise* blood pressure. A recent study confirms this. Researchers at Albert Einstein College of Medicine at Yeshiva University gave a group of untreated hypertension patients one of the leading blood pressure drugs in order to monitor the medications' effectiveness. Patients received either a diuretic, a calcium channel blocker, a beta blocker, or an ACE inhibitor.

The results were surprising. Nearly 8% of the patients—including 16% on the beta blockers and ACE inhibitors—actually experienced *higher* blood pressure levels, according to the study published in the *American Journal of Hypertension.*

"Our findings suggest that physicians should use renin levels to predict the most appropriate first drug for treating patients with hypertension," says the study's lead author Michael Alderman, MD, professor of epidemiology and population health, and of medicine, at Einstein. "This would increase the likelihood of achieving blood pressure control, and reduce the need for patients to take additional antihypertensive medications." [26] (Renin is an enzyme produced by the kidneys that participates in blood pressure regulation.)

EVEN WORSE THAN MEDICATIONS?

The medical industry has outdone itself with this one—a new procedure in which a doctor threads a catheter through your groin and all the way up to your kidneys to burn away nerves that control blood pressure. [27] These nerves help manage kidney function, but they're also responsible for switching your body into "fight-or-flight" mode during stressful situations, which in turn pushes your blood pressure up. The theory is that in certain people, these nerves don't switch off, and their hypertension remains resistant to antihypertensive drugs.

So if it works, what's the problem? The problem is the cure may be worse than the disease. Side effects can include excessive bleeding at the puncture site, injured blood vessels, rapidly developing blood pressure or heart problems, and complications from the medications used during the catheterization.

This is an invasive and potentially dangerous procedure. The only people who are absolutely sure to benefit from it are the doctors who can charge enormous sums for performing it. There are better, holistic, completely safe and natural ways to control blood pressure, as you'll see in this book.

SHOULD YOU THINK TWICE ABOUT MEDICATION?

After taking all these drawbacks into consideration, you may want to reevaluate your decision to rely on drug therapy. Drugs should be viewed as a temporary measure that can bail you out of an emergency situation. If your blood pressure is dangerously high, for instance, taking a drug until you get your numbers under control not only makes sense—it could save your life.

But you shouldn't consider the problem solved by any means. Rather, you should use your "close call" as motivation to uncover the underlying cause of your elevated blood pressure, so you can correct it.

Hypertension drugs are like your car's spare tire. They are helpful in getting you out of a jam, but are not ideal for permanent use. Remember that hypertension rarely presents itself alone. It is often a symptom of other health problems, such as insulin resistance, sick arteries, a poor diet, or a sedentary lifestyle. Consider your elevated blood pressure to be a wake-up call; and begin investigating what's *causing* the problem, along with the diet and lifestyle steps you can take to correct it.

No matter which medications your doctor prescribes to treat your high blood pressure, you'll need to make certain lifestyle changes to lower your blood pressure—and keep it there. (We'll describe some of the most effective self-help steps you can take later in this book.)

AN OVERVIEW OF CURRENT BLOOD PRESSURE DRUGS

There are at least 10 separate classes of medications used to treat high blood pressure, with numerous products in each category. The drug (or drugs) that your doctor selects for you depends on numerous factors, including ease of use, side effects and coexisting medical conditions, which might dictate preferential use of one medication over another.

Official treatment guidelines call for any anti-hypertensive drug to be started at the lowest, and therefore safest, dose (although this isn't common practice). At a relatively low dose, a physician is able to carefully monitor your response to the drug over the course of several weeks. If your blood pressure remains elevated, the dose of the medication then can be gradually increased. (Of course, this, too, rarely happens in the real world.)

If treatment with higher doses of a medication fails to reduce blood pressure to target levels, the physician has two options: (1) the particular medication may be discontinued and a different class of antihypertensive medication started; or (2) a second class of medication may be added to the first. This second approach is often used because different classes of anti-hypertensive drugs lower blood pressure in different ways, so the action of one may complement the action of the second. Sometimes it may be necessary to add a third drug.

Many of the newer blood pressure medications are taken once or twice a day. All blood pressure drugs produce side effects, some worse than others. Be sure to discuss these with your physician, but do not stop your investigation there. So many new drugs have recently entered the treatment arena that the average physician finds it difficult to stay current. We encourage you to go online and enter a Google search for "side effects of [your drug's name]." Survey several responses and discount those from the manufacturer. Pay particular attention to independent sources such as www.medicinenet.com and www.rxlist.com. (Be wary of WebMD—its search engine is sketchy and its advice is strictly from drug company product inserts, pharmaceutical websites, and official Big Medicine sources.)

See Appendix A (beginning on page 307) for a description of all the various types of anti-hypertension drugs now in use.

IF YOUR DRUG THERAPY IS SUCCESSFUL

Once your blood pressure is under control, your doctor may want you to take a daily aspirin to reduce your risk of cardiovascular disorders because aspirin produces anti-inflammatory effects. (A number of natural substances and supplements also have the same action.)

To reduce the number of daily medication doses you need, your doctor may prescribe a combination of low-dose medications rather than larger doses of one single drug. In fact, two or more blood pressure drugs often work better than one. Sometimes finding the most effective medication—or combination of drugs—is a matter of trial and error. If you are committed to taking the drug route, you'll have to be patient as your doctor explores the right drug(s) and dosage(s) for you.

IF YOUR BLOOD PRESSURE WILL NOT BUDGE

Some patients find that their blood pressure is difficult to get under control, even with multiple medications. If your blood pressure remains stubbornly high despite taking at least three different types of high blood pressure drugs (one of which should be a diuretic), you may have "resistant hypertension."

Quite simply, resistant hypertension is blood pressure that doesn't respond easily to treatment. This classification also refers to patients who are taking four different types of medications simultaneously, even if their blood pressure *is* under control.

Having resistant hypertension doesn't mean your blood pressure will never come down. In fact, if you and your doctor can identify what's causing your resistant blood pressure, the chances of normalizing it are much better. Your doctor or healthcare provider should be able to determine whether the medications and doses you're taking are right for your condition, but he may have to fine-tune your treatment to discover the best combination and doses.

INTERACTIONS WITH FOODS, SUPPLEMENTS, AND OTHER MEDICINES

Your doctor should review all other medications you're taking for other conditions. Some medications, foods, and nutritional supplements can worsen high blood pressure or prevent your antihypertensive medications from working effectively.

Be very honest with your doctor about all the medications and/or supplements you are taking—and any other chemicals you consume as well, especially smoking or recreational drug and/or alcohol consumption. Your health and very life are on the line, so you will only hurt yourself by misrepresenting your habits.

Important: that you must take your medications exactly as directed, or your blood pressure and health may suffer. If you skip doses due to financial concerns, side effects you're experiencing or because you simply forget, talk to your doctor about your situation. Never stop taking your medication or alter your dosage without your doctor's knowledge. [28]

WHY OLD BP DRUGS WORK BETTER THAN NEWER ONES

Few people realize that blood pressure drugs are updated every few years. This is not necessarily because the new drugs are better (often they are not), but rather for financial advantages to the drug manufacturers. Patents expire after seven years, and pharmaceutical companies need to develop new products to replace older ones because they can't compete with cheaper generic versions of their drugs.

Studies show that these newer medications tend to be no more effective than the older versions—and often, they are far more dangerous. If you must take antihypertensive medication, ask your doctor for an older product or generic version. Then, do everything in your power to improve your blood pressure by natural means so you can get off these drugs. (Later in this book, we'll show you how.)

Most people stay on blood pressure drugs far too long (usually for life). This is often unnecessary because hypertension is one of the easiest medical conditions to heal and improve naturally.

SHOULD YOU TRY A DIURETIC FIRST?

One of the oldest and most reliable type of blood pressure medication is the diuretic. In generic form, their cost can be as low as a penny a day—and they are perhaps the safest blood pressure drug you can take. Unfortunately, new treatment guidelines are silent about these effective compounds. We suspect that drug companies may have a hand in this obvious silence because diuretics are their least profitable—and oldest—product.

A CONVERSATION WITH MICHAEL ALDERMAN, MD

On this topic, we came across a provocative online conversation with Michael Alderman, MD, past president of the American Society of Hypertension. Dr. Alderman is also a professor of medicine and population health sciences at Albert Einstein School of Medicine, Bronx, New York, and has conducted several important studies on high blood pressure. (We've referred to Dr. Alderman previously in this text because he is a recognized expert in the field.) He is being interviewed by *Medical Consumer* (represented as "*MC*" here). We've excerpted the section most relevant to diuretics.

MC: You said that treatment should start with diuretics. Is it a stepped approach that is recommended, starting with diuretics, and if they don't work, you move up to beta-blockers, and so forth?

Dr. Alderman: Yes, for most people, I think that's right. However, there are specific situations, such as kidney disease characterized by leaking protein, where other drugs are useful, for example, the angiotensin-converting enzyme inhibitors (e.g., Capoten, Vasotec) and the A2 receptor blockers (e.g., Atacand, Avapro).[29] Clinical trials say that's the best. But for the garden variety, uncomplicated hypertension (this includes about 70% of all people with hypertension), starting with a diuretic is right. And there's no evidence that there is anything better, though you have to worry a little bit about diabetes and loss of potassium with diuretics. Reasonable monitoring, however, should cover that risk. [30]

CHECKING IN WITH J. M. WRIGHT, MD, PHD

The conversation about diuretics and doses now switches to J. M. Wright, MD, PhD, a professor of anesthesiology, pharmacology and therapeutics at the University of British Columbia in Canada.

MC: Women seem to be more prone to harm from drugs in general than men. Why?

Dr. Wright: My theory is that women, on average, weigh significantly less than men, and we (doctors) usually give the same doses to men and women. So women, in general, are getting a higher dose per (their body weight). And that's going to play out in terms of more harm than in men. In all the clinical trials, the same dose of the drug is given to men and to women.

MC: I'm familiar enough with your work to know that you would probably agree with their promotion of lower doses of these drugs because so many people with high blood pressure stop taking their drugs due to adverse effects.

Dr. Wright: Yes, we do agree that lower doses are almost as effective as the standard doses.

MC: What about the point that the five drug classes prescribed for high blood pressure are largely interchangeable? Do you agree with that?

Dr. Wright: Ideally, you would want to be on an antihypertensive drug that has been shown to reduce morbidity (non-fatal stroke, non-fatal heart attack) and mortality.

MC: That leaves you with the least expensive drug of all—thiazide diuretics.

Dr. Wright: The morbidity and mortality evidence is, by far, stronger for the thiazide diuretics than for any other drug classes.

MC: Do you think it's reasonable—based on the findings from your new review—for drug-treated people with blood pressures lower than 140/90 to ask their doctors to reduce the dose?

Dr. Wright: Yes, it is reasonable. Patients who have been referred to me often say, "Do I really need all these drugs?" And my reaction usually is, "We probably should start thinking of cutting back."[31]

BLOOD PRESSURE DRUGS LINKED TO CANCER

A new study has found that women taking blood pressure drugs have a 2.5 times higher occurrence of breast cancer.

The research, published in the *Journal of the American Medical Association Internal Medicine,* found that postmenopausal women who use a type of blood pressure medication called a calcium-channel blocker were at a higher risk for cancer. This was the first study of its kind to examine the effects of blood pressure medications and cancer. [32]

"We looked at these drugs because people who use them to manage their blood pressure are usually on them for the rest of their lives," said the study's lead author, Christopher Li, MD, PhD, of the Fred Hutchinson Cancer Research Center in Seattle.

Drugs to control high blood pressure are the most commonly prescribed type of medication in the US. Channel blockers alone accounted for 98 million prescriptions filled in 2010.

Calcium-channel blockers include the drugs *amlodipine* (Norvasc), *diltiazem* (Cardizem LA, Tiazac), *isradipine* (DynaCirc CR), *nicardipine* (Cardene SR), *nifedipine* (Procardia, Procardia XL, Adalat CC), *nisoldipine* (Sular), and *verapamil* (Calan, Verelan, Covera-PM).

Women who used calcium-channel blockers for more than 10 years had a significantly higher risk of developing breast cancer compared with women not taking these drugs, the researchers concluded. [33]

CHAPTER FOUR

THE BLOOD PRESSURE MISTAKE MOST DOCTORS MAKE

Here's a shocking statistic that's sure to make your eyes pop…

One out of every four people in the US (that's 25%!) with an official diagnosis of hypertension actually *does not* have high blood pressure at all!

That is a fact—and you could be one of them—even if you saw your elevated readings with your own eyes, and even if you've been taking one or more blood pressure drugs for several years now.

A new study reveals that 25% of all hypertension patients may be taking drugs for a condition they don't actually have.

IS YOUR DOCTOR UPSETTING YOUR BLOOD PRESSURE?

Taking your blood pressure reading is one of the simplest, most basic tests that your doctor administers. It is also the most important.

Unfortunately, it is the test that your physician gets wrong most often.

This is not because the doctor or the nurse has bad technique. Instead, his/her very presence could be causing your blood pressure levels to jump.

This quirky phenomenon is so common, it even has a name. It's called "white coat hypertension," and you've probably heard of it. A new study confirms that it not only causes dramatic increases in a patient's blood pressure levels, but that it happens a lot more frequently than anyone realized.

NEW STUDY DOCUMENTS "WHITE COAT" PHENOMENON

Researchers from Duke University and the Durham VA Medical Center had a group of male hypertension patients (they were receiving drug therapy) check their blood pressure readings in a doctor's office, at home, and at a research lab. The readings were taken four different times during the 18-month study: At the start, at six months, at 12 months, and at 18 months.

When the researchers examined the readings, they received a troubling surprise. Only 33% of the patients had readings that were either consistently under control or consistently out of control at all three locations.

For the other two-thirds, the readings varied wildly. The highest blood pressure levels were recorded at the doctor's office—and more than 50% of the patients saw increases of 10 points or more.

Publishing their results in the *Annals of Internal Medicine*, the researchers noted that systolic readings (the top number) averaged 145 in the doctor's office, but only 130 in the research lab. This 15-point difference can mean the difference between a hypertension diagnosis requiring drug therapy and a clean bill of health.

This study suggests that as many as 20 million hypertension patients could be taking drugs and modifying their diet and lifestyle for a condition they don't have. Could you be one of them? There's only one way to know for sure—and we'll tell you about it in a moment.

TAKING DRUGS FOR A CONDITION THEY DON'T HAVE

Some people see that white jacket and stethoscope coming toward them and their blood pressure immediately starts to rise. Yet once they're safely back home, their blood pressure goes back to normal again. One in four people may be misdiagnosed with hypertension due to this anomaly.

Their doctors prescribe drugs and may continue to prescribe new meds and tinker with the dosage or prescribe multiple drugs, because when the patient's blood pressure is checked in the doctor's office, his reading stays high, regardless of the meds he's on. Doctors may mistakenly conclude that the patients is "drug-resistant" when temporary white coat hypertension is the real cause.[34]

In a study published in the journal *Hypertension*, Spanish researchers analyzed data of more than 68,000 patients being treated for hypertension, and determined that 8,295 of them seemed to be "resistant to antihypertensive drugs." But when they investigated further, and gathered more data by using a diagnostic method called ambulatory blood pressure monitoring (a device that measures the effect these drugs are having intermittently throughout the day and night), the researchers discovered that while 62.5% of the 8,295 patients were truly resistant to drug therapy, 37.5% of the cases were innocent victims of the white coat effect. [35]

IS YOUR HYPERTENSION THE "WHITE COAT" KIND?

The easiest, surest way to find out if you truly have hypertension (and not the white coat variety) is to monitor your own blood pressure at home. This is the fascinating finding from an analysis of 37 international clinical trials that examined thousands of men and women with high blood pressure and also published in a recent issue of the medical journal *Hypertension*.

The studies revealed that patients who track their own blood pressure with home monitors received the most accurate readings. The researchers explained that these lower readings seen as a result of home monitoring eliminated the "white coat" effect, which can falsely increase patients' blood pressure and land them on drugs.

HOME MONITORING HELPS LOWER BLOOD PRESSURE

Standard medical care is no match for a home blood pressure monitoring program for keeping hypertension in check, according to a randomized trial published online in *Circulation: Cardiovascular Quality and Outcomes.*

Over 50% of patients monitoring themselves at home reached their blood pressure goals after six months, compared with those receiving the usual medical care (54% versus 35%).

At six months, the average blood pressure of patients in the home monitoring group was significantly lower than in the usual care group (128/79 versus 137/83 mmHg), reported David J. Magid, MD, MPH, and colleagues from Kaiser Permanente Colorado in Denver.

The benefits of the home monitoring program were even better for patients with diabetes and/or chronic kidney disease (52% reached their target goal compared with 22% in usual medical care).

Patients in the home monitoring group used the American Heart Association's web-based Heart360, a free online tool for tracking heart health (www.Heart360.org). From the site, users can upload blood pressure data and send it to their health providers. Heart360 also provides patients with educational information and allows them to track progress.

Those being home-monitored experienced a 12.4 mmHg larger drop in systolic (top number) blood pressure and a 5.7 mmHg larger drop in diastolic blood pressure than those in the usual care group. Patients with diabetes and/or chronic kidney disease had an even larger drop: 15.4/7.3 mmHg. [36]

GETTING YOUR MEDICATION DOSE REDUCED OR COMPLETELY ELIMINATED

Here's another important benefit of taking your own blood pressure: Home monitoring was also shown to be very effective at having the patients' medications adjusted to lower doses—or to have the drugs completely withdrawn. That can mean freedom from those nasty side effects and needless expense.

And home monitoring is valuable in another way: Keeping track of your blood pressure on a regular basis provides positive reinforcement for the good things you do, such as exercise, a better diet, and specific nutritional supplements that can lower blood pressure and keep you off drugs. When you see the positive effect these good habits are having on your readings, you're much more likely to stay with your healthy habits—and even add other positive behaviors. This, too, can result in having a drug dose reduced or completely eliminated.

CHOOSE THE RIGHT MONITOR

Picking the right monitor is essential. While there are numerous models for sale today, many of the cheaper units aren't worth the money because they don't provide accurate readings. We've examined a wide variety of products and found that, while the high-end models provide reliable data, they are just too expensive for the average person's budget. You can easily locate a decent monitor for around $50.

To be sure your monitor is reliable, take it with you to your next doctor's appointment and check its reading against the numbers the nurse gets on her device (officially called a sphygmomanometer). If both readings jibe, you can feel confident in taking your own at home.

TAKE YOUR OWN READINGS

We suggest that you check your blood pressure daily and keep a log of your results (we've provided a space to do this in the Success Planner). Follow the manufacturer's directions for operating the monitor. We suggest you take three or four readings, a minute or two apart, and in alternating arms. Don't fret about the time—it's only about six minutes for all of the readings. A pittance when you consider the risks of shortcutting.

Monitor both arms. A new study has discovered that a difference in blood pressure readings between the right and left arm in people with hypertension can indicate an increased risk of cardiovascular disease and death. Even though hypertension guidelines recommending that blood pressure be checked in both arms date back to the 1930s, few doctors do it because of the extra time required. Now, this study finds that a difference of more than 10 mmHg in the systolic (top) reading between arms can signal a significantly higher risk of a fatal heart attack or stroke. If you notice such a difference when monitoring yourself, bring this to your doctor's attention immediately. [37]

Check your blood pressure at different times throughout the day. Whether you have hypertension or not, it's a good idea to monitor your blood pressure a few times during the day. You should check yourself first thing in the morning, after lunch, after your workout, and before bed. You may be surprised at how your readings fluctuate throughout the day.

Enter the average of each reading in your health log so you have a record. This way you can tell at a glance how a particular food, beverage, or nutritional supplement affects your blood pressure. This is a good habit to get into if you have hypertension, and it allows you to discuss your highs and lows with your doctor at checkup time.

CHAPTER FIVE

THE PRE-HYPERTENSION PLOY

Here's Jim's curious blood pressure story…

One night in May, 2003, I went to sleep with perfectly normal blood pressure, 120/80. I awoke the next morning and my blood pressure and my cardiovascular health were suddenly "in danger."

No, my blood pressure hadn't shot up overnight because of a nightmare or a pepperoni pizza party. Rather, government health officials had pulled a fast one: They revised the official blood pressure guidelines to include a new category called "pre-hypertension."

Because of these new guidelines, anyone with a blood pressure top number (systolic) of 120 or over, or a bottom number (diastolic) of 80 or over—once the hallmark of "perfect blood pressure"—receives a diagnosis of "pre-hypertension" and should start worrying about the very real possibility of having a heart attack or stroke; or at least that's what Big Medicine wants you to think.

WHO ME? WERE THEY KIDDING?

You'd be hard-pressed to find anyone more "health obsessed" than me. I weigh exactly the same as when I played football in college (only now, I have more muscles). My waistline is the same 31 inches. My health stats are enviable. Glucose level: Perfect. PSA: Perfect. Cholesterol and triglycerides: Both perfect. Even though my birth certificate says I'm 65, my biological age (according to Dr. Keith Roach's Real Age testing at www.realage.com) is a youthful 38.

How could I suddenly have a blood pressure problem?

I wasn't alone. Almost 25% of all Americans over 18 now fit this new category (along with another 25% who already have been diagnosed with hypertension). Millions of us in our 30s, 40s, 50s, and 60s, who thought we were paragons of health, were crestfallen when these new guidelines were released.

I guess we were not trying hard enough to be healthy.

THE GOVERNMENT SOUNDS A WAKE-UP CALL

"This is a wake-up call," warned Sheldon Sheps, MD, who served on the National Heart Lung and Blood Institute (NHLBI) committee that drafted the new blood pressure guidelines. "We've changed what 'normal' is, because we now know that blood pressure in the pre-hypertension range is not normal." [38]

Huh?

These new recommendations resulted from the NHLBI examining more than 30 clinical studies worldwide that showed the risk of heart disease and stroke starts to rise with readings as low as 115/75—and the risk doubles for each increase of 20/10 millimeters of mercury.

The NHLBI committee believes that raising the threshold for healthy blood pressure will drastically reduce the number of deaths from cardiovascular disease, stroke and kidney disease. Lowering high blood pressure may also reduce the advance of dementia and cognitive impairment, which is more common in people who suffer from hypertension. [39]

Their research found that people with blood pressure levels between 120/80 and 140/90 have twice the risk of heart disease as those with lower blood pressure. And people with blood pressure above 140/90—the official definition of hypertension—have four times the risk of heart disease. [40]

"We've also learned that people age 55 and older who currently have normal blood pressure have a 90% risk of developing high blood pressure down the road," says Aram Chobanian, MD, Dean of Boston University School of Medicine, who chaired the guidelines committee.

Those of us now classified with pre-hypertension were told we needed to make aggressive lifestyle changes, which included losing excess weight, becoming more physically active, limiting alcoholic beverages, quitting cigarettes, and following a heart-healthy diet (including reducing sodium consumption). Doctors were also urged to take high blood pressure more seriously and treat it more aggressively, often with more than one drug. [41]

MORE PATIENTS, MORE DRUGS?

Can you imagine the whoops and cheers that arose from drug manufacturers when the NHLBI announced these new guidelines? Overnight, the market for blood pressure drugs doubled! An estimated 50 million additional Americans became potential customers.

"The vast majority of these newly diagnosed pre-hypertensive patients eventually will end up on drugs," Dr. Alderman predicted at the time.[42] That's because the lifestyle recommendations mentioned above will not be adopted by the majority of patients, because their healthcare providers have no incentive (or, often, the knowledge) to adequately educate them.

Remember, health insurance providers don't reimburse physicians for "education." Few patients, therefore, will have the opportunity to adopt and stick with these nondrug remedies. So, the pharmaceutical companies gained new customers by default—and anti-hypertensive drugs have become a $17 billion-a-year industry.

DRUG INDUSTRY COLLUSION?

With so much money to gain, it's natural to wonder if the manufacturers of blood pressure drugs helped to influence the NHLBI's decision. It certainly wouldn't be the first time. In a 2006 *New York Times* article, reporter Stephanie Saul revealed that three major pharmaceutical companies—Merck, Novartis, Sankyo—donated hundreds of thousands of dollars to the American Society of Hypertension to schedule lecture dinners at which the main topic of conversation was an "expanded concept of high blood pressure," i.e., lower numbers for treatable hypertension.

Saul states that doctors were quite aware that this "redistricting" of hypertension numbers potentially put millions of people on drugs that would not otherwise be popping them faithfully each day. By changing the definition of normal, more people were taking drugs on doctor's orders. And why not? Physicians, too, make lots of money on this pre-hypertension ploy, with the more patients they see and appointments they book.

The *Journal of Internal Medicine* published a study that demonstrates that these "expanded concepts of high blood pressure" (that's a cute euphemism, isn't it?) result in many people taking drugs they don't need. Mind you, this is a respected medical journal connecting the dots.

The researchers studied 20,000 people, using "pre-hypertension era" data to determine if people at the new borderline category were really at risk. The evidence confirmed they were not. For people under the age of 50, the researchers found that a systolic reading could reach as high as 200 before there was a genuine health risk. And, for the diastolic reading, any number under 100 was acceptable. For those older than 50, researchers did not note any health risk at all until patients reached a diastolic pressure of 140.

This study confirms that the "imminent danger of pre-hypertension" may well be a lot of baloney. As the physicians of yesteryear realized, blood pressure is an individual thing. What may be high for one person may be just fine for another. We are not, after all, machines.

Unfortunately, when a doctor tells a person that his blood pressure is high and requires drug treatment, most people comply without question and then stoically suffer the resultant side effects. And that's just what the drug companies want people to do.

NO SCIENTIFIC EVIDENCE SUPPORTS THESE NEW GUIDELINES

Dr. Alderman emphasizes the absence of any new scientific evidence to support the NHLBI claim that artery damage and an increased risk of heart disease begins at blood pressure in the new pre-hypertensive range. Here's his conclusion:

> Since I went to medical school (and I graduated in 1962)…the level at which we called people hypertensive is arbitrary, and that level has constantly been reduced since 1910.

The effect of moving that level from 140 to 120 is to include 50 million Americans into some thing labeled pre-hypertension…So now we have medicalized 100 million (additional) Americans…" [43]

Now, eight years later, thanks to a recent meta-analysis of existing hypertension research by the celebrated Cochrane Collaboration, we know that forcing blood pressure below the 140/90 level *does* not prolong survival—nor does it reduce the risk of stroke, heart attack, heart failure, or kidney failure. [44] (The Cochrane Collaboration is widely considered to be among the most reliable sources for scientific judgments about whether some intervention—a diet, a surgical procedure, a diagnostic technique—will actually do what doctors hope it does.) [45]

In other words, the 2003 NHLBI revised guidelines on pre-hypertension was bogus—and still is. We recommend that you bring this up with your physician the next time he tries to put you on a blood pressure drug if you're reading comes in at 140/90 or lower, and if you have no other risk factors for cardiovascular disease.

Of course, that's small consolation for the millions of patients who followed doctor's orders back then, put their health at risk and suffered miserable side effects, by taking unnecessary medication to "manage their pre-hypertension."

WHO KNEW?

So far, despite the findings from the Cochrane Collaboration review, the NHLBI still has not rescinded its proclamation on pre-hypertension. So, it is safe to assume that the average physician is still routinely handing out drug prescriptions to patients who don't need it.

Who knows if the NHLBI will ever acknowledge that its 2003 revised guidelines were a mistake.

But the medical community *did* know.

As early as 2000, the *European Heart Journal* went on record to say: "No randomized clinical trial has ever demonstrated any reduction of the risk of either overall or cardiovascular death by reducing systolic blood pressure to below 149 mmHg."

And in a research paper presented at the American Stroke Association's 29th International Stroke Conference (in February 2004) entitled "Hypertension, But Not Pre-hypertension, Increases Stroke Risk," attendees received an analysis of data from the National Health and Nutrition Examination Survey (NHANES I) showing that people defined as having "pre-hypertension" according to this new blood pressure category, do not appear to be at increased risk of heart attack or stroke. Indeed, the new pre-hypertension category was criticized as having created a new "disease," with consequent and needless anxiety for the public. [46]

CREATING NEW DISEASES FOR PROFIT?

What is more likely is that the makers of blood pressure drugs tore a page from the playbook of the cholesterol drug manufacturers—a marketing strategy that has raked in billions since the National Cholesterol Education Program (NCEP) updated its clinical guidelines for cholesterol levels in 2001. Those revised guidelines had the effect of turning elevated cholesterol into a new disease category, with the result of *tripling* the number of people who should take prescription drugs to lower their cholesterol, from 13 million to 36 million. This was a boon for the makers of cholesterol-lowering drugs known as statins.

Pre-diabetes. A similar strategy was employed in the creation of the "pre-diabetes" category. In 2002, the American Diabetes Association felt this new term was a clearer way of explaining what it means to have higher than normal blood sugar levels—that you are likely to develop diabetes and may already be experiencing its adverse health effects.

Pre-osteoporosis. "Osteopenia" is the term that describes the state of bone mineral density (BMD) that is below average, but not so low as to be considered osteoporosis. The condition was first defined in 1992 and has only recently been thought of as a medical problem requiring treatment.

It is a little-known fact that the pharmaceutical giant Merck aggressively popularized osteopenia to expand the market for its blockbuster drug, Fosamax, which had $3 billion annual sales until the patent recently expired. Merck accomplished this by pressuring manufacturers of bone density scanners to create a low-cost version of their diagnostic machine so that larger numbers of women could be tested. Merck also created a bogus nonprofit organization called the Bone Measurement Institute and used it to successfully lobby Medicare to cover the cost of bone scans. This opened the door to large-scale screenings and millions of diagnoses for the new condition, "osteopenia." Merck profited handsomely from this expansion of its Fosamax market. [47]

"There's a powerful economic incentive for pharmaceutical firms to expand the boundaries of the use of different therapies," says Caleb Alexander, MD, a pharmacoepidemiologist at the University of Chicago. "Whether you consider treatments for osteoporosis or treatments for depression or treatments for high cholesterol…pharmaceutical firms stand to benefit if the therapies for these diseases are broadly used—even if they're used among people who have very mild forms of these diseases."

This is why drug companies and pharmacy chains routinely sponsor free screenings for blood pressure, cholesterol, diabetes, and other medical conditions. They know the odds of identifying a health problem or "irregularity" among people tested are on their side. And they, more than anyone else, stand to benefit should treatment or "preventative treatment" be necessary. Diagnosis is good for pharmaceutical and medical commerce, which helps explain why there's so much "free" testing going on today.

IS HIGHER BLOOD PRESSURE NORMAL WITH AGING?

Before the advent of Big Pharma, physicians considered blood pressure "normal" if it was either 140/90 or 100 plus the person's age over 90. This was because doctors recognized that blood pressure naturally rises as people in Western cultures get older. [48] "This is adaptive, not hypertensive," writes Thomas Cowan, MD, author of *The Fourfold Path to Healing*. It's a normal response to arterial 'wear and tear' as one ages."

"In medical school, we were taught that the top (systolic) number was normal if it was less than 100 plus the age of the patient," Dr. Cowan explained. "Thus, 170 would be normal systolic reading for a 70-year-old man. The bottom (diastolic) number always was considered normal if it was under 90."

"About 10 years ago, a number of studies seemed to show that the bottom (diastolic) number was more important than the top (systolic) number in predicting adverse outcomes such as stroke and kidney disease," he notes. "For years, physicians tended to ignore the systolic pressure and focused on normalizing the diastolic pressure. But, lately, a few studies have shown that both numbers are important for predicting outcomes. Also, we no longer say that 100 plus the patient's age is normal. Rather, 140 is said to be the safe systolic limit, regardless of the age of the patient." [49]

But the NHLBI, perhaps with the encouragement of hypertension drug makers, didn't think so back in 2003 when it revised the nation's blood pressure guidelines.

"We've learned that people age 55 and older, who currently have normal blood pressure, have a 90% risk of developing high blood pressure down the road," says Aram Chobanian, MD, Dean of Boston University School of Medicine, who chaired the guidelines committee.

"We have a lot of concern about this rise in blood pressure over the course of our lifetimes, and to try to prevent that from happening, we have identified a 'pre-hypertension' group in which lifestyle changes can make a difference," Dr. Chobanian says. [50]

THE NHLBI DEFIES MOTHER NATURE

But maybe high blood pressure is just an inevitable consequence of aging, as physicians around the world have believed since the beginning of modern medicine?

Not so, said Dr. Chobanian and the NHLBI. "There are populations in the world where age-related rises in blood pressure are minimal," he responded. "In areas of Mexico, certain areas of the South Pacific, and other parts of the world with very low salt intake, there's not anywhere near the age-related rise in blood pressure that we see in the United States." [51]

We find this response quite incredible for two reasons.

First, that an aggressive national (and now global) policy to drive down what may be completely natural and safe elevations in blood pressure among the elderly is based on nothing more than someone's anecdotal interpretation of epidemiology seems quite absurd.

Could it also be that the pace of life in those low blood pressure areas of Mexico and the South Pacific was less hectic than the pace of the US? Or could their health be affected by the mineral content of their drinking water? Or could the absence of sugar, sodas, or refined carbohydrates in their diet be making the difference? Or perhaps any number of other possibilities that the NHLBI overlooked? For goodness' sake, this is the chairperson of a very influential committee setting health standards for our nation who is jumping to these unwarranted conclusions.

Second, that Dr. Chobanian offhandedly tossed in the dietary salt reference merely *assumes* that sodium is responsible for the higher level of blood pressure in the US. (In Chapter Seven, you will see a convincing argument that this simply isn't the case.)

Our point is: If national health policy is decided in such a casual, unscientific manner, all of us had better think twice, and thoroughly investigate the science, before following *any* official health pronouncements.

Or dare we suspect that such a flimsy argument is merely a smokescreen explanation to cover up the real motivation for revising the accepted blood pressure levels: Helping the pharmaceutical industry sell more drugs to gullible, trusting Americans.

Makes you wonder, doesn't it?

CHAPTER SIX

RISK FACTORS FOR HYPERTENSION

If you know your own risk factors for developing hypertension, you can use the information in this book to change some and eliminate very damaging patterns. Here are common factors that contribute to hypertension.

- Arterial inflammation.

- Atherosclerosis (hardening of the arteries).

- Poor diet.

- Overweight.

- Inactivity.

- Smoking.

- Excess alcohol consumption.

- Aging.

- Genetics.

- Uncontrolled stress.

- Insulin resistance or diabetes.

- Women's use of hormone replacement therapy (HRT).

- Air pollution.

- Heavy metal toxicity including lead, mercury, arsenic, and cadmium.

WHAT CAUSES HYPERTENSION

So what's causing the underlying problem that is raising your blood pressure?

Think of hypertension as your body sending you a red flag warning that says, "Hey, we are developing a problem down here!"

Whether that problem is being caused by cigarette smoke, an inflammatory diet, or any of the other risk factors described below, your body is crying out for *healing,* not drugs. Forcing down your blood pressure with drugs is like turning up your home's air conditioning because a fire in the basement is making the living room uncomfortably warm. Once that fire gets out of control, you are probably going to lose the entire house.

The same dire consequences can befall your cardiovascular system. If one of those plaques erupts, it may trigger a blood clot that can obstruct the arteries that feed the heart or brain. This cuts off the oxygen supply to these vital organs, causing a heart attack or stroke, resulting in serious damage or sudden death. In fact, half of all heart attacks are fatal and have no prior warning signs.

There is a close link between hypertension and atherosclerosis (hardening of the arteries) and either one can contribute to the development of the other. Certain populations should pay particular attention to these relationships. For example, 60% of patients with high blood pressure also have diabetes. In another instance, hypertension disproportionately affects African-Americans, who tend to develop hypertension at a younger age than the general population and are more susceptible to complications from the disorder, such as stroke and heart disease. [52] We will examine these and other co-relationships in this chapter.

First, let's take a look at the recognized risk factors and general medical advice...

Arterial Inflammation. Doctors are slowly realizing that inflammation is a common risk factor for numerous diseases, including heart disease, Alzheimer's disease, arthritis, and many others. In fact, they are discovering that nearly every degenerative disease humans develop has a link to inflammation.

Here's how it occurs in the case of cardiovascular disease and hypertension. Because the endothelial tissue that lines the inside walls of your arteries is so delicate, it is easily damaged. Common irritants include cigarette smoke, glucose (sugar), insulin, excess blood pressure, lead toxicity, and air pollution. These irritants "burn" and "etch" the endothelium as if acid had been poured on it, triggering an immune response, which initiates the healing process.

To repair these microscopic burns and scratches, your body lays down fatty deposits called plaques, which are later fortified with calcium. This calcium is what narrows arteries and renders them inflexible (causing hardening of the arteries, or atherosclerosis). Both factors elevate blood pressure.

Atherosclerosis. Let's remember one thing: hypertension *is not* a disease. As we stated earlier, it is really a signal that your arteries are sick and need healing. This is commonly experienced around middle age, when most adult Americans develop the early (or late) stages of atherosclerosis. [53] The main effect is congestion of the arteries and veins, resulting from plaque accumulation, being overweight, or chronic inhalation of toxic substances (especially air pollution, auto exhaust, and household mold). Another cause is a lack of nutrients necessary for healthy blood pressure and artery health. [54]

In addition, hardened arteries—and the elevated blood pressure they help create—increase the workload on the heart, making it beat harder until it is exhausted with the effort and can't go on any longer. This "giving up" is referred to as congestive heart failure.

Hypertension eventually damages blood vessels everywhere in the human body, including those in the kidneys. If that happens, the kidneys may stop excreting waste and extra fluids, which in turn causes blood pressure to go up even more. Eventually, the kidneys will fail completely, necessitating either dialysis (filtering the blood through a machine to remove toxins) or an organ transplant. [55]

Poor diet. Certain foods, such as sweets, soda pop, and refined carbohydrates (baked goods using white flour, chips, crackers, breakfast cereals) break down into glucose immediately after eating them and elevate your blood sugar. This high blood sugar signals the body to release insulin into the bloodstream to reduce the concentration of glucose. The combination of insulin and blood sugar, if chronically elevated, inflames your arteries and leads to atherosclerosis and hypertension, along with the same risks of heart disease, heart attack, and stroke described above. Your body also uses up nutrients that help keep blood pressure under control when it has to process and function on "junk" food.

Weight gain and hypertension. If you've experienced excessive weight gain, chances are you have hypertension. [56] Population studies show that high blood pressure is directly proportional to body weight—and that the number of people who are obese corresponds with the prevalence of hypertension around the world, although this relationship differs among races. As the magnitude of weight gain increases, blood pressure also rises. In general, being overweight or obese is by far the biggest risk for developing high blood pressure.

In fact, as much as 50% of overweight men and women with high blood pressure may be hypertensive as a result of their weight, according to research presented at the American Heart Association's 2007 Conference of the Council for High Blood Pressure Research.

"This is important because it means…the high blood pressure was not a form of essential hypertension, but was hypertension secondary to body weight," said Roberto Fogari, MD, lead investigator of the study and professor of medicine at the University of Pavia, Italy. [57]

A 14-year observational study conducted by the Mayo Clinic found that even people of normal weight who had a high waist-to-hip ratio (i.e. they had belly fat) were at an increased risk for death caused by a cardiovascular event. Central obesity, that is fat stored around the midsection, increases the mortality risk even for people of normal weight. A larger waist size may also increase hypertension. [58]

While the association between weight gain and hypertension is widely recognized, the exact nature of this relationship is still being studied. Some researchers believe high insulin levels are the cause. Others blame it on stiffening arteries due to glycation, particularly if you have an accumulation of belly fat.[59] (Glycation is an uncontrolled chemical reaction of sugars with proteins that can damage blood vessels.) But a far more plausible explanation is described in Chapter Eight.

Fitness level. Lack of exercise is one of the most important risk factors for hypertension—and statistics confirm this. Those who are less active are found to be 30% to 50% more likely to develop hypertension than those who are active. [60]

In the ongoing Kuopio Ischemic Heart Disease Risk Factor Study, researchers studied the fitness level of 2,682 men between the ages of 42 and 60. Nearly 11 years later, the scientists followed up with 585 of the original study participants. A declining fitness level was shown to be a strong predictor of heart problems. [61] Men who lost more than 15% of their cardio-respiratory fitness over a 10-year period faced a near doubling of their risk of acute myocardial infarction (heart attack) over the subsequent decade and more than twice the risk of dying of any cause. Fitness is important at any age. This study proves that it's even more important as we age.

Alcohol. In small amounts, alcohol can actually lower your blood pressure by a couple of points. But more than one drink a day for women of any age and men over the age of 65, or two daily drinks for men under 65, can cause blood pressure to rise. [62, 63] In addition, if you're on blood pressure medication, be sure to ask your doctor if you should be drinking alcohol at all.

Excess caffeine. It is well known that drinking caffeinated beverages constricts blood vessels, which raises blood pressure temporarily (for about an hour after consumption). But if you chain-drink coffee or tea continuously throughout the day, your blood vessels never get a chance to relax, and that's not healthy. Studies show that caffeine in moderate amounts is fine, particularly if you are a habitual coffee drinker and your body has already built up a tolerance to the stimulant.

In fact, coffee or tea can be beneficial for your cardiovascular system. Both are high in antioxidant content, which lessens arterial inflammation, helps prevent fat and calcium deposits from accumulating on artery walls, and can even reduce blood pressure over time. (Did you know that coffee is the leading source of antioxidants in the American diet?) However, caffeine can drain your cortisol levels, the most important hormone in the body. Our advice is to limit your consumption to no more than four cups per day—less if your blood pressure spikes after drinking it.

Age. The older you get, the more likely your blood pressure will rise due to hardening of the arteries, especially the systolic (top) number. But this isn't necessarily something to worry about, because it's normal for arteries to lose a certain amount of their elasticity with age. Before the advent and influence of Big Pharma, most physicians knew this and weren't really concerned about elevated blood pressure in the elderly (except in extreme cases). In fact, rising blood pressure is so common with advancing age that one is tempted to consider this normal. For instance, in the famous Framingham Heart Study, hypertension eventually developed in more than 90% of the participants who had normal blood pressure at age 55. [64]

Genetics. If hypertension runs in your family, you're at greater risk for having it. However, this doesn't have to be your destiny. Hypertension is largely a lifestyle condition, and your diet and behavior are more important than your genes. Heredity means that your body will more readily respond to the behavioral factors that cause high blood pressure (poor diet, smoking, being overweight, inactivity, stress, etc.), but conditioning plays the deciding role.

If your mother lived on chocolate or your father smoked, you are more likely to display these traits—not because of your genes, but because you "modeled" (or learned) their behaviors as you grew up. The good news is that these behaviors can be un-learned (and must be!) if you want to escape the fate to which these behaviors lead.

Stress. Did you catch the worry bug? Do you fret over every little thing that pops up in your day or life? Uncontrolled stress can cause or worsen hypertension. When you're feeling stressed, worried, or chronically agitated or angry, cortisol (the stress hormone) and adrenaline (the fight-or-flight hormone) are activated. These cause the heart to beat faster, make arteries constrict, stimulate your appetite, and disrupt your sleep. Each of these factors can elevate your blood pressure and trigger unhealthy behaviors that make things worse. Uncontrolled stress, worry, and anger are the fast track to cardiovascular trouble, including heart attack and stroke.

Smoking. Cigarette smoking raises blood pressure and accelerates the hardening of arteries, but does not directly cause hypertension. Nonetheless, it is an indirect risk factor for hypertension. This effect is caused by nicotine, which constricts blood vessels, and this effect occurs with each cigarette smoked. The rise in blood pressure is most prominent with the first cigarette of the day. In one study of non-hypertensive smokers, researchers recorded an average rise in systolic pressure of 20 mmHg after the first cigarette. [65]

Smoking inflames and injures blood vessel walls, thus speeding up the hardening of the arteries,[66] which may persist for a decade after quitting. [67] About 30% of all heart disease deaths in the US are directly related to cigarette smoking, because smoking causes coronary artery disease (CAD). [68]

Indeed, your risk of heart attack increases with the number of cigarettes you've inhaled. The longer you've smoked, the greater your risk. People who smoke a pack of cigarettes a day have more than twice the risk of heart attack than non-smokers. Women who smoke and also take birth control pills increase by several times their risk of heart attack, stroke, and peripheral vascular disease. [69]

Smoking increases the risk of atherosclerosis in several ways. It decreases the level of protective HDL cholesterol and increases the level of triglycerides, which are pro-inflammatory. Smoking also boosts the level of carbon monoxide in the blood, which damages the delicate lining of arteries. As mentioned, nicotine constricts arteries, and if an artery is already partially blocked, this constriction further decreases the amount of blood reaching the tissues and heart muscle. (It should be noted that secondhand smoke also produces these negative effects.) [70]

Diabetes. Hypertension and diabetes share several common risk factors, including:

- Obesity.

- Inactivity.

- Elevated insulin.

- Elevated blood sugar levels.

- Inflammatory diet.

- Air pollution and lead toxicity.

Diabetes often contributes to the development of hypertension because it damages artery walls and leads to atherosclerosis; thickens the blood, forcing the heart to work harder; and decreases the flexibility of the walls of the arteries. Fundamentally, diabetes means having excess insulin in the bloodstream, and one of insulin's roles is to control arterial tension. Changes in the way the body processes insulin have been shown to raise blood pressure. [71]

Standard medical treatment for both conditions does little to heal or reverse them. As with hypertension medications, the medications that doctors prescribe for diabetes merely manage symptoms while the underlying problem worsens. Doctors are satisfied if your numbers (blood sugar or blood pressure) are within an acceptable range, so they rarely try to correct the problem that's causing these symptoms. (With diabetes it's often your diet.) If you have diabetes and want to see how you can dramatically improve your condition, check out *The 30-Day Diabetes Cure* at www.30daydiabetescure.com.

Women's use of hormone replacement therapy (HRT). A recent study[72] of more than 40,000 post-menopausal women (average age 63 years) in Australia revealed that the use of HRT significantly raised a woman's risk for developing high blood pressure. The youngest group, ages 45 to 55 years, showed the most pronounced association. Overall, the risk was 3% higher among women on HRT than in those who had never used it. The longer HRT was used, the higher the risk. However, this study was seriously flawed in that no one checked hormone levels (especially in saliva). Hormone supplementation can be dangerous and giving it blindly is ill advised. No one is yet certain if HRT actually *causes* elevated blood pressure, but the likelihood is high enough for researchers to suggest that physicians should take this newly discovered risk into account when prescribing HRT for their patients, and try to minimize the time they use it.

Air pollution and lead. The medical journal *Circulation* reported that even a very small level of lead toxicity dramatically increased the risk for strokes, heart attacks, and death in adults. This is because the aorta, which is the body's main artery, is a primary area where lead accumulates. Since the aorta supplies oxygenated blood to the entire body, it's no surprise that even small amounts of lead are a big danger, increasing the risk of cardiovascular events and death.

In this study, a fractional level of lead toxicity of only 2 micrograms per deciliter increased the risk of heart attack by a whopping 151%. Lead increased the risk of stroke by 89%.

Lead-based paints were not banned in the US until 1978, so many Americans alive today have lived in homes and apartments that were painted with lead paint. Lead paint was also used to paint children's toys in the past. In fact, even in these times, when we know better, some toys made in China have been found to contain lead-based paints.

Plumbing fixtures used to be soldered with lead joints. This type of plumbing is still in use in many older homes and even in municipal water systems (another very good reason to filter your drinking water—see more on how in Chapter Fifteen).

In addition, industrial pollution sends lead dust into the air we breathe and deposits lead into our soil and water. Lead "sinkers" are common in tackle boxes, and unknowing fishermen can absorb lead through their skin every time they weight a line. Lead is found in batteries, radiation shields, some ceramic glazes on cups and dishware, certain art supplies, and in sewer sludge.

Even some cosmetics contain lead. A study published in 2007 found lead present in 33 different brands of red lipstick, including one "natural" brand. Worse yet, lead has even been found in some dietary supplements.

Traditional healthcare providers often overlook the symptoms of lead poisoning. Common symptoms such as hair loss can easily be blamed on aging, and lead-induced anemia is often treated with iron supplements. This can lead to even greater damage in the body, including adding excessive iron to a body already trying to cope with excess lead.

Lead can also be deposited in the bones. *The Journal of the American Medical Association (JAMA)* reported back in 2003 that there was a strong correlation between lead levels and high blood pressure in post-menopausal women. Aging may cause bones to decalcify. Women are especially at risk for this loss of bone density. As the bones decalcify, they release any stored lead into the circulatory system where it can cause further damage. [73]

One of the most frightening things about lead poisoning is that the symptoms can be very mild, and even go unnoticed, until the victim suffers a heart attack. That's one of the reasons lead poisoning is called, like hypertension, "the silent killer."[74]

You can read more about detoxifying your body and your environment—as well as chelation therapy—in Chapter Fifteen.

OTHER HYPERTENSION RISK FACTORS THAT DOCTORS OVERLOOK

If you have high blood pressure, ask your doctor to check for these often-overlooked risk factors:

Hormonal imbalances. The human body is regulated by two major hormones (thyroid and cortisol) and four minor ones (estrogen, progesterone, testosterone, and DHEA). The best way to measure thyroid accurately is a blood test for TSH, free T4 and free T3. The most accurate way to measure cortisol is via saliva. Your doctor can also run various tests that will identify your levels of the minor hormones mentioned above. Having your hormones in balance is crucial to controlling and reversing hypertension.

Testosterone deficiency. Middle-aged men with metabolic syndrome—a cluster of symptoms including high blood pressure, insulin resistance, a potbelly, and low HDL (good) cholesterol— often have testosterone deficiency. Be sure your doctor checks your levels of "free testosterone," which is the testosterone available for immediate use by your body. Supplementation with bioidentical testosterone (available by prescription only from compounding pharmacies) may normalize your blood pressure, as well as your blood sugar, HDL cholesterol and reverse your weight gain.

Sleep apnea. In this condition, fatty tissue in the throat obstructs airways during sleep, interrupting your breathing for brief periods throughout the night. When you breathe normally, air enters and exits the lungs freely through an open airway. If the airway becomes obstructed to any degree—as is often the case for people suffering from sleep apnea—the amount of pressure needed to draw air though the airway is increased. Over time, these pressures can lead to pulmonary hypertension.

Here's how to tell if you have sleep apnea: "If you snore, are overweight, your spouse says you stop breathing during the night, and/or you're tired during the day—you have sleep apnea," reports Craig Schwimmer, MD, clinical assistant professor at the University of Texas Southwest Medical School and medical director of the Snoring Center in Texas. Another symptom is awakening suddenly and gasping for breath. And even thin people can have sleep apnea.

Solutions for sleep apnea include:

- Losing weight.

- Using a mouth guard appliance prepared by your dentist.

- Sleeping on your side instead of your back or stomach.

- Using a continuous positive airway pressure machine (CPAP) during sleep.

The CPAP remedy is cumbersome, involving the wearing of a special mask during sleep. Fewer than 50% of people prescribed a CPAP stick with it. If the other approaches don't work for you, a better, more permanent solution is a quick outpatient surgery called the *pillar procedure,* in which small polyester rods are placed in your soft palate to make it stiffer and keep it from fluttering.

Food allergies. Do you have food allergies or sensitivities? Food allergies can release "antibody antigen complexes" into your blood vessels, causing blood pressure to rise. Wheat, dairy, seafood, soy, and nuts are common allergenic foods. If your pulse or body temperature tends to rise after eating, ask your doctor to check you for food allergies using any of the diagnostic tests listed below.

- **The Skin Prick Test** involves placing a small amount of an allergen on the skin, pricking the skin, and waiting for a reaction.

- **The Intradermal Skin Test** is similar, but it directly injects allergens underneath the skin.

- **Patch Tests** require taping an allergen to the skin for 48 hours and waiting for a reaction.

- **Blood Tests** measure how many immunoglobulin (Ig E) antibodies to a particular allergen are in the blood.

- **Elimination Diet.** If all this talk of needles makes you a little weak in the knees, you can experiment with an elimination diet. This is a special eating plan that eliminates all of the suspect foods from your diet for about two weeks and then reintroduces them, one every few days, after which you and your healthcare provider will monitor your blood pressure to see if the reintroduction of a specific food produces adverse results. Although the elimination diet is time consuming, its ability to pinpoint exactly which foods are affecting your blood pressure makes it the best way to identify your personal problem foods.

THE 800-POUND GORILLA IN THE ROOM

These are the major risk factors for hypertension, widely recognized by doctors and health officials. But we are certain there is an even greater risk factor for hypertension, which the vast majority of physicians are overlooking. And while we've only alluded to it in this chapter, we are convinced that this culprit is the single most important underlying cause of hypertension—and also of arterial disease, insulin resistance, metabolic syndrome, and obesity.

Little attention is given to this under-the-radar risk factor, but from all the studies and research we've reviewed, it is Public Enemy Number One with regard to blood pressure dysfunction and poor health. It's so serious, in our opinion, that we've reserved the entirety of Chapter Nine for the purpose of exposing this risk, explaining its connection to hypertension and showing you how to protect yourself.

CHAPTER SEVEN

THE SODIUM SCARE

Does eating too much salt cause hypertension and, ultimately, stroke and heart attack?

The correct answer is going to completely surprise you—especially if you have been trying to follow the current official medical guidelines to cut your sodium consumption in half.

Most doctors fervently believe that sodium causes or contributes to blood pressure problems; so they regularly admonish their patients to cut back their salt intake. Their rationale is that sodium consumption forces the body to retain water, which increases the overall volume of fluid the heart must pump, thus raising blood pressure while also stressing the kidneys. Time and again we are reminded about how potentially "toxic" the salt level in the US diet can be.

The Institute of Medicine of the National Academies of Science (IOM), the scientific organization that sets the nation's standards for recommended levels of nutrients, currently advises that American adults keep their intake of salt between 1,500 mg (recommended adequate intake) and 2,300 mg (the amount above which health problems appear). People aged 70 and over may require less than 1,200 mg. [75]

Given how widespread and consistent the warnings are, you'd think there would be tons of scientific studies demonstrating the health dangers of salt. But the truth is, there isn't a single double-blind, placebo-controlled trial to back up these warnings. *Not one*.

THE SALT SCARE ISN'T BASED ON SCIENCE

If there was even a shred of scientific evidence, Michael Alderman, MD, would know of it. Besides being a professor of cardiovascular medicine, he is a past president of the American Society of Hypertension. In a 2003 interview with the Center for Medical Consumers, Dr. Alderman admitted that there is no scientific evidence relating sodium restriction to cardiovascular benefit. [76]

This finding is echoed by David McCarron, MD, a nutritionist and professor at the University of California, who stated, "There currently is no reliable scientific evidence to support the recommendation that we should reduce our sodium consumption for cardiovascular health." Dr. McCarron claims the recommendation to reduce sodium intake is based solely on personal opinion and the misguided demonization of salt by health authorities, such as the CDC.

To prove this, Dr. McCarron led a study that measured the daily salt intake of more than 19,000 subjects from about 30 countries.[77] The results confirmed three surprising conclusions:

1. Americans consume no more salt than people in other countries.

2. Salt consumption in the US has *not* increased over the past 25 years.

3. No matter how salty your food may be, your body naturally regulates its absorption, so you wind up with a consistent level overall.

According to Dr. McCarron's statistics, Americans *aren't* consuming more sodium—and salt isn't the health-destroyer that doctors and health officials claim.[78] It is a high-salt diet in combination with low intake of other nutrients that is the problem, as you'll see below. And Drs. McCarron and Alderman aren't the only medical professionals who think so.

SALT REDUCTION DOESN'T REDUCE HEART RISK

In fact, a very recent review of the existing research—including six randomized clinical trials on the effects of sodium on cardiovascular disease—shows that the IOM's recommended reductions in salt intake do *not* reduce mortality or the incidence of cardiovascular disease. The meta-analysis was performed by the Cochrane Collaboration, a highly respected nonprofit organization composed of international scientific experts. [79]

While the research did show that decreasing salt consumption by 50% did reduce blood pressure modestly, it produced no reduction in overall fatalities or the risk of heart attack and/or stroke. The Cochrane review stated that "Cutting down on the amount of salt has no clear benefits in terms of likelihood of dying or experiencing cardiovascular disease," while a press release sent by the Cochrane Library clearly stated: "Cutting down on salt does not reduce your chance of dying." [80]

Incidentally, this latest review follows a Cochrane meta-analysis of 57 studies conducted a few years ago that also found no benefit from lowering salt intake, while a separate Cochrane review found cutting back on salt will only shave a point off your blood pressure.[81]

In other words, both Cochrane reviews concluded that cutting back on salt consumption to levels that the IOM is recommending will result in *zero reduction* in mortality or cardiovascular events. If this is true—and many consider the Cochrane group to be one of the most dependable sources of clinical interpretation—you might ask, "Why bother?"

What benefit is a meager reduction in blood pressure if it doesn't lead to a lower risk of death and disease? And is this worth reducing your salt consumption by half (which is very difficult for most people to achieve in the real world)? What this really illustrates is that minor reductions in your blood pressure are not nearly as important as your doctor has been telling you, according to the most reliable science.

SOMETIMES SALT RESTRICTION CAN BE DEADLY

Not only would you be correct to doubt the value of going to all that trouble, but your prudence might save your life. That's because some studies show that restricting salt actually may *increase* the risk of premature death by as much as 500%. Three separate clinical trials that tested low-sodium diets on patients with kidney disease and heart failure linked the salt-restricted diets to higher risks of hospitalizations, cardiovascular events, and death.

Researchers from the University of Leuven in Belgium tracked nearly 4,000 people age 60 years and younger for eight years and found absolutely no link at all between sodium consumption and blood pressure levels. Overall, they found a death rate of 4.1% from heart conditions among those with the lowest sodium intake, 1.9% among those with moderate intake, and 0.8% among those with the highest intake of salt.

This means that patients with the lowest salt intakes were more than five times more likely to die of cardiovascular disease (CVD) than those who consumed the most, according to this study published in the *Journal of the American Medical Association (JAMA)*. [82]

These findings were further confirmed by a study that analyzed seven years of diet and health data from nearly 9,000 people. The researchers found that those with a lower intake of salt did indeed have a *higher risk* of cardiovascular disease (CVD). Their conclusion? "For the general population, higher sodium intake is unlikely to be independently associated with (a direct cause of) higher CVD or all-cause mortality from any cause." [83]

Low blood levels of sodium (a medical condition called *hyponatraemia*) represent another potential health problem. German researchers found that elderly people who avoided salt in an effort to deter high blood pressure were secretly suffering from this low-salt disorder, as well as higher risk of hospitalizations, cardiovascular events, and even death.

Dr. Alderman explains how this is possible: "When you lower sodium intake in some people, it lowers blood pressure. But for most people, it doesn't. And in a few people, it actually *raises* blood pressure." [84]

He adds, "Lowering salt to reduce blood pressure has other effects. It stimulates the renin angiotensin system and raises the pulse rate. Both of these things adversely affect the heart. And it decreases insulin sensitivity—that's bad for you, too."[85] (Keep this observation of Dr. Alderman's in mind: Reducing salt consumption decreases insulin sensitivity; or in other words, increases your body's need for more insulin.)

Bottom line: A low-salt diet alone won't significantly lower your blood pressure, protect your heart, or increase your longevity. In fact, just the opposite might be true. We realize that this flies in the face of everything you've heard in your doctor's office and from the mainstream media, but it's hard to dispute the science.

THE GLOBAL CAMPAIGN FOR SALT REDUCTION

Nevertheless, the US government and Big Medicine are continuing to pressure food manufacturers to reduce the sodium content of their products. And they are continuing to badger consumers into limiting their daily salt intake to 1,500 mg.

Indeed, the medical community flatly rejected the Cochrane findings and echoed their stubborn opinion that "…all the other evidence clearly demonstrates that a reduction in the whole of the UK population and worldwide is immensely important," said Professor Graham MacGregor, chairman of World Action on Salt and Health (WASH). "A reduction in population salt intake will have major beneficial effects on health along with major cost savings in all countries around the world," said the WASH researchers. [86]

The American Heart Association, too, insisted its position on sodium reduction would not change. "The American Heart Association strongly recommends that…reducing sodium now—even for people who have normal blood pressure—can reap enormous long-term benefits by reducing the risk for developing high blood pressure and helping those with high blood pressure manage their condition more effectively."[87]

Weighing in on the controversy, the popular online physician Joseph Mercola, MD, has written, "The data supporting universal salt reduction have never been compelling, nor has it ever been demonstrated that such a program would not have unforeseen negative side effects. This was the verdict, for instance, of a review published in *JAMA*." [88]

The study he's referring to was conducted by University of Copenhagen researchers who analyzed 114 randomized trials of sodium reduction. They concluded that: "A 'measurable' benefit in individuals with normal blood pressure of even a single millimeter of mercury could only be achieved with an 'extreme' reduction in salt intake." Commenting on the findings, Drummond Rennie, a *JAMA* editor and a physiologist at the University of California (UC), San Francisco, said: "You can say without any shadow of a doubt, that the National Heart Lung and Blood Institute (NHLBI) has made a commitment to salt education that goes way beyond the scientific facts." [89]

PREVIOUS STUDIES ARE BEING IGNORED

Numerous other meta-reviews of the existing evidence, whether first published by pro-salt or anti-salt researchers, have shown that significantly reducing salt consumption—say, by cutting average salt consumption by 50%—will result in a meager drop in blood pressure of only 4 to 5 mmHg in hypertensives and 1 to 2 mmHg in non-hypertensives. This yields little improvement for people with stage 1 hypertension, in which systolic blood pressure is already elevated at least 20 mmHg over what's healthy and stage 2 hypertension, in which pressure is elevated by at least 40 mmHg. In either instance, reducing salt intake makes little difference.[90]

If excessive salt consumption *is not* causing the current hypertension problem, as these clinical trials clearly show, then what is? (Keep reading. We'll shed more light on this in Chapter Nine.)

ARE MORE STUDIES NEEDED?

What of those "further studies" that the Cochrane group is recommending? WASH's MacGregor dismissed them as "…impractical…because of logistical and financial constraints and the ethical issues of putting a group of people on a high salt diet for so many years."[91] So much for science, right?

It appears that the strongly held opinion of Big Medicine will (once again) trump science. Indeed, just weeks after the Cochrane announcement, the *British Medical Journal* announced a new *global* push to sharply reduce dietary salt intake. [92]

If this sounds hard to believe, you aren't familiar with how medical politics "works" (we use the word loosely). Too many times we have seen opinions, half-truths and bad science become public policy. The cholesterol theory of heart disease leaps foremost to mind (see Chapter Ten). When asked how this is possible, Dr. Alderman—a true insider who's been in the trenches of the Salt Wars for much of his career—explains: "The NHLBI has been heavily invested in sodium restriction for 30 years. It's hard to change [their] views."

What Dr. Alderman is saying is that policy-setting doctors and health officials don't like to admit they are wrong. Even in the face of facts proving the contrary, they tend to stick to their guns. And more often than not, this stubbornness drives public health policy and treatment guidelines.

This is true regarding many official medical dictums, including the cholesterol theory of heart disease, calcium supplementation and osteoporosis, low-fat diets and obesity, glucose-lowering and diabetes, and on and on. In each of these instances, strong scientific findings reveal that the standard medical advice has been mistaken. Despite the evidence, the medical establishment continues to cling to its faulty beliefs like a captain going down with his ship.

TOO MUCH SODIUM ISN'T THE PROBLEM—
RATHER, IT'S TOO LITTLE POTASSIUM

The irony here is that "the salt crisis" that has doctors so alarmed has less to do with salt alone and more to do with the mineral potassium. Scientists have known for some time that sodium and potassium have an intimate and mutually dependent relationship in the human body.

This relationship, known as "the sodium-potassium pump," functions much like a revolving door. The pump keeps sodium ions outside of your cells and potassium ions inside.

Sodium attracts water, so when there's too much sodium and not enough potassium, cells become over-hydrated, or "bloated." This raises the volume of the blood and, in turn, raises blood pressure. Normally, adequate levels of dietary potassium would prevent or reverse this situation by pumping out the sodium, thus canceling its negative effect on blood pressure. But the typical American diet is notoriously potassium deficient, and therefore increasingly prone to hypertension.

DIETARY POTASSIUM CORRECTS THE SODIUM PROBLEM

Nutritionists have known for quite some time that raising potassium levels will lower blood pressure. Dutch research reported in the September 13, 2010, issue of the *Archives of Internal Medicine (AIM)* confirmed that raising potassium to the recommended level of 4.7g per day was shown to decrease mortality from stroke and heart disease by up to 15% and 11% respectively. More potassium also reduces salt sensitivity, the researchers reported.[93]

Confirming this beneficial effect, a 15-year study found that people with the lowest ratio of potassium-to-sodium in their diets had a significantly higher risk of death from cardiovascular disease compared with those with the highest ratio. These findings were published in the July 11, 2011, issue of *AIM*. [94,95]

So what are the best ways to boost your potassium intake?

One simple way is to replace processed snacks with fresh fruit. For example, a doughnut contains 210 mg of sodium and 120 mg of potassium. Swap this for a fresh orange (not juice), and you'll have just 1.6 mg of sodium and 150 mg of potassium. An ideal ratio of sodium to potassium in your snacks—and your overall diet—is between 1:2 and 1:3, meaning you should be consuming two to three times more potassium than sodium.

Increasing potassium intake is also easily accomplished by consuming more fresh vegetables and dairy products, which are all excellent sources of potassium. (In Chapter Twelve, we'll tell you about other foods and nutrients that help and heal hypertension.)

WHERE HAS ALL THE POTASSIUM GONE?

Americans, in general, are potassium-deficient—and there are three reasons for this:

1. Fewer people are eating fresh fruits, vegetables, and whole grains—all of which are rich in natural potassium. This high potassium content is one reason that the Hypertension Healing Foods you'll read about in Chapter Twelve are so effective.

2. More people are consuming processed foods. Processing completely removes or significantly diminishes potassium from these food products.

3. Ironically, some antihypertensive drugs, such as diuretics, flush potassium from the body. But this prescribing to help control hypertension can deplete the body of the potassium it needs to reduce blood pressure, thus making blood pressure more difficult to control. In fact, antihypertensive drugs are making blood pressure worse for many patients, as you will see in a moment.

Bottom line: "Don't torture yourself trying to achieve super-low levels of salt intake," says Jacob Teitelbaum, MD, in his book coauthored with well-known health author and holistic health coach, Bill Gottleib, *Real Cause, Real Cure* (Rodale, 2011). Lowering your salt intake further won't really help your blood pressure, and as you've seen, can actually increase your risk for the very health problem you're trying to prevent or improve.

Dr. Mercola puts it more succinctly: "Just switching to low-sodium processed foods is not going to do much to improve your health."

BREAKING NEWS: LOW-SALT DIETS MAY BE DANGEROUS

As science writer Gary Taubes, author of *Why We Get Fat* (Knopf; 2011) recounted in a recent *New York Times* opinion piece, over the last 40 years, despite all the claims about the danger of dietary salt made by the CDC, the USDA, the Institute of Medicine (IOM), and the National Institute of Health (NIH), there appears to be no credible evidence to support the hypothesis. [96] So today, all of these institutions rely on the results from a single 30-day investigation called the DASH Sodium study, which suggests that drastic reductions of salt intake would modestly decrease blood pressure. That's a far cry from saying it would prevent hypertension or even reduce it in any significant way.

Italian researchers have done a series of clinical trials that suggested reducing salt consumption among patients with heart failure actually made them more likely to die! Since then, other studies looking at nearly 100,000 individuals in some 30 countries have supported the findings of the Italians. In fact, the data suggests that people who consume less salt are more likely to have heart disease. [97]

Reducing your salt consumption can raise blood pressure? Yes, indeed. A very convincing article in the July 8, 2011, issue of *The Scientific American* entitled "It's Time to End the War on Salt" explains how this is possible: "…when salt intake is cut, the body responds by releasing renin and aldosterone, an enzyme and a hormone, respectively, that increase blood pressure."

The article also cited a 2006 *American Journal of Medicine* study that compared the reported daily sodium intakes of 78 million Americans with their risk of dying from heart disease over the course of 14 years. It found that the more sodium people ate, the less likely they were to die from heart disease. And a 2007 study published in the *European Journal of Epidemiology* followed 1,500 older people for five years and found no association between urinary sodium levels and the risk of coronary vascular disease or death. [98]

Despite these and other findings, when the Department of Agriculture and the FDA recently held a hearing to discuss how to motivate Americans to eat less salt, the consensus was to keep marching blindly forward, as if no new, contradictory evidence existed. This is unfortunate, if not tragic. When leaders hide their heads in the sand, the people who believe in them most often end up paying the price.

NATURAL VS. PROCESSED SALT

Ordinary table salt is highly processed and composed of 97.5% sodium chloride and 2.5% chemicals, such as iodine and moisture absorbents. It is also processed under extreme heat, which alters the natural chemical structure of the salt.

By contrast, natural salt, such as Himalayan salt and naturally dried sea salt, is 84% sodium chloride and 16% other naturally occurring minerals, including many beneficial trace minerals such as silicon, phosphorous, and vanadium. Natural salt is important to many biological processes, including blood pressure regulation.

However, for every gram of excess sodium chloride that your body has to neutralize, it uses up 23 grams of cellular water. Hence, eating too much processed salt will cause fluid to accumulate in your tissues, which can contribute to hypertension, if sufficient potassium isn't present.

Neither of us consumes processed table salt, preferring the superior flavor of raw sea salt. One of our favorite products is Celtic Brand Sea Salt (www.celticseasalt.com).

CHAPTER EIGHT

THE BIG FAT LIE

If you have hypertension, chances are your physician has recommended or prescribed one or more of the anti-hypertensive medications described in Appendix A (beginning on page 307) for you. This drug approach is routine these days, even though official treatment guidelines advise doctors to recommend at least six months of diet and lifestyle modifications before resorting to medication (except in emergency situations, when a patient's blood pressure is dangerously elevated).

If your doctor has given you lifestyle advice, it has probably been something along the lines of "Eat a low-fat diet, consume fewer cholesterol-containing foods (a code phrase for animal products), lose some weight, get more exercise, and cut back on the salt."

This is not because he has personally researched any of this advice. Rather, the official guidelines from the National Heart, Lung, and Blood Institute (NHLBI) tell all physicians to recommend that patients with hypertension eat a diet low in salt, cholesterol and fat. Their goal is to limit total fat intake to no more than 30% of total daily calorie intake and cholesterol to no more than 300mg per day. [99]

WHY THIS ADVICE IS WRONG—AND DANGEROUS

Losing weight and physical activity are definitely worthwhile. But, as hard as it may be for you to believe this, the rest of the routine advice is in direct contradiction to the latest research. Following these "official" suggestions will not only fail to improve your blood pressure, but can have dangerous consequences for your overall health. Here's why:

Sodium restriction. In Chapter Seven, you read why restricting sodium provides only a modest benefit to blood pressure and has no beneficial effect on cardiovascular disease or overall mortality. Regardless, the NHLBI remains adamant about making sure physicians emphasize this point to all patients, especially those with elevated blood pressure. This is much ado about nothing.

Cholesterol consumption. It is now well known in the medical and scientific communities that dietary cholesterol has almost no effect on blood cholesterol levels. This is because your liver manufactures cholesterol as needed, providing 90% of it—while your diet provides less than 10%. When your blood levels of cholesterol are elevated, your liver simply reduces its output. So the cholesterol in the foods you eat exerts almost no effect on your blood levels of cholesterol. (There is also overwhelming evidence that your cholesterol level has nothing to do with your risk of heart disease. We'll tell you more about this in Chapter Ten.)

Low-fat diet. This may be the worst medical advice of all. Reducing your consumption of any one of the three macronutrients (protein, fat, and carbohydrates), will result in an increased consumption of another—or both—unless you also cut calories, which is nearly impossible to sustain successfully in the long term. Therefore, the standard low-fat diet too often becomes a high-carb diet because people tend naturally toward carbs and sugar when other high-calorie foods, such as fat, are off limits.

As you'll see, consuming too many refined carbohydrates elevates blood sugar and insulin, thus leading to a host of health problems, including inflammation, insulin resistance and Type 2 diabetes, heart disease, many cancers, and hypertension. So it's hard to understand why the American Heart Association (AHA), the American Diabetes Association (ADA) and the NHLBI continue to push this dietary advice on patients and the general public, when according to reliable research, it may be *causing* the very health problems they are trying to alleviate.

As Gary Taubes points out in his book *Why We Get Fat*, replacing the saturated fat in your diet with carbohydrates—say, by swapping a breakfast of bacon and eggs for cornflakes, skim milk, banana slices, orange juice, and toast (hold the butter)—will indeed lower LDL (bad) cholesterol. But it will also lower your HDL (good) cholesterol, increase your triglyceride levels, and raise your risk of metabolic syndrome and heart attack.[100]

Now what happens when you trade that low-fat cornflake breakfast for the high-fat bacon and eggs? Studies dating back to the 1970s show it will *raise* your HDL cholesterol—an indicator of improved heart health—and lower your risk of heart attack. [101]

WE HAVE BEEN MISINFORMED ABOUT DIETARY FAT

If this sounds counterintuitive, it's only because we've repeatedly been told for nearly 50 years that a low-fat diet is good for us. This has become a cultural belief, although there is no credible research to support it. In fact, when researchers finally got around to testing this, the results demonstrated no benefit from a low-fat diet. This should have sent shockwaves through the medical community and changed public health policy. Unfortunately, it did not.

Several such clinical studies have been conducted in the last 10 years comparing the low-fat diet still recommended to this day by the AHA and the British Heart Foundation with those high in fat—and especially saturated fat. [102] These trials are considered the best ever done on the effect of eating high-fat diets on risk for heart disease and diabetes. In each of these trials, participants were instructed to eat as much fat and protein foods as they wanted—including meat, fish, and poultry—but to restrict carbohydrates to no more than 50 grams per day. Their results were compared with subjects who ate fewer overall calories and avoided fat and saturated fat. The results were remarkably consistent across all studies.

Here's what happened to those who ate mostly saturated fat and protein:

1. Their HDL (good) cholesterol went up.
2. Their triglycerides (fat in the blood) went way down.
3. Their blood pressure went down.
4. Their total cholesterol remained about the same.
5. Their LDL (bad) cholesterol went up slightly.
6. They lost about the same amount of weight as the low-fat group.
7. Their risk of having a heart attack decreased significantly. [103]

One of these research trials, named the *A TO Z Weight Loss Study*, was conducted at Stanford University and cost the US government two million dollars; the results were published in *JAMA* in 2007.

Here's what the Stanford researchers said about the results: "Many concerns have been expressed that low-carbohydrate weight-loss diets (which are) high in total and saturated fat, will adversely affect blood lipid levels and cardiovascular risk. These concerns have not been substantiated in recent weight-loss diet trials. These studies have consistently reported that triglycerides, HDL cholesterol, blood pressure, and measures of insulin resistance were not significantly different or were more favorable for the very-low-carbohydrate groups." [104]

FAT IS NOT THE PROBLEM

That is a public reversal of an earlier opinion from Walter C. Willett, MD, PhD, MPH, a well-respected professor, chairman of the department of nutrition at the Harvard School of Public Health, and a principal investigator in the Nurses' Health Study (NHS), one of the largest, long-term investigations into the effects of diet on human health. [105] "If Americans could eliminate sugary beverages, potatoes, white bread, pasta, white rice, and sugary snacks," Dr. Willett advises, "we would wipe out almost all the problems we have with weight and diabetes and other metabolic diseases."

"Dietary fat used to be public enemy No. 1," says Edward Saltzman, MD, associate professor of nutrition and medicine at Tufts University. "Now a growing and convincing body of science is pointing the finger at carbs, especially those containing refined flour and sugar."[106]

"Put these people on a low-carb diet, and they'll not only lose weight, which always helps these conditions, but their blood levels will improve," says Stephen Phinney, MD, PhD, a nutritional biochemist and an emeritus professor at UC Davis, who has studied carbohydrates for 30 years.

In a 12-week study published in 2008, Dr. Phinney and his colleagues put 40 overweight or obese men and women with metabolic syndrome on a 1,500 calorie per day diet. Half went on a low-fat, high-carb diet. The others went on a low-carb, high-fat diet. The low-fat group consumed 12 grams of saturated fat a day out of a total of 40 grams of fat, while the low-carb group ate 36 grams of saturated fat a day—three times more—out of a total of 100 grams of fat.

Despite all the extra saturated fat that the low-carb group consumed, at the end of the 12 weeks, their triglyceride levels, an indicator of risk for heart disease, had dropped by 50%. Levels of HDL cholesterol increased by 15%, confirming earlier research. In the low-fat, high-carb group, triglycerides dropped only 20%, and there was no change in HDL. [107]

The take-home message from this study and others like it—contrary to what doctors still claim—is that dietary fat intake is not directly related to blood fat. Rather, the amount of *carbohydrates* in the diet appears to be the real villain.[108]

SHOULD DOCTORS BE MAKING DIETARY RECOMMENDATIONS AT ALL?

The results of this and the earlier research should have given the NHLBI, the AHA, and the ADA plenty of reasons to investigate their presumptions about the benefits of a low-fat diet. Instead, the existing studies showing the benefits of high-fat diets—even the Stanford study, which cost taxpayers a bundle of cash—went unheeded. This response reminds me of the late Senator Earl Landgrebe's (R, Indiana) unforgettable line at Richard Nixon's Watergate hearing: "Don't confuse me with the facts."

This illustrates an important point to remember. Most of us believe that modern medical advice is science-driven, and that treatment protocols, as well as official health advice, are grounded in solid research. We assume that if a doctor proclaims something or prescribes something, then he must be acting on facts. Unfortunately, this isn't always the case.

Too many times—as we've already seen with "official" advice regarding cholesterol, carbohydrates, sodium, "heart-healthy" margarine, and dietary fat in general—the treatments and advice we are receiving from the medical establishment are based on outdated science, medical politics, drug industry influence, oversimplifications (for the sake of public understanding), and/ or blind belief.

HOW CAN THIS BE?

The unavoidable truth is that it takes money—big money—to conduct a research study these days, and the only major funding sources that can afford this are federal government agencies and the pharmaceutical industry. Competition for these funds is fierce among researchers, and motivation to make a name for oneself is strong. Leading and publishing a study is how scientists gain recognition and peer respect, broaden their reputation, and raise their prestige. The next stop from there can be a cushy position with the NIH or a drug company, or a promotion up the academic ladder.

Obviously, bucking strongly held status quo policy positions (such as those on saturated fat, cholesterol, or cholesterol-lowering drugs) is not going to make an ambitious researcher very popular; so there is a powerful incentive to go along with these accepted ideas. As one insider put it, "It's very difficult to get something published that goes against established dogma."

This isn't how scientific inquiry is supposed to work. In an ideal world, pure science follows the evidence and accepts the obvious conclusions, regardless of who it offends or what beliefs it upends. But these days, medical and nutritional researchers don't operate in accord with the dictums of pure science. And the tragic consequences can be that scientific discovery is slowed considerably, flawed health advice becomes public health policy, and millions of people are prescribed dubious pharmaceutical "solutions" that don't improve their conditions and may actually make them worse.

A perfect example of this breakdown between science and popular health advice is what the public is told about dietary fat and oils.

GOOD FATS, BAD FATS: THE REAL SKINNY

Fat is the target of much scorn these days. But as you're about to see, this scorn is born not of facts, but rather of confusion, bias, and misinformation.

The first thing you should know is that fat is an important part of the human diet. It delivers health benefits we can't live without. Dietary fat supplies essential fatty acids (EFAs) such as linoleic acid and alpha-linolenic acid, which are the building blocks of fat molecules. Your body is incapable of producing them on its own, which is why they're called "essential." Therefore, you must obtain these fats from food.

Fat transports vitamins A, D, E, and K—the fat-soluble vitamins—into and around your body. It is necessary for maintaining healthy skin and plays a central role in maintaining proper eyesight and brain development in babies and children.

Fats also provide the building blocks for cell membranes, as well as a number of important hormones. And fat is necessary for the conversion of carotene to vitamin A, for mineral absorption and for a host of other important biochemical processes. [109]

Finally, fat satisfies our hunger much better than carbs because it takes longer to breakdown. In this way, it delivers a slow, steady stream of energy, unlike the roller coaster of energy ups and downs you feel from eating carbs. And while carbohydrates are supposedly the ideal "comfort food," new research finds that dietary fat makes us feel good by brightening our mood.

So why does fat get such a bad rap? Despite its many health benefits, fat is frequently blamed as the cause of weight gain and obesity. The explanation usually given is that, at nine calories per gram, fat packs more than twice the calories by volume of carbohydrates and protein. But it's a mistake to equate dietary fat with accumulating body fat simply because of its caloric content. As everyone knows, you can gain weight by overeating carbs or protein, even if you eat a minimum amount of dietary fat.

Just as there are good and bad carbs, there are fats that are good for you and others that are not. This chapter will help you understand which is which.

After more than five decades of repetitive indoctrination, most people believe they can tell a good fat from a bad one and are making the correct choices. In fact, it's become common "knowledge" that saturated fats are "bad" and should be replaced by polyunsaturated fats (PUFAs), which are "good." This advice, no matter how popular, is unhealthful and dangerous.

A large body of scientific evidence indicates that the vast majority of people, doctors included, are *wrong* about which fats are healthful and which are harmful. If this is true (and we are absolutely convinced that it is), then the politically correct advice doctors have been giving us about dietary fats could be responsible for making us sicker and shortening our life spans. Before we explain why this is probably the case, let's examine the types of fat available in our diet.

UNDERSTANDING THE FATS IN YOUR DIET

Fats (or more correctly, fatty acids) are a class of organic compounds that are insoluble in water. They are distinguished by chains of carbon atoms, with hydrogen atoms filling the available bonds. Fats are classified into two main categories: saturated and unsaturated, based on the degree their carbon bonds are occupied by hydrogen atoms. For example, a fat is considered "saturated" when all of its available carbon bonds are occupied by hydrogen atoms.

Unsaturated fats are further broken down into two subgroups: polyunsaturated and monounsaturated. In addition to these naturally occurring fats, there is a category of manmade fats referred to as trans-fats or trans-fatty acids.

Saturated fats. A fatty acid is considered saturated when all available carbon bonds are occupied, or "saturated" by hydrogen atoms. Because of this saturated occupation, these fats are highly stable (meaning they resist easy oxidation or rancidity). In practical terms, this means they do not readily breakdown, even when heated at high temperatures. They are usually solid or semi-solid at room temperature. Saturated fats are found in animal fats and tropical oils, such as coconut and palm.

Saturated fat, we've been told, is the "bad fat" that clogs our arteries and causes heart attacks. Since the late 1970s and early '80s, doctors have said we should reduce our consumption of it (in the form of meat, eggs, and full-fat dairy products) and replace saturated fat with "healthy" polyunsaturated fats and oils. This was because early studies showed that saturated fat raises our cholesterol levels, and that PUFAs (polyunsaturated fatty acids) from liquid vegetable oils reduce them. While this is true, doctors were not telling us the full story back then—and they still are not.

Monounsaturated fats. Somewhat less stable than saturated fats, monounsaturated fatty acids have one double bond in the form of two carbon atoms double-bonded to each other and lacking two hydrogen atoms. Your body makes monounsaturated fatty acids from saturated fatty acids and uses them in a number of ways. Monounsaturated fats (also called MUFAs) tend to be liquid at room temperature. Like saturated fats, they are relatively stable and do not oxidize easily.

The most common monounsaturated fat in our food is oleic acid, the main component of olive oil. MUFAs are also present in small amounts in meat and whole milk products, and in larger amounts in nuts, and high-fat fruits such as olives and avocados. Other sources include the oils from almonds, pecans, cashews, peanuts, macadamias, and grape seeds. [110]

Polyunsaturated fats. These fatty acids have two or more pairs of double bonds and consequently lack four or more hydrogen atoms. The unpaired electrons make these fats highly reactive and easily oxidized. They spoil easily (especially omega-3 fatty acids) and must be treated with care. Contrary to popular belief, PUFA oils should never be heated or used in cooking because they become unstable and are prone to oxidation. How many times have you cooked with corn oil or canola oil believing you are making a healthy choice for your family?

The two polyunsaturated fats found most frequently in our foods are omega-6 and omega-3. (The omega number indicates the position of the first double bond.) More about why this is important, later. Since your body is unable to make these fatty acids, they are called "essential" fatty acids (or EFAs) and must be obtained from our foods. PUFAs are liquid at room temperature. They include oil made from corn, fish, flaxseed, hemp, pumpkin seed, safflower, sesame, soybean, and sunflower.

Doctors have been keen on getting more of the "good" unsaturated fats into our diet because some studies have shown they help decrease inflammation, reduce heart disease, reduce blood clotting (and/or thick blood), and help regulate blood pressure. Just as with saturated fats, the public hasn't gotten the full story about unsaturated fats and oils, either. And as you'll soon see, the result has been a worsening of our health because PUFA vegetable oils encourage the very diseases that doctors claim they prevent.

Omega-6 and omega-3. We realize you may be tiring of all this science, but stick it out just a little longer because your knowledge about these different types of fats—and how they affect your body—will translate directly into better health for you and your family. For example, you've probably heard that omega-3 fats (fish oil being the most heralded example) are good for you and exert a healing effect on a variety of medical conditions. Allow us to explain why.

PUFAs are divided into two types: omega-6 and omega-3 fatty acids. Ideally, these two should appear in the diet in a nearly equal proportion because they both compete for the same pathways. When there is an excess of omega-6 and an insufficiency of omega-3, the imbalance can interfere with production of important prostaglandins. These are hormone-like substances that mediate inflammation, among other factors, in the body. This disruption can result in a tendency to form blood clots, can cause widespread inflammation (particularly in arteries), trigger higher blood pressure, promote irritation of the digestive tract, depress immune function, lead to cancer, and encourage weight gain. [110]

As it turns out, most polyunsaturated vegetable oils (the very oils that doctors recommend we turn to because of their superior "health benefits") contain large amounts of omega-6 linoleic acid and very little omega-3 linolenic acid. This imbalance diminishes the healthful omega-3s available to your body.

But the problem is not limited to PUFA in fats and oils. Our modern diet is overloaded with foods rich in omega-6, particularly grains, and eating too many of them will overpower the meager amounts of omega-3s we get from certain foods. Examples of foods high in omega-6s include:

- Grains (such as wheat and corn) and soybeans, plus the many processed foods made from them.

- Feedlot animals raised for meat, which are fed a diet of corn, other grains, and soybeans.

- Cage-confined laying hens and their eggs.

- Dairy cows and their milk products.

- Farm-raised fish (especially salmon), which are fed a diet of pellets made from grain and soybeans.

On the other hand, meat, dairy, and poultry products labeled "free-range" contain far more omega-3s than those that are conventionally raised. (This is also true for wild-caught Alaskan salmon and other cold water fish.) For example, eggs from free-range hens that are allowed to feed on insects and green plants contain 10 times more omega-3 fats than do the eggs of cage-confined chickens fed only corn and grains. [112] In addition, the ratio of omega-6s to omega-3s in free-range eggs is in the ideal one-to-one range—but eggs from grain-fed hens, on the other hand, can contain as much as 19 times more omega-6s than omega-3s. [113]

This may not sound very important to the average consumer, but keeping this in mind when you are shopping can have important implications for your health. Omega-3s protect your cells from free radical damage and put the kibosh on chronic inflammation—while omega-6 foods deplete your body of omega-3s and therefore increase inflammation. High levels of omega-6s are linked to the increased risk of diabetes, [114] asthma, heart disease, and learning disorders. [115]

One big reason we are seeing so many of these health problems today is that Americans are eating too many omega-6 foods and not enough omega-3s. While the ideal ratio for good health should be 1:1, we currently are consuming closer to 20:1 or even 50:1. This is way out of balance and a huge cause of inflammation-driven diseases, leading to a host of ailments, among them coronary artery disease and hypertension.

But here's the most important reason to be concerned about eating too many omega-6 foods and not enough omega-3s: Harvard researchers report that omega-3 deficiency is now the sixth leading cause of death in the US. [116]

One of the biggest reasons so many Americans are running around with critically low levels of omega-3s is that we're eating too many grain-based commercial food products that are loaded with omega-6s. Just look at the ingredient labels and you'll be surprised by the number of prepared foods made from wheat, soybeans, corn, and rice—the "Big Four" agricultural crops. Even commercially grown vegetables now contain fewer omega-3s due to modern agriculture methods. [117]

By far the most worrisome omega-6 products in your supermarket are PUFA vegetable oils because they contain very little omega-3 linolenic acid, large amounts of the omega-6 linoleic acid, and oxidize easily in the body, generating massive amounts of harmful free radical molecules. Tragically, most people aren't even aware there's a problem because doctors, the AHA and the US Department of Agriculture (USDA) are still advising the American public to shun "unhealthful saturated fats" in favor of these omega-6 PUFA vegetable oils.

Trans-fat. While there remains much disagreement about the healthfulness of saturated and unsaturated fats, the one fat everyone agrees is bad for you is trans-fat. This is by far the worst fat for your heart, blood vessels, and your entire body—yet for decades it has lurked in tens of thousands of US food products. Trans-fats are hidden under coded names such as "partially hydrogenated vegetable oil" and "vegetable shortening." Savvy shoppers who recognize those codes know that they refer to harmful trans-fats and they avoid products containing them.

Ironically, it was again doctors, the AHA, and the USDA who initially encouraged Americans to consume these trans-fat foods. The biggest offenders were margarines made from hydrogenated PUFA oils and labeled as "heart healthy" because some studies showed that the vegetable oils (which margarines were made from) lowered cholesterol. Little did these official sources realize they were promoting one of the most toxic foods ever to hit our food supply.

Researchers from Harvard School of Public Health have estimated that eliminating trans-fats from the American diet could have prevented approximately one in five heart attacks and related deaths per year. [118] (We have no estimate of the number of cancer fatalities trans-fats have caused, but the figure could even be higher than all cardiovascular disease-related deaths.)

Hydrogenation is the process that turns PUFA vegetable oils, normally liquid at room temperature, into fats that are solid. Margarine and shortening are the best-known examples. This process was of great interest to the food industry because hydrogenated oils do not spoil as easily, so products containing them have a much longer shelf life. They are also much cheaper than animal fats.

Profit was the main consideration for the introduction of these substances into our food supply; their effects on human health were never deeply investigated by the food industry. Fortunately, most—but not all—of these foods are now gone from the marketplace.

As you might imagine, most trans-fats are pure poison to the body, even though your digestive system doesn't recognize them as such (otherwise they would be vomited out like other poisons). Instead of being eliminated, trans-fats are incorporated into cell membranes, which actually become partially hydrogenated.

The health problems with trans-fats are numerous and serious. They block your body's utilization of essential fatty acids and cause a variety of harmful effects, including sexual dysfunction, elevated cholesterol, and depression of the immune system.

As far back as the 1940s, researchers identified a strong link between cancer and the consumption of hydrogenated fats, yet the results were presented as though the real culprit was saturated fat. This occurred because in those days it was common practice for saturated fats to be lumped together with trans-fats in databases that correlated dietary trends with diseases. Little wonder that natural saturated fats achieved such a bad reputation. [119]

Mary Enig, PhD, of the Weston A. Price Foundation, was one of the first to recognize the dangers of trans-fats and to alert the public about them. She testified before Congress on the matter in the 1970s, yet her warnings went unheeded, and a deluge of products containing trans-fats were unleashed on unsuspecting consumers with tragic consequences. According to Dr. Enig's research, trans-fats:

- Lower HDL (good) cholesterol (the more fat in the diet, the lower the HDL levels go).
- Raise LDL (bad) cholesterol.
- Elevate apolipoprotein-B (ApoB)—which leads to increased artery blockages.
- Raise the risk for diabetes by increasing insulin resistance.
- Weaken the body's immune response.

- Decrease testosterone levels in males.
- Increase the number and size of fat cells. [120]

It took nearly 40 years for our government and the health community to heed Dr. Enig's warnings. As of January 1, 2006, trans-fats had to be listed on food labels along with other fats. But there's a catch: The FDA allows products claiming to have "zero trans-fat" on their labels actually to contain up to a half gram. (Canada sets the standard of "zero" as under 0.2 grams.) This is dangerous because trans-fats accumulate in your body, so purchasing multiple "zero trans-fat" products can provide a nasty collective dose. Our advice is that you consider any amount of trans-fat to be unhealthful and that you read food labels carefully to spot it. Do not buy anything containing "partially hydrogenated vegetable oil," "vegetable shortening" or "margarine."

Unfortunately, many foods, such as those sold in bakeries, cafeterias, schools, and restaurants, don't come with labels. Because consumers can't tell whether these unlabeled foods contain trans-fats, many cities and states have passed, or are considering passing, laws to eliminate trans-fats in these foods. California became the first state in the nation to phase out trans-fats from restaurants and from baked goods. New York City became the largest city in the nation to require its restaurants, cafeterias, and schools to go trans-fat-free. Other cities and towns, such as Boston, are following NYC's lead.

Regardless of where you live, you must be vigilant. Trans-fats are commonly found in many processed foods including commercially baked goods, icing, margarine, and "snack" foods like potato chips, cookies, crackers, and microwavable popcorn. They are even commonly used in some vegan and kosher products, which many people think of as more healthful. Trans-fats are also widely used in fast foods and fried foods, such as French fries and fried chicken. Since most of these are unhealthful anyway, your smartest strategy is simply to avoid them. Even the alternative—foods fried in PUFA oils—is no better, because the oil becomes rancid so easily from the high heat of frying.

So that's a recap of the conventional medical advice regarding the fats you should and should not be consuming; at least that's what doctors have been telling us for quite a while. But are they correct? Has this health advice decreased the incidence of heart disease and hypertension? Are we healthier for it? And is this advice supported by solid scientific research? Let's take a look.

WHY DOCTORS ARE WRONG ABOUT SATURATED FATS

How many times have you heard that saturated fats, usually contained in animal products, are the "bad fats" you should consume less of, while polyunsaturated fats, commonly found in plants, are the "good fats" you should consume?

This advice, which has been around since the early 1950s, states that saturated fat raises your LDL cholesterol levels and thereby contributes to clogged arteries, increasing your risk of heart attack and stroke. Since the main sources of saturated fat are meat, eggs, milk, and dairy products as well as saturated vegetable fats, such as coconut oil, palm oil, and cocoa butter, restricting these foods should have resulted in less heart disease and other cardiovascular problems in the US, including hypertension.

If consuming saturated fat is a leading risk factor for heart disease, as we've been told, why is this health problem a relatively *modern* phenomenon? We humans have been eating animal products for our entire history (about 500,000 to 2.4 million years), yet heart disease was rare until the 1900s. It wasn't until the 1950s that heart disease rates began to spike, and by the mid-70s, it had become the leading killer in America.

What could explain the emergence of this new epidemic? Had consumption of meat products and saturated fats dramatically increased during these decades? As it turns out, with the exception of the World War II years when meat, eggs, and dairy foods were rationed, saturated fat consumption remained steady. Even after the mid-1970s, when the AHA and the US government began urging the American public to reduce consumption of saturated fat (which we did), heart disease rates did not decline—though one would expect them to fall if foods containing saturated fat were responsible.

From the end of World War II, when the USDA statistics became more reliable, to the late 1960s, while coronary heart-disease mortality rates supposedly soared, *per-capita* consumption of whole milk dropped steadily; and the use of cream was cut by half. We ate dramatically less lard (from 13 pounds per person per year to 7 pounds) and less butter (8.5 pounds versus 4) and more margarine (4.5 pounds to 9 pounds), vegetable shortening (9.5 pounds to 17 pounds), and salad and cooking oils (from 7 pounds all the way to 18 pounds). As a result, during the worst decades of the heart-disease "epidemic," vegetable-fat consumption per capita in America doubled (from 28 pounds in the years 1947–49 to 55 pounds in 1976), while the average consumption of all animal fat (including the fat in meat, eggs, and dairy products) dropped from 84 pounds to 71.

WHAT THEY ARE NOT TELLING YOU ABOUT SATURATED FATS

While it's true that saturated fats do indeed raise LDL ("bad") cholesterol, they also raise HDL cholesterol (a marker for cardiovascular health) just as much, if not more. This is a good thing because elevated HDL seems to be protective and is associated with a lower risk of heart disease. You see, while this LDL—the "bad" cholesterol—is purportedly laying down plaque on your artery walls (as most doctors believe, though there is recent research to contradict this), the extra HDL from saturated fat is removing it. Increasing both LDL and HDL is at worst a "wash"—and may actually provide an individual with a net benefit. This is why informed physicians consider the ratio of HDL/LDL to be a more reliable predictor of future heart disease than LDL alone.

If this is true, then why do doctors tell us that diets low in saturated fat protect against heart disease?

The fact is, *they do not.* In 2000, the Cochrane Collaboration conducted a "meta-analysis" of the scientific literature on these so-called cholesterol-lowering, low-saturated-fat diets. The Cochrane researchers examined 27 clinical studies involving more than 18,000 participants. Their published data states that diets low in saturated fats have no significant effect on mortality, or even on deaths due to heart attacks. [121]

The famous Framingham Study came to a similar conclusion several years before. As Gary Taubes reports: "…the Framingham Study wasn't the only one that failed to reveal any correlation between the fat consumed and either cholesterol levels or heart disease. This was the case in virtually every study in which diet, cholesterol, and heart disease were compared within a single population, be it in Framingham; Honolulu, Hawaii; Chicago, Illinois; Tecumseh, Michigan; Evans County, Georgia; the island of Puerto Rico; or [the] nation of Israel."[122] All of these studies failed to show a causal relationship between dietary fat, elevated cholesterol, and heart disease.

Indeed, it may surprise you to learn that over the past decades, researchers have spent billions of tax dollars trying to prove the connection between saturated fat and heart disease, yet with the exception of four small, seriously flawed trials, these studies have failed to provide any definitive proof.

The most famous example of failed research attempts appeared in the early 70s when the NHLBI spent $115 million on a huge, decade-long clinical trial to test its stubbornly held belief that eating less saturated fat would curb heart disease. The clinical trial, known as the Multiple Risk Factor Intervention Trial (commonly referred to as MRFIT, or "Mr. Fit"), failed to show that a single heart attack had been prevented. When the disappointing results were published in 1982, *The Wall Street Journal* headline announced, "Heart Attacks: A Test Collapses."[123]

You'd think this mistaken belief would have been put to rest with MRFIT. But stubborn opponents of saturated fat convinced the government to include the proposition in the $725 million clinical trial known as the Women's Health Initiative (WHI), the largest and most expensive dietary investigation ever conducted in the US. The results, published in 2006, show that a diet low in total fat and saturated fat had no impact in reducing heart attack and stroke in some 20,000 women who had adhered to the regimen for an average of eight years.[124]

THE HEALTH BENEFITS OF SATURATED FAT

These studies and others failed to unearth any evidence that saturated fat causes heart disease for one simple reason: Saturated fat is not only innocent, but it actually may be *beneficial* to human health.

Sally Fallon Morell, MA, founding president of the Weston A. Price Foundation, along with Dr. Mary Enig, have been fighting the undocumented bias against saturated fats for several decades. In a paper titled "The Skinny on Fats," they cite numerous documented health benefits of saturated fats in the human diet, among which are:

- Saturated fats make up 50% of cell membranes and give cells their necessary stiffness and integrity.

- They play a vital role in bone health and are essential for calcium to be effectively absorbed and incorporated.

- They lower apolipoprotein-B (ApoB), a significant factor in the development of heart disease.

- They protect the liver from toxins, including alcohol.

- They help fortify the immune system.

- They are necessary for the proper utilization of essential fatty acids—especially omega-3s.

Animal fats are not the only saturated fats in the human diet. Tropical oils, such as coconut and palm, also are highly saturated. Coconut oil, for example, is 92% saturated. Far from being pariahs, these oils are recommended for cooking because their molecular structure is very stable and helps them resist oxidation even when exposed to high heat. This is sometimes referred to as having a "high smoke point," which makes them ideal for high heat cooking and frying.

It's also important to remember that all fats and oils, whether of vegetable or animal origin, contain some combination of saturated fats, monounsaturated fats, and PUFAs. No food or oil is made up of 100% of any one type of fat. For example, as Gary Taubes points out, more than half of the fat in a porterhouse steak (stearic acid) gets converted in your body to the same type of monounsaturated fat that's found in olive oil (oleic acid). [125]

Some foods considered "deadly" under the saturated-fat-is-bad dogma actually turn out to be very healthful when you analyze their fat content. More than 66% of the saturated fat in that porterhouse will definitively improve your cholesterol profile—especially compared with the French fries or baked potato sitting next to it. [126] Yes, it will raise your LDL; but as we've already seen, it will also boost your protective HDL, which seems to be a far better predictor of heart health.

The same is true for lard (the fat that humans have been cooking with for thousands of years). Taubes suggests that when you look strictly at the science, you can't avoid coming to the conclusion that consuming lard actually *lowers* your risk of heart disease. I know this sounds crazy, but that's indicative of how brainwashed we've been over the last four decades by misinformed doctors who have refused to heed the research on saturated fats. If you pay attention to the most reliable science we have, lard is far healthier for you than the refined vegetable oils that doctors are telling us to use.

THE DANGERS OF POLYUNSATURATED FATS

For thousands of years of human history, the fats in the human diet were either saturated or monounsaturated (MUFAs), primarily in the forms of butter, lard, poultry fat, and the harder animal fats called tallow; as well as coconut oil and small amounts of olive oil. This changed dramatically around the 1940s in the US with the introduction of refined PUFA vegetable oils, which were derived from corn, soy, safflower, and later rapeseed (now called canola). When plotted on the same timeline, this radical alteration in our diet corresponds to a profound decline in human health along with the rise of heart disease and many cancers. This correlation simply can't be explained by coincidence.

By the mid-1900s, margarines produced from corn oil and cottonseed oil had supplanted butter in the American diet; hydrogenated vegetable oil (called "shortening") had replaced lard; and corn and safflower oils became the medium that we fried and sautéed our foods in. Up to 30% of our calories were now coming from PUFA oils—an amount that scientific research warns us is far too high. [127]

During this same period, statistics show a significant rise in heart attacks, stroke, hypertension, and cardiovascular disease in general, plus a variety of newly emerging cancers—diseases that were all relatively unknown just 50 years before. Full blame can't be laid at the feet of these polyunsaturated oil products because Americans were also consuming unprecedented quantities of sugar, sweets of all types, baked goods made with white flour, refined carbohydrates, and products containing trans-fats. However, it's safe to say that refined vegetable oils played their role in America's declining health. PUFA oils, for instance, have been linked to increased incidence of cancer, heart disease, immune system dysfunction, liver damage, digestive disorders, weight gain, Alzheimer's disease, and cataracts, to name just a few.[128]

These oils appeared on the market not because science suddenly had discovered that saturated fats were unhealthful and PUFAs were better for us (this rationale was to emerge decades later). The motivation behind the introduction of these wholly new food products was purely financial.

American farmers were producing huge crops of corn, soybeans, and cotton, and food manufacturers were eager to discover new ways to profit from these commodities. For example, this era witnessed an explosion of new food products made from corn—including cornflakes, corn chips, cornmeal, corn dextrose, corn whiskey, cornstarch, and the list goes on.

Of the 10,000 items in the typical grocery store during the mid-1900s, at least 2,500 of them utilized corn in some form during production or processing.[129] Topping this list were corn oil and margarine. Needless to say, consideration of the health effects of these new food products got lost in the frenzy of production and sales.

REFINING RENDERS PUFAS EVEN MORE DANGEROUS

It didn't take long for independent scientists like Dr. Enig and others to recognize the dangers of polyunsaturated oils. The worst of these is their tendency to oxidize, or turn rancid, when subjected to heat or light because of their unstable molecular structure. (PUFA oils contain long-chain fatty acids, which are exceptionally fragile and unstable.) Rancid oils are generators of free radical molecules, which are extremely chemically reactive. In the body, these rogue molecules attack cell membranes, trigger inflammation, exhaust the body's antioxidant reserves, and damage DNA, which can trigger cancerous mutations. Free radical damage to blood vessels initiates the buildup of plaque, which, as we've already seen, hardens arteries, elevates blood pressure, and ultimately leads to heart attack and/or stroke. [130]

Eating food that contains even slightly rancid PUFA oils is extremely unhealthful, since the oil will oxidize at a much higher rate once it enters the body. Your body temperature is high enough to cause oxidation and the formation of free radical molecules. While damage from PUFAs affects every part of the body, the thyroid gland is particularly vulnerable. Symptoms include slow metabolism, low energy, and increased inflammation, which can manifest as achy muscles and sore joints. And the process of removing and refining PUFA vegetable oils makes them even more dangerous and unhealthful.

While these PUFA oils occur naturally in fruits, nuts, and seeds, they must first be extracted—and therein lies the danger. Prior to the early 1900s, this extraction was achieved by slow-moving stone presses, which didn't damage the delicate oil. Mass production radically changed this.

By the early 1900s manufacturers began processing oils in factories where the oil-bearing seeds were crushed and heated to 230 degrees F. The oil was then squeezed out under massive pressure, which generated even more heat and exposed the oil to damaging light and oxygen. Finally, to extract the remaining 10% of the oil from the crushed seeds, a toxic chemical solvent called hexane was added. Then, BHT and BHA, preservatives that scientists at the time suspected might cause cancer and brain damage, were often added to these oils to replace vitamin E and other natural preservatives destroyed by heat. These were the "heart healthy" vegetable oils that doctors endorsed and corporations marketed to trusting and gullible American consumers. This process, you should know, is largely unchanged today.

Safer PUFA oils. There is a safe, modern extraction technique that makes polyunsaturated oils safe for consumption. Instead of high-heat extraction, it "drills" into the seeds and removes the oil, along with its precious antioxidants, under low temperatures with minimal exposure to light and oxygen. These oils are more stable than conventional PUFAs and will remain fresh longer if they are stored in the refrigerator in dark bottles. When shopping, look for labels that say "expeller-expressed" and "unrefined." These are the only polyunsaturated vegetable oils you should buy and consume. Store them in a cool, dry place and in non-transparent glass bottles. Still, the very best way to ensure you're receiving high-quality polyunsaturated fats is to consume the whole foods that contain them, such as ground flaxseed, chia and hemp seeds, walnuts, sunflower and pumpkin seeds, and freshly ground whole grains such as oats and quinoa.

NEW STUDY SHOWS THAT
DOCTORS' ADVICE ON FATS WAS WRONG

Just as we were about to go to press with this book, newly discovered results from a 1973 study (yes, 1973!) indicate that medical advice urging people to replace saturated animal fats with omega-6 polyunsaturated vegetable fats (PUFAs) and "heart-healthy" margarine made from safflower oil is linked to an *increased risk* of death among patients with heart disease.

The study, known as the Sydney Diet Heart Study, was a randomized controlled trial conducted from 1966 to 1973, measuring the effect of PUFA vegetable oils and saturated fats from animal sources on heart disease. Results of this trial have not been previously available because the data has been "missing."

A team of American and Australian researchers have recovered and analyzed the original data, using modern statistical methods to compare death rates from all causes, and coronary heart disease, in particular.

Their findings have sent shockwaves through the medical and cardiovascular communities. Their analysis shows that heart patients who substituted PUFA safflower oil for saturated fat had a higher risk of death from all causes, especially from cardiovascular disease and coronary heart disease.

Advice to substitute polyunsaturated vegetable oil for saturated fats in order to reduce the risk of heart disease has been a cornerstone of dietary health guidelines for the past 50 years—especially from the American Heart Association. Now, researchers analyzing the Sydney Study results say that these guidelines need to be revisited and revised.

An editorial in the *British Medical Journal* that accompanied the publication of these results characterized the AHA's guidelines on fats as "misguided" and stated that these new results "underscored the need to properly align dietary advice and recommendations with the scientific evidence base." [131]

We have no doubt that subsequent studies will confirm that the dietary advice about fats handed out by doctors—just like their guidelines for a carbohydrate-centric diet—has caused untold suffering, disease, and deaths in our population for more than half a century.

THE MOST HEALTHFUL FATS AND OILS
FOR YOUR BLOOD PRESSURE, ARTERIES, AND HEART HEALTH

The right fats and oils are important parts of a healthful diet and will protect you from illness, premature deterioration, and degenerative diseases. They do this by helping your body and brain function at peak performance levels, by boosting your energy levels, keeping you slim and fit, preserving your body's muscle mass, and increasing your longevity.

Please remember: If you follow the "average" health advice making the rounds today, you will have "average" health (and you only need to look around you to see what that is).

Our advice: Follow the science, think for yourself, do your own research, and don't be afraid to separate yourself from the herd. The following tips for choosing truly healthful dietary fats and oils are based on the latest scientific findings from highly reliable sources we have come to trust.

Avoid "low-fat" food products. Americans have become positively fat phobic, and this contributes to a host of ills and out-of-control weight problems. There are more than 15,000 low-fat and non-fat food products on supermarket shelves that represent massive trickery and create widespread confusion in the marketplace. Not only are these reduced-fat foods lacking in flavor, but many have had their fat content replaced by sugar and artificial sweeteners, refined carbohydrates, chemical flavorings, and binding agents. These substitutions often make the foods *more* fattening than their full-fat versions. In most cases, the fat-reduced versions contain as many calories—or more.

Don't be afraid of fat—especially saturated fat. All the science we've seen has convinced us that it's a healthful food. Choose whole butter, cream, artisan cheeses, and whole dairy products rather than low-fat or fat-free versions. Remember that your body needs fat to be slim and healthy—just make sure it's the right kind. You're much better off with full-fat products because fat satisfies your hunger much better than carbohydrates, so you wind up eating less in the long run.

Completely eliminate trans-fats from your diet. Avoid margarine and other butter substitutes—and that includes so-called "healthy spreads" by Smart Balance, Earth Balance and others. Check food labels carefully before purchasing food items. If you see the words "partially hydrogenated" or "hydrogenated" on food labels, put the products back on the shelf.

Say "no" to refined vegetable oils. You're better off without refined PUFA oils, such as safflower, canola oil, seed oils, soybean oil, and corn oil. Despite what their advertising says, these are *not* health foods.

Don't fry or sauté with them. Don't drizzle them on your salads. Don't use them in baked goods. Don't even buy them. In fact, there's absolutely no use for these refined PUFA oils other than lubricating a rusty hinge. Pay particular attention to ingredient labels when buying processed food products. Many vegetable oils end up in packaged and processed foods. Because they are loaded with omega-6 fatty acids, refined PUFA oils lead to deficiencies in beneficial omega-3s that prevent inflammation. Research has also linked PUFA consumption to several cancers.

They also make you fat. One group of blood lipids profoundly affect some important processes in the nervous system, including pain sensation, mood, memory, and appetite. They work by attaching to receptor sites—areas that fit perfectly with connecting molecules of the right shape—on the surface of cell membranes. These particular lipids have the same shape as cannabis (marijuana) molecules, so they're called *endocannabinoids.*

Endocannabinoids that drive appetite come from an omega-6 fatty acid called arachidonic acid (AA) and, just like marijuana, when AA activates certain cells in the nervous system, you get the "munchies." That promotes overeating, which can quickly lead to overweight.

So where does your body get this stuff? To start with, it's plentiful in beef, pork and poultry. But it also derives from an omega-6 oil, called linoleic acid (LA), which abounds in PUFA oils.

An exciting new study, [132] however, suggests that adding beneficial omega-3s to your diet can actually put your body back into balance and reverse the "obesogenic" effects of AA. When mice in the study consumed diets rich in LA, predictably, they gained weight. But mice that consumed the same diet with one change, the addition of omega-3, stayed thin. The same may work for you. Cutting back PUFA oils will make the effect even stronger.

Choose butter over margarine. Since the 1950s, we have been told that butter raises our cholesterol and is bad for the heart. Don't believe it. The truth is that margarine eaters have 100% more heart disease then butter eaters.[133] Doctors and health officials have also told us that the saturated fats in butter clog our arteries. But according to a study published in the British medical journal, *Lancet,* the fats found in artery plaques are predominantly unsaturated. [134] Go figure.

Butter is a natural fat, made from cream—each is good for you, provided the cows have been allowed free access to pasture grass for their entire lives. This type of butter is rich in the fat-soluble vitamins A, D, E, and K; plus the important trace minerals magnesium, zinc, chromium, selenium, and iodine. Just make sure you purchase butter produced from milk that is free of hormones, steroids, and antibiotics, and comes from pasture-raised cows.

Twenty years after the disastrous Food Pyramid of the 1990s, Dr. Walter Willett admits his mistake about advocating margarine over butter: "Unfortunately, as a physician back in the 1980s, I was telling people they should replace butter with margarine because it was cholesterol free, and professional organizations like the AHA were telling us as physicians that we should be promoting this. In reality, there was never any evidence that these margarines, that were high in trans-fat, were any better than butter, and as it turned out, they were actually far worse than butter." [135]

Eggs are a perfect food. Doctors have been flip-flopping about eggs for several decades. In 1956, the AHA blamed America's rising rates of heart disease on consumption of butter, lard, beef, and eggs. (Eggs, we were told, contain entirely too much cholesterol to be included in the human diet.) The famous cardiologist Dudley White, MD, was one of the few physicians at the time who rejected this notion, noting that heart attacks were non existent in 1900 (when egg consumption was three times what it was in the 1950s).

Eggs are now back in fashion, although doctors still advise us to go easy and not to consume them more than one or two times per week. This is simply more bad advice. As reported in the *International Journal of Cardiology* in 2005, participants who ate two eggs a day for six weeks showed no increase in total cholesterol, no increase in LDL (bad) cholesterol, and no narrowing of the arteries. [136]

Eggs are also a weight-watcher's dream. Two extra-large eggs contain just 160 calories and 14 grams of protein. In fact, researchers at St. Louis University found that people who ate eggs instead of a bagel (with equal calories) for breakfast ate fewer total calories at both lunch and dinner. The egg-eaters lost 65% more weight than the bagel-eaters. [137]

Finally, eggs are a great source of the vision-protecting compounds lutein and zeaxanthin, carotenoids that are especially vital for people who suffer vision loss as a complication of diabetes. The risks of cataracts and macular degeneration are both significantly lower in people who eat eggs regularly. [138]

Shop for eggs labeled "omega-3 fortified," produced by hens allowed to range free to feed on grasses and wilds herbs rich in omega-3 essential fatty acids. These eggs have three to six times the omega-3s of other grocery eggs. Omega-3s are essential for both cardiovascular and mental health.

The truth about red meat. Forget about meat's "bad reputation," which it got simply because it contains saturated fats. In one Danish study, researchers found that subjects who ate more saturated fat, especially in butter and high-fat dairy products, actually gained less weight around their midsections than those eating low-fat diets. The same was true of participants who ate more red meat; their waist measurements were smaller than those who ate less. (Waist size is strongly linked to hypertension, as well as an increased risk for heart disease, cancer, insulin resistance, and diabetes.) [139]

While some studies show that eating red meat isn't healthful, when you look closer, it's apparent that this research doesn't distinguish between good quality beef and processed meats such as cold cuts, bacon, beef jerky, and other meat products that are loaded with cancer-causing nitrites and other harmful chemicals. There's a big difference between a sirloin from a pasture-raised cow and the slab of pepperoni or a can of Spam processed in a factory.

Research, attempting to link poor health to a diet high in saturated fats from animal sources, rarely (if ever) mentions the source of that meat. We believe that most of the clinical data indicating that red meat consumption is linked to heart disease and cancer has more to do with the poor quality of the meat products and with the chemicals they contain, rather than red meat consumption per se. A daily serving of one hot dog, for example, raised the risk of diabetes by double-digits—43% per serving, and bacon by 49%—far more than the red meat alone did.

The incidence of stroke (a serious complication of CVD and hypertension) increases with the consumption of these processed meats. A recently published study of 40,291 Swedish men over a period of 10 years found that a higher intake of processed meat—but not fresh red meat—is associated with an increased risk of stroke. This is the largest research project to date examining the relationship between stroke and red meat consumption.

The findings suggest that meats consumers often believe are healthier, such as low-fat deli turkey, ham, and bologna, may actually increase stroke risk if intake is high enough. The study appeared in the August 2011 issue of the *American Journal of Clinical Nutrition.* [140]

Another overlooked factor in many of these red meat studies is that people who consume lots of meat products tend to eat fewer fruits, vegetables, and whole grains. This makes it hard to tell which causes these diseases—eating meat or not eating fruits and vegetables.

On the other hand, there are studies that have focused exclusively on grass-fed, naturally raised cattle and bison and free-range chickens. All find that these provide excellent sources of high-quality protein, are higher in beneficial fats, and are less likely to spread dangerous bacteria that thrive in crowded feedlot conditions.

Grass-fed beef is also lower in calories—one of its many health advantages over its industrialized, grain-fed, factory feedlot counterpart. You might be thinking, *"Meat is meat. How can one piece of beef have fewer calories than another?"* It may surprise you to learn that lean, grass-fed beef and bison contain about the same number of calories as *chicken* (about 200 calories per cup)—and half the calorie content of a fast-food hamburger (about 400 calories per cup).

Naturally raised meats also contain healthful fats. Grass-fed beef is high in omega-3s, which, as you know, are essential fatty acids (EFAs) that lower inflammation and are beneficial for cardiovascular health, proper blood sugar metabolism, and reducing cancer risk. Your brain also benefits from these EFAs. People with a diet high in omega-3s are less likely to fall victim to depression, schizophrenia, attention deficit disorder, and Alzheimer's disease. In fact, pasture-raised cattle contain up to four times more omega-3s than grain-fed beef—and nearly as much as some cold-water fish species.

Where do grass-fed animals get so much of their omega-3 fat? Some 60% of the fatty acids in pasture grass are omega-3s, which accounts for the high level in grass-fed beef. When cattle are taken from the pasture to the feedlot to eat a diet of omega-6 corn and other grains, the cattle's beneficial EFA plummets. The longer they stay on the feedlot, the lower their omega-3 drops.[141] Cattle need to be both grass-fed and grass-finished to have good quantities of omega-3s. This means they spend their entire lives grazing in pastures, from birth to death. Not many brands of beef fit this bill…but supermarkets are slowly including grass-fed, free-range products in their meat sections. It's worth seeking out.

Believe it or not, lard is a healthful fat. Most people cringe at the word. But lard is a healthy, natural "saturated" fat that you should welcome into your kitchen. Lard is rendered fat from pork and is mostly monounsaturated. It's also one of the few food sources rich in vitamin D—the vitamin that many scientists are raving about these days. Cooking with lard is not only health-ful, but it will also add rich flavor to many foods. Like beef products, however, the lard you use should come from free range (not corn fed) pigs, not only because they have a more healthful diet, but also because they are exposed to more sunlight, allowing them to produce plentiful vitamin D. [142]

Poultry fat is healthful, too. The fat composition of chickens, turkeys, and ducks is very similar to that of beef. So, like beef fat, poultry fat can reduce your risk of cardiovascular disease. And before you wonder if there's a difference between dark meat fat and white meat fat, there isn't: they're both equally healthy fats.

Coconut and palm oils for high heat. These tropical oils are saturated fat from vegetable sources. Both contain lauric acid, which has strong antifungal and antimicrobial properties. Because their molecular structure is extremely stable, they can be used for stir-frying, sautéing, braising, and baking. Macadamia nut oil is also excellent for high-heat cooking. One of our favorite brands is Mac-Nut (www.macnutoil.com).

Extra virgin olive oil. This is natural "medicine" for your arteries. Olive oil is the mainstay of the Mediterranean diet and has been used for thousands of years for its mind-boggling health and healing benefits. It's a rich source of antioxidants, relieves the pain and inflammation of arthritis, normalizes blood fats and cholesterol, lowers blood pressure, and makes arteries resistant to plaque formation.

These healthful qualities are greatest in extra virgin olive oil (EVOO). It is produced by crushing olives between stone or steel rollers, otherwise known as "cold-pressing." EVOO is the first pressing of the olive and contains the highest concentration of beneficial nutrients. All other grades are inferior to it. Cold-pressing preserves the integrity of its monounsaturated fatty acids and its impressive phytochemicals. Don't purchase EVOO in large containers, but rather buy smaller amounts so they keep better. Store EVOO in the fridge and maintain a small supply in an opaque container at room temperature for daily use.

Olive oil is most healthful when freshly pressed. After 12 months, its inflammation-fighting potency is significantly diminished, as well as the unique flavor. Unfortunately, supermarket olive oils don't carry the pressing date on the label, so it's impossible to tell how fresh they are. These oils actually can be quite old. For this reason, you can purchase olive oil fresh-pressed from a buyer's club. Immediately after pressing, the oil is air-freighted to your home. (If you've ever been lucky enough to taste fresh-pressed EVOO, you know there's no comparison to the stuff they sell at the supermarket—even at the high-priced "natural" stores.) We've thoroughly researched and tested various sources, and the one we prefer is The Fresh-Pressed Olive Oil Club (www.freshpressedoliveoil.com).

Olive oil can be used for light sautéing, either alone or mixed with a little butter. Too many cooks use it for high-heat frying, which breaks down its molecular structure and renders it easily oxidized in the body. To impart the flavor of olive oil to cooked dishes, add it midway through the simmering stage. EVOO is best enjoyed fresh in salad dressings and for drizzling on cooked vegetables. However, it is important not to use olive oil as your only fat because your body needs the nutrients found in animal fats. Too much monounsaturated fat, without a balance of saturated fats, can cause problems. Vegetarians should become familiar with cooking with ghee (clarified butter), which has a high smoke point and is rich in essential fatty acids more commonly found in animal fats.

Best omega-3 sources. When it comes to the most healthful fat, nothing compares with omega-3. Seafood is the richest source of the omega-3 fatty acids, which consist of DHA (docosahexanoic acid) and EPA (eicosapentanoic acid). These unsaturated fats are essential for cognitive function, mood maintenance, and cardiovascular health. According to a 2005 study [143] in *Archives of Internal Medicine*, omega-3 fats have prevented more cardiac deaths and overall mortality than the cholesterol-lowering drugs called statins.

Remember to purchase only wild-caught fish because farm-raised fish contain very little omega-3. And since farm-raised fish are grain-fed, they can be loaded with pro-inflammatory omega-6s. Wild Alaskan salmon is an excellent seafood choice. (One of the most reliable suppliers of high-quality seafood is the Vital Choice fishery. It delivers frozen or canned wild salmon and other seafood via Federal Express, and its quality is consistently high and reliable—with cost comparable to your local Whole Foods market—www.vitalchoice.com.) Economical sources of omega-3 include canned anchovies and sardines. With a little creativity, these fish make for tasty, healthful meals in a tight economy. For recipe ideas, visit Jim's My Healing Kitchen website at www.myhealingkitchen.com.

There also are a few plant sources of omega-3s that you should know about, such as walnuts and flaxseeds. Your body is able to synthesize DHA and EPA from the alpha-linolenic acid (ALA) contained in walnuts and flaxseed, but less than 10% is actually converted. Still, these are very healthful foods and should be included regularly in your diet.

We have said it before, but it's worth repeating: Since the Western diet contains an overabundance of omega-6s, it's important that you get enough omega-3s into your diet. That's why supplementing your diet with omega-3 fish oil makes sense because this helps create the healthy balance between these two essential fatty acids.

Personally, we both have a problem with fish oil supplements (including krill oil) because they encourage over-fishing and disrupt the oceanic food chain. Now that stocks of large fish have become depleted, fishing fleets are harvesting smaller varieties of omega-3-rich seafood, including sardines, anchovies, and krill (a tiny shrimp-like creature that's especially rich in astaxanthin, a powerful orange-colored antioxidant that gives omega-3 its healing properties and bright hue). But, because these smaller creatures are the main food source for larger fish (some whales and dolphins, for instance, feed exclusively on krill), harvesting the smaller varieties is upsetting the ocean's ecology and depriving entire species of their food supply.

Fish don't produce the omega-3 fatty acids found in fish oil. Instead, they get their astaxanthin from marine plankton. Marine plankton is not only one of the richest sources of omega-3, but it's also an ocean-friendly product that won't disrupt the food chain. That's because phytoplankton is grown in large land-based, freshwater tanks—guaranteeing that it's completely free of contaminants, heavy metals, mercury, and ocean pollution.

This environmentally conscious omega-3 product is relatively new but rapidly gaining popularity because of its many advantages over conventional fish oil supplements. You'll find several brands on the market, but one of the more reliable products is Oceans Alive Marine Phytoplankton, available from many different websites and health food stores.

CHAPTER NINE

THE SECRET CAUSE OF HYPERTENSION

In addition to salt, medical organizations such as the American Medical Association (AMA) and the American Diabetes Association (ADA) are in the habit of blaming hypertension on dietary fat (especially the saturated fats found in animal products). If we, as a nation, reduced our consumption of these fatty foods, they tell us, hypertension would decrease in the US and there would be fewer cases of heart disease, heart attack, and stroke. This is why these medical societies have steered the country toward a low-fat diet since the 1970s.

In 1984, this low-fat diet advice became official doctrine when the National Heart, Lung, and Blood Institute (NHLBI) launched an all-out public health campaign to convince Americans that low-fat diets "afford significant protection against coronary heart disease." [144]

The public was told to eat less fat, particularly less saturated fat, which we did, or at least tried to do. As a result, according to US Department of Agriculture (USDA) statistics, consumption of saturated fat steadily declined in the years that followed. But instead of getting leaner, Americans got fatter. [145] Indeed, the US saw a marked *increase* in overweight individuals and obesity during this period.

Furthermore, as you've seen in the previous chapter, the incidence of heart disease and heart attacks didn't decline as health officials expected it would. This is documented in numerous studies, including one that appeared in *The Journal of the American Medical Association (JAMA)*. [146]

THE CULPRIT RIGHT UNDER OUR NOSES

While everyone has been focusing blame on obesity, stress, dietary fat, and excess salt as the culprits responsible for today's epidemic of hypertension and other cardiovascular problems, the real troublemaker has gone unnoticed by Big Medicine.

This is truly mind-boggling because researchers had identified this obvious risk factor and written it into the medical literature as far back as 1860. How and why it doesn't appear on modern medicine's radar screen is one of the most disturbing mysteries of our time. But the evidence pointing to this single cause is very strong indeed, indicating that it may be responsible for the 90% of hypertension that doctors maintain is *idiopathic* (has no known cause).

Much recognition and gratitude is due to author Gary Taubes, for tracking it down and bringing it to the public's attention in his book, *Good Calories, Bad Calories*. His account reads like a spellbinding detective novel; as such, it follows the evidence and takes care to question every unsubstantiated assumption. Taubes' research is thorough and convincing, making it all but impossible for any open-minded reader or investigator to doubt his ultimate conclusion: That something in the modern diet, other than fat or sodium, is responsible for today's high rates of hypertension and cardiovascular disease.

That "something" is the refined carbohydrate.

HOW CARBOHYDRATES RAISE BLOOD PRESSURE

Throughout the 1980s and 1990s, Americans jumped on the low-fat bandwagon *en masse*, led by food manufacturers who filled supermarket shelves with tens of thousands of new "reduced-fat," "lite" and "fat-free" products. Ironically, this low-fat and fat-free craze produced the largest collective weight gain ever recorded in US history. If eating fat made us fat, how could this possibly be?

The answer lies in what food manufactures substituted for the fat they removed from their products: carbohydrates and, in particular, sugar and other sweeteners. It makes sense that if you remove one of the macronutrients (protein, fat, or carbohydrate) from a food, you have to increase the quantity of another to compensate. This is exactly how low-fat products are made.

When manufacturers remove some or all of the fat from a food product, they replace it with refined carbohydrates. In making low-fat yogurt, they replace fat with high fructose corn syrup (HFCS) or an artificial sweetener. We may believe we're eating a heart-healthy, low-fat snack that will help us lose weight, but the truth is, these foods make us fatter, endanger our health, and raise the risk of heart disease because of added sugar and artificial sweeteners.

We won't go into all the details here of how sugar and HFCS make, and keep us, fat. (If you are interested in the details, see our book *The 30-Day Diabetes Cure*, www.30daydiabetescure.com.) However, we do want to explain how sugar and sweeteners cause problems in your arteries that can lead to heart disease, stroke, and sudden death—and how these same refined carbohydrates directly elevate blood pressure to dangerous levels.

In his book, Taubes points to early scientific evidence that carbohydrate-rich diets raise blood pressure by causing the body to retain water. This was first noted by the German chemist Carl von Voit in 1860. It was corroborated in 1919 by Francis Benedict, director of the nutrition laboratory of the Carnegie Institute in Washington, DC, who described the phenomenon this way: "With diets predominantly carbohydrate, there is a strong tendency for the body to retain water, while with diets predominantly fat, there is a distinct tendency for the body to lose water." [147]

Benedict was referring to the weight loss during the first few weeks of any diet that restricts either calories or carbohydrates (especially the latter). This initial weight loss is mostly water, not body fat, as many veteran dieters know. Less well-known is the corresponding effect of this water loss: lowering of blood pressure.

Consuming a carbohydrate-rich diet causes the kidneys to hold onto salt that is already in the body, rather than excrete it. In reaction, the body retains water to maintain the sodium concentration of the blood. This is the same result (water retention) that occurs when we consume more sodium. "Removing carbohydrates from the diet works, in effect, just like the antihypertensive drugs known as diuretics, which cause the kidneys to excrete sodium, and water along with it," early researchers noted. In fact, this drop in blood pressure is so considerable that it led critics of low-carbohydrate diets to worry publicly about the "low blood pressure resulting from... losses of...fluid, sodium, and other minerals." [148]

By the early 1970s, researchers also discovered that a high-carbohydrate diet causes fluid retention because it increases insulin levels. They found that high insulin levels signal the kidneys to retain sodium rather than excrete it.[149] So widely accepted was this notion, that by the mid-1900s, diabetes textbooks were discussing the likelihood that chronically elevated levels of insulin were causing hypertension in Type 2 patients. Unfortunately, no one considered this might also be true for non-diabetics.

LOW-FAT DIETS MAKE HYPERTENSION WORSE

Today, it is well known that a low-carbohydrate diet makes your body lose water, and thus reduces blood pressure. Conversely, a high-carbohydrate diet makes your body retain both salt and water, which raises blood pressure. So it is strange that doctors still recommend a standard low-fat, high-carb diet to patients who are both overweight and hypertensive. This is self-defeating because low-fat diets have not proven to be effective ways to lose weight, and consuming more carbohydrates causes water retention and higher blood pressure. [150]

Diets high in carbohydrates also stimulate chronically high insulin levels because insulin is needed to move sugar from the blood into cells. The more carbs consumed, the more sugar there is to transport, and the more insulin is needed. And insulin has a direct influence on raising blood pressure. Harvard researchers found that insulin stimulates the nervous system with the same "fight-or-flight" response triggered by adrenaline, thus increasing the heart rate and constricting blood vessels, resulting in an increase in blood pressure. "The higher the insulin level, the greater the stimulation of the nervous system," the researchers note. "If insulin levels remain high, the result would be constantly elevated blood pressure." [151]

High insulin is one reason hypertension appears so frequently with diabetes. But high insulin levels—and hypertension—can be present in anyone who eats a high-carb diet. It is not limited to people with diabetes.

Obesity, too, is associated with higher insulin levels. But because it is now generally recognized that obesity raises blood insulin (and not the other way around), doctors have tended to overlook high levels of insulin as a cause of hypertension in normal-weight people. This is a huge oversight and quite likely the "unidentified cause" that mystifies doctors in the majority of hypertension cases today.

THE CARBOHYDRATE CONNECTION TO HYPERTENSION

As you'll recall from the Introduction, hypertension is a "disease of civilization," as epidemiologists first noted in the late 1920s. Back then, missionary and colonial doctors found that the blood pressure in native populations was much lower than in Western societies. (It is well noted that hypertension was nonexistent in these cultures, and that blood pressure was observed to drop with age—the opposite of what happens in developed nations.)

With exposure to Western lifestyles and diets, however, these native populations began to experience an average rise in blood pressure and increase in the incidence of hypertension. Researchers attributed this to the higher salt consumption typical in the Western diet. Incredibly, virtually no one noticed that the same cultures that consumed little or no salt, also had no sugar, white flour or other refined carbohydrates in their diets. So, the absence of hypertension could have just as easily been attributed to the lack of sugar and refined carbohydrates rather than high salt consumption.

It's truly amazing that the medical community missed this correlation because the most obvious and dramatic change in the human diet over the past 10,000 years—besides the emergence of agriculture—has been the introduction of refined carbohydrates and sugar into our diet. These substances, in particular, have created such profound and sudden havoc in blood sugar metabolism and insulin production that they have upset the homeostatic balance of the entire body. [152]

THE LINK TO OTHER "DISEASES OF CIVILIZATION"

Many "diseases of civilization," including obesity, diabetes, heart disease and hypertension, are intimately related, and they are even considered risk factors for each other. As we've seen with metabolic syndrome, an individual who develops one of these medical conditions is more likely to develop others.

Hypertension, for instance, is a major risk factor for both heart disease and stroke. It is also a risk factor for obesity and diabetes. Yet, this works the other way around, too. If you're diabetic and/or obese, you're more likely to have hypertension.

For people with diabetes, having hypertension accounts for up to 85% of their increased risk of heart disease. And since insulin levels are chronically elevated in hypertensives, having hypertension—whether or not you are overweight or have diabetes—usually also means you have insulin resistance.

Finally, hypertension is so common in the obese and obesity so common among hypertensives, that many textbooks speculate that being overweight causes hypertension. [153]

The pattern that many doctors are seeing (at least those who are willing to honestly look) is that the higher the blood pressure, the higher the cholesterol and triglyceride levels; and the greater the body weight, the stronger the risk of diabetes and heart disease.[154] This is why doctors are beginning to look for "co-morbidities" in patients. This is also why having metabolic syndrome is a far more reliable indicator of your overall mortality risk than high cholesterol or hypertension, alone.

What we find truly significant is that one factor, the over-consumption of sugar and refined carbohydrates, seems very likely to be the root cause of so many of these related conditions. And that one simple action—eliminating these troublesome foods from your diet—could significantly improve, if not resolve, these multiple health problems.

Imagine! With one simple dietary change you could reduce your risk for hypertension, insulin resistance, pre-diabetes and diabetes, cardiovascular disease, and, quite possibly, Alzheimer's disease plus many cancers (because a growing body of research links both to over-consumption of sugar and refined carbohydrates, as well). These are today's leading degenerative diseases. They cripple and they kill. Think how you could rig the current health odds in your favor with this single dietary decision.

The evidence is too strong to ignore, or at the least, to not aggressively investigate further. These multiple "diseases of civilization" seem to have their root in the "diet of civilization," which features a disproportionate and unhealthful percentage of refined sugar, flour and polyunsaturated vegetable oils—"foods" that trigger chaos throughout the body's metabolic and hormonal systems.

IS CURRENT DIETARY ADVICE MAKING THE SITUATION WORSE?

Big Medicine's refusal to acknowledge this connection (or at least to aggressively investigate it with an open mind) seems to be prolonging our collective poor health and misery. It makes no sense at all that such influential groups as the American Medical Association, the American Diabetes Association, the American Cancer Society, the National Institutes of Health, the Centers for Disease Prevention, the Institute of Medicine of the National Academy of Sciences, the National Heart Lung and Blood Institute, and the US Department of Agriculture (to name but a few powerful medical groups in the US) continue to recommend a low-fat/high-carb diet as the dietary path to optimal health. As with the salt-hypertension hypothesis we debunked in Chapter 7, much of the conventional advice we're receiving these days seems contraindicated, given the trove of research findings already in our possession.

Why aren't medical textbooks encouraging the restriction of sugar and refined carbohydrates in people with diabetes? Or at least pushing for new research to explore the connection between refined carbs and disease?

New guidelines from the USDA regarding sugar consumption allow individuals up to 25% of their daily calories from added sugars, including high-fructose corn syrup (HFCS). Incredibly, this happens to be the same amount of sugar that's been demonstrated to cause heart disease, according to a recent study published in the *Journal of Clinical Endocrinology & Metabolism.* [155]

Furthermore, these ill effects occur rather quickly. After just two weeks of consuming 25% of their daily calories from either sucrose or HFCS, subjects were already experiencing heart-damaging effects. Their triglyceride levels rose to dangerously high levels, and they had a dramatic increase in a subclass of LDL cholesterol called apolipoprotein-B (ApoB)—an increase that is directly linked to the formation of artery plaque. [156] Keep in mind that these are the same official guidelines that advise us to restrict fats to as little as 20% of our diet.

HOW SUGAR CAUSES HEART DISEASE

Previously, we explained how inflammation damages the delicate lining of artery walls, setting in motion the formation of plaque and calcification that hardens arteries and raises blood pressure. Though you most likely will not hear it from your doctor (most MDs still believe what they have been taught and told—that saturated fat and cholesterol are responsible for heart disease), the greatest causes of artery inflammation are sugar, sweeteners like HFCS, and refined carbohydrates, such as processed grain products.

While it is long overdue, the AHA and the cardiology community have lately started to suspect that sugar, sweeteners, and especially HFCS may be an unrecognized cause of heart disease. Unfortunately, they claim the relationship is indirect, saying that sugar and HFCS in foods and beverages cause obesity, which is a risk factor for heart disease. In fact, the evidence shows that the link is far more direct.

Sugar causes inflammation. As Mehmet Oz, MD, explained on Oprah's nationally televised special about diabetes, entitled "America's Silent Killer," dietary sugar and sweets damage arteries directly: "It's like tiny glass shards scraping the linings of the arteries, which the body then hardens over by forming little scabs."[157]

An occasional dessert or a teaspoon of sugar in your coffee will not have this harmful effect, of course. But Americans consume massive quantities of sugar and sweeteners—about 150–175 pounds per person annually. The human metabolism simply cannot cope with this amount. All this sugar raises the body's blood sugar (glucose) levels, which, over time, leads to obesity, diabetes, heart disease, stroke, cancer—and, along the way, hypertension.

One common factor in these diseases is inflammation. Elevated blood sugar levels are as inflammatory as smoking cigarettes; some researchers believe it's even worse. Excessive sugar consumption also is a major factor in other medical conditions such as asthma, acne, migraines, and arthritis.

But it is not only sugar and HFCS that cause so much inflammation. All refined carbohydrates—white bread, baked goods, chips and crackers, pasta, pastries, and white rice—quickly turn into glucose during the digestion process and elevate blood sugar.

Insulin worsens inflammation. Elevated blood sugar triggers a surge of insulin into the bloodstream (insulin is the hormone responsible for removing glucose from the bloodstream and delivering it to cells where it can be metabolized into energy). When blood levels of insulin are chronically high due to chronically elevated blood glucose, cells become resistant to insulin (called insulin resistance or pre-diabetes) and more of the hormone is needed to clear the bloodstream.

Making matters worse is the fact that insulin is also highly inflammatory. Together and separately, glucose and insulin inflame and damage arteries, triggering the formation of hardened artery plaques, clogged kidneys, hypertension and, ultimately, heart attack and/or stroke.

Glycation. In addition to inflaming arteries, excess glucose directly damages arteries in a process called glycation, in which sugar and protein molecules cross-link to form a tangled mess of hardened tissue. Glycated tissue is dry, brittle, and weaker than it once was. For instance, skin that was previously supple starts to sag and wrinkle. Glycation accelerates the aging of your body's cells, tissues, and organs—including your arteries, heart, and brain.

To picture this, think about what happens to the runny part of a raw egg, which is almost entirely protein. When heat is applied, the white of an egg is changed into a solid, rubbery substance. This is what glycation does to healthy tissue and organs. When the proteins in blood vessels are glycated, they harden just like the egg white, leading to hypertension by making arteries less flexible.

This glycated tissue, technically referred to as advanced glycation end products (AGEs), also throws off a barrage of free radical molecules that oxidize healthy tissue in the same way that exposure to oxygen "browns" a freshly cut apple and speeds its deterioration. Unless there is a sufficient storehouse of antioxidant vitamins in the body, these free radicals will run amuck, eventually penetrating the DNA itself and initiating the development of cancer.

A healthy heart and arteries are nearly impossible to maintain in an environment containing so much glucose and insulin. This is why heart disease and heart attack are the leading cause of death for people with diabetes, being responsible for a stunning 75% of all diabetic fatalities.

The good news is that there are many ways (all of them natural) to prevent and even reverse some of this damage, which you will discover in the chapters ahead.

WHY ARE WE ON SUCH A SUGAR BINGE?

Why are we consuming so many sugary foods and sweetened beverages? The reason is clear: they are so pleasing to our taste buds and because our brains are wired to seek them out. Back in the early days when humans were hunter-gatherers, naturally sweet foods were a considered a real treat. Our preference for sweet foods hasn't changed, even though the nature of our food supply has been altered dramatically.

Americans have a major crush on sugar, which is making us sick and killing us in record numbers. On average, we consume 22 teaspoons of the stuff every day in baked goods and desserts, in candy and soda pop, and straight from the sugar jar—spooned into our coffee and tea. That adds up to an unbelievable 150 to175 pounds of sugar and sweeteners for every man, woman, and child in our nation. This is an increase of 500% over the last 100 years! Add to this another 50 pounds per year of high fructose corn syrup (HFCS), the sweetener in soda pop, and it's easy to understand why diabetes, hypertension, obesity, and heart disease are national health epidemics.

Sugar, HFCS, and other sweeteners pervade our food supply. Food manufacturers add them to everything, including ketchup, mayonnaise and products that don't even taste sweet. If you don't believe this, just start examining food labels more closely. You'll notice that sugar, HFCS, sweeteners, and artificial sweeteners are added to practically every food item in the supermarket. (Sugar has many names—including raw sugar, turbinado sugar, sucrose, glucose, dextrose, maltodextrin, brown sugar, and maltose.)

HFCS is now found in every type of processed food and beverage you can name. Invented by the Japanese in the 1970s as a low-cost alternative to sugar, its presence in the American diet has increased by a staggering 10,673% (!) between 1970 and 2005, according to the USDA. It is now the number one source of calories in our diet. [158]

Sugar addiction. It may surprise you to learn that sugar and sweeteners are as physically addictive as cocaine. So says Richard Johnson, MD, professor of medicine at the University of Colorado, where he runs the kidney division and is in charge of blood pressure research. He is also author of *The Sugar Fix*, an excellent book that explains the dangers of sugar and HFCS.

In his book, Dr. Johnson explains how sugar satisfies the same reward center of the brain as cigarettes, alcohol, sex, and drugs. And don't think for a minute that food and soft drink manufacturers don't realize this. They know they need only add sugar or sweetener to a new food product to ensure its popularity.

Health experts and doctors are still telling us that being overweight, obesity, heart disease, hypertension, and even diabetes are caused by eating too much dietary fat—even though this has been thoroughly debunked and disproved by science. The fact is, fat consumption has steadily *decreased* in the US since the late 1970s; yet our collective weight has continued to blimp up and rates for heart disease and hypertension have not declined.

Soda pop and hypertension. Excess sugar consumption and hypertension go hand-in-hand, and the number one culprits are soda pop and other sweetened beverages. Researchers tracked the diets of nearly 2,700 people and found that those who drank sugar-sweetened beverages had higher blood pressures—both systolic and diastolic numbers. The highest blood pressure levels occurred in those who consumed the most fructose and glucose, which are both found in HFCS.

Another study examined the nutritional data of 4,500 people, none of whom had hypertension. After consuming 74 grams of HFCS a day (the equivalent of two and a half cans of soda pop), these previously healthy people had a 77% greater risk of developing blood pressure readings of 160/100 mmHG or higher. The negative effect that sweets have on blood pressure happens rather quickly. One study found that men eating a high-fructose diet began to see their blood pressure numbers rise after just two weeks.

Average soda pop consumption in the US is about two cans per person per day, according to the National Soft Drink Association. This means that much of the hypertension in this country could be eliminated if people simply swore off soft drinks. Now that is a "Pepsi challenge" worth taking!

How HFCS raises blood pressure. Dr. Johnson's research reveals that the human body processes HFCS and other sugars in a manner that also raises blood levels of uric acid immediately after ingestion. Elevated levels of uric acid are usually associated with gout, but high levels are also present in people with hypertension and kidney disease. Uric acid drives up blood pressure by inhibiting nitric oxide in your blood vessels. Nitric oxide helps blood vessels maintain their elasticity and facilitates their expansion (dilation). Thus, suppression of nitric oxide by HFCS consumption leads to increases in blood pressure. This is confirmed by 17 studies, which find that elevated uric acid levels lead to hypertension.[159] Too much uric acid is also a factor in kidney disease, insulin resistance and diabetes, obesity, fatty liver disease, elevated triglycerides and LDL, and cardiovascular disease. [160]

What about fruits and fruit juices? Because fructose (fruit sugar) occurs naturally in fresh fruits, people with high blood pressure, insulin resistance, diabetes, weight issues, and high cholesterol should go easy on them. Their fiber and antioxidant content can help neutralize some of the detrimental effects of the fructose, but they should still be eaten in moderation. Fruit juices, on the other hand, are nearly as harmful as soft drinks, because they have lots of fructose and little fiber. Consuming lots of fructose-laden fruit juice can play havoc with your biochemistry and physiology.

If you have hypertension, ask your doctor to check your uric acid level. A level of 4 mg/dL for men and 3.5 mg/dL for women indicates a very low risk for fructose toxicity. The higher your level, the more you should limit or even avoid fructose until your uric acid level normalizes.

The problem with beer. Dr. Johnson found that drinking beer also elevates uric acid levels, and therefore blood pressure. The classic "beer belly" is characteristic of metabolic syndrome, which includes abdominal obesity, elevated triglycerides, low HDL, high blood pressure, and insulin resistance. People with hypertension should strictly limit—or completely eliminate—beer consumption. Dry white wine and distilled spirits are less harmful alternatives because they have relatively lower fructose content.

Resetting your sugar metabolism. According to Dr. Mercola, the more sugar, fructose, and HFCS you consume, the more sensitive your body becomes to them, and the more your body absorbs. Going "cold turkey"—adopting a very low fructose diet—for two weeks can "reboot" your sugar metabolism. The less of these sugars you consume during this period, the weaker your cravings for them will become.

REFINED CARBS: AS BAD AS SUGAR

It isn't only sugar and sweets that have us hooked. Ever since the popularity of these foods began to skyrocket in the 1950s, we've become increasingly obsessed with refined carbohydrate foods. Unfortunately, refined carbohydrate foods produce the same effect on our blood sugar and insulin levels as if we were eating table sugar straight from the jar. They are equally responsible for all sorts of cardiovascular disease, including hypertension.

In *Good Calories, Bad Calories,* Gary Taubes cites abundant research linking today's predominant low-fat/high-carb diet to heart disease. Many of these studies fly in the face of conventional medical advice, which promotes the low-fat diet as the road to heart health. But Taubes makes a compelling case that indicts refined carbohydrates as Public Health Enemy Number Three (just behind sugar and HFCS).

A TALE OF TWO CARBOHYDRATES

Carbs come in two forms. To make things easy, we're going to use the "fast"and "slow" terminology because the pertinent factor is the speed at which your body breaks down any food into glucose during digestion.

Refined. Also referred to as "simple carbs," or "fast carbs" (referring to the speed at which the carbohydrate food breaks down into blood sugar, or glucose, during digestion). Fast carbs are highly refined grain and vegetable-based food products that have had their fiber, nutrients and oils removed during processing. As a result, fast carbs convert *quickly* into glucose in your bloodstream. Fast carbs are also called "simple carbs" because they consist of only a few carbohydrate molecules. Sugars, for instance, a subcategory of fast carbs, may contain only two carbohydrate molecules, such as sucrose and fructose. Because they are so small, they can be broken down into glucose fast.

Whole. Also termed "complex" or "slow carbs." Slow carbs are whole foods that haven't been refined. As a result, they still contain their full nutrition and fiber. This fiber content *slows down* the food's conversion into glucose in your bloodstream. Slow carbs have a more complicated molecular chain, which is why they are also called "complex carbs."

By the way, don't confuse "slow carb" with "low carb," which simply refers to the amount of carbohydrate, fast or slow, in a given food product.

HOW TO TELL A FAST CARB FROM A SLOW CARB

A slow-carb food is easy to recognize because it appears in its natural state—or very close to the way it looked when it was growing. Fast carbs, on the other hand, are usually found in boxes, bags, cans, and the frozen food section of your supermarket.

But, sometimes it is tricky. Some fruits (especially those that have been dried, such as raisins) possess high sugar content and should only be eaten in moderation. Fruit juice, which has been stripped of its fiber, turns into glucose almost immediately after you drink it.

USING THE GLYCEMIC INDEX

When in doubt, you can refer to the Glycemic Index (GI), a system devised to determine how fast or slow a carbohydrate food enters the bloodstream and elevates your blood sugar level. Fast carbs rank very high on the GI. In general, foods with a high GI ranking are fast carbs and should be avoided.

An even more reliable way to determine whether a food is a fast carb is its glycemic load (GL), which not only gives its GI rating, but also tells how much carbohydrate is actually in the food. Here is where the science can get a little confusing, because a food might have a high GI number but a small amount of actual carbohydrate in relation to its fiber (which slows it down). This means that some whole foods, like carrots or potatoes (which are high in fiber), might have a high GI number but a low GL ranking. The GL reveals the true impact a food has on your glucose metabolism.

For the glycemic listing of the top 100+ foods, see Appendix B, on page 312.

THE TOP 10 WORST CARBS

1. White bread, toast, bagels, English muffins, bread sticks.

2. Fruit juice, soda pop, energy drinks, and all sweetened beverages.

3. Waffles, pancakes, French toast.

4. Pastries, coffee cake, muffins, donuts, cupcakes, cake, and cookies.

5. Jams and jellies, especially those with added sugar or sweeteners; fruit pies.

6. Boxed breakfast cereals and "instant" hot cereals, including instant oatmeal.

7. Chips, crackers, and many grain-based processed snacks.

8. Tortillas made from white flour.

9. French fries.

10. White rice and white flour pasta products—including macaroni.

WHY FAST CARBS ARE BAD FOR YOUR BLOOD PRESSURE

They instantly raise your blood sugar. Your body responds to the fast carbs in white-flour foods such as bread, pastries, and pasta as if you just ate table sugar. They turn into glucose immediately upon digestion, spike your blood sugar, and trigger your body's insulin response. Each of these factors drives up your blood pressure, but the harm doesn't stop there.

The continuous presence of insulin in your bloodstream, due to elevated glucose levels caused by the repeated consumption of fast carbs, conditions your cells to ignore the insulin. Consuming muffins, toast, breakfast cereal, waffles, pancakes, sandwich bread, sodas, chips, cookies, mac n' cheese, spaghetti, french fries, beer, soft drinks, and sweet desserts makes your cells resistant to insulin. As a result, it takes more and more insulin to clear the glucose out of your bloodstream. And as you've learned, more insulin means higher blood pressure and greater inflammation.

How effectively your body uses insulin is directly related to your risk of developing high blood pressure, reported researchers from Wake Forest University Baptist Medical Center. "We found you can predict who's at higher risk for developing high blood pressure based on their insulin resistance," said David Goff Jr., PhD, MD, the lead researcher for the Insulin Resistance Atherosclerosis Study (IRAS)[161] conducted in 2000. Numerous other studies, before and since IRAS, have confirmed this connection.

When Dr. Goff's study began, all 809 middle-aged adults had normal blood pressure and varying levels of resistance to insulin. Five years later, researchers found that participants who were most resistant to insulin had a higher incidence of high blood pressure. "The one-third of participants with the highest levels of insulin resistance had rates of hypertension that were 35% higher than the one-third with the least resistance," said Dr. Goff. "These findings point out that reducing the body's resistance to insulin may help prevent hypertension and cardio-vascular disease." [162]

Fast carbs make you fat. Insulin's main job is to get glucose out of your bloodstream any way it can. So when your muscle cells refuse to accept any more blood sugar, insulin transports it into liver cells, where it is converted into fat (called triglycerides). This fat accumulates in fat cells, primarily around your belly (in men) and your hips (in women). This is why insulin is called "the fat storage hormone."

As long as insulin is present in the bloodstream, storage fats will not break down into fatty acids and become available for use as fuel. So you'll have a hard time losing body fat. And because stored fat will not be readily available to you as an alternative source of energy when you run low on glucose, you will tend to become hungry, and overeat. This is a vicious cycle that very few people, doctors included, understand clearly.

Contrary to what almost everyone believes, overeating *does not* cause obesity. Instead, the obesity causes overeating. This is because the fatty acids that should be feeding your body between meals and during sleep remain locked away in your fat cells because of insulin's constant presence (due to continuous consumption of fast carbohydrates). This vicious cycle is what really leads to overeating and accumulating fat storage.

Fast carbs trigger inflammation. They create inflammatory proteins called *cytokines*, which aggravate the body's inflammation response. More inflammation is the last thing you want in your body because it raises your risk of practically every serious chronic and degenerative disease—including arterial disease, heart attack, and stroke. Inflammation also makes your joints and back painfully sore. It causes your arteries to clog up with plaque. It destroys brain cells. It raises your risk of all cancers. And last but not least, it elevates your blood pressure. You can pretend to ignore all of this as you chomp on your morning bagel, but denial won't stop the inflammation.

Fast carbs are loaded with damaging fats. Most processed foods, including buns, rolls, breakfast cereals, soft breads, crackers, and chips, contain refined PUFA vegetable oils, such as soy, corn, cottonseed, or canola oil, which are high in omega-6 fatty acids. As you may recall, they often contain trans-fats (labeled as "hydrogenated oil" or "vegetable shortening"). Omega-6s deplete omega-3 essential fatty acids—which fight inflammation—resulting in higher inflammation throughout the body.

So when you consume baked goods such as burger buns, snack cakes, and dinner rolls, you're getting a double whammy: a spike in glucose from the fast carbs and more inflammation due to the excessive omega-6 content. Too much omega-6 also elevates your levels of triglycerides and cholesterol, increases insulin resistance, impairs normal cellular repair, and raises your risk of diabetic complications.[163] And although there has been some progress by food manufacturers, trans-fats—the unhealthiest fats ever invented—are still present in baked goods, crackers, and snack foods and are also frequently used to deep-fry fast foods such as French fries, fried chicken, fish, and chips. [164]

Fast carbs lack fiber. When you're fighting hypertension and heart disease, fiber is your best ally. High-fiber carbohydrates (such as beans and fresh vegetables) contain fewer calories because the fiber component is not digested by your body. Fiber is the *roughage* component of vegetables, fruits, whole grains, and beans that give these foods their bulk. Because the ratio of calories-to-volume is so high, you can eat until you are full without gaining weight—in fact, you find yourself *losing* pounds steadily by eating these foods. It is easy to see why: An apple is more filling than the juice of the apple, which contains about the same number of calories.

Refined carbs, such as bread products, are the black sheep of the carbohydrate family. Because they've had their fiber removed, they're a more concentrated source of calories. Since their volume has been reduced by processing, it is easy to eat more of them before your stomach tells your brain, "I'm full." That's just one reason they are so fattening: They are very easy to over-consume.

A bigger problem results when many of these refined carbs are combined with other high-calorie ingredients, as in the case of bakery goods. When white flour is mixed with eggs, oil, milk, and sweeteners, its calorie content jumps, but its volume (the amount it takes to fill your stomach) increases only slightly. The sugar combined with the refined flour carbs also triggers an instant spike in your glucose levels. As you now know, this signals the release of insulin, which unfortunately facilitates the rapid conversion of carbohydrates into fatty triglycerides and belly fat.

Fast carbs may trigger hidden allergies. Bread products are loaded with gluten, a compound found in wheat, rye, oats, and barley, which can be difficult to digest and cause inflammation of the intestines. A full-blown allergic reaction to gluten is called *celiac disease.* Doctors are beginning to realize that millions of Americans may have an undiagnosed sensitivity or an outright intolerance for gluten. Estimates are that 30% of the US population is adversely affected in some way by gluten. Symptoms of gluten sensitivity include fatigue, weakness, general achiness, abdominal bloating, and chronic diarrhea. Gluten intolerance has also been linked to osteoporosis, anemia, cancer, lupus, multiple sclerosis, and other autoimmune diseases, as well as psychiatric and neurological conditions such as depression, migraines, and schizophrenia, according to various studies published in the *New England Journal of Medicine.*

You may not even suspect you have gluten intolerance until you start paying attention to how you feel after eating gluten-containing foods. Eliminating these foods is the first step to improving your health and well-being, especially if you suffer from an already debilitating disease like diabetes.

Fast carbs take the place of nutritious foods. If you are consuming a lot of bread-based foods, you're probably eating fewer of the Hypertension Healing Superfoods you'll discover in Chapter Twelve. Remember: You always have the choice. The next time you reach for a piece of toast, thick sandwich, plate of pasta, dinner roll, cupcake, brownie, Danish, or morning muffin, ask yourself, "What could I be eating instead that would help heal my blood pressure and blood sugar problems?"

In Chapter Twelve, you will discover a pleasing variety of answers to this important question. You will learn about the delicious, super-nutritious foods that can lower your blood pressure; reduce your inflammation; help you lose weight naturally; slash your triglycerides, cholesterol, blood sugar and insulin levels; give you more energy; perk up your mood; improve your general health; and ultimately, lengthen your life. [165]

DOES YOUR BODY EVEN NEED CARBS?

Almost everyone believes so. Even many doctors believe that your body and brain need carbohydrates because they are its main source of "high octane" fuel. They also claim your body prefers carbs above protein and fat (the other two macronutrients) because it metabolizes glucose before the other two. These are the justifications they provide for recommending your diet be composed mostly (50% to 60%!) of carbohydrates.

But carbohydrates are not necessary for a healthful human diet. Indeed, as Gary Taubes reminds us in *Why We Get Fat,* "...there is no such thing as an 'essential carbohydrate'" (as opposed to the other two macronutrients, fat and protein, which are indeed essential). Furthermore, glucose is not the body's "preferred" fuel as many nutritionists claim. The fact is, under normal circumstances your body burns fat and glucose on an almost 50/50 basis. However, if you're consuming a carbohydrate-rich diet, your metabolism focuses on clearing the bloodstream of carb-derived glucose *first* because this is what the insulin response dictates.

If there were no carbohydrates in your diet, your brain and central nervous system would be able to function quite nicely on molecules called "ketones," which the liver produces when it breaks down fatty acids. Ketones also can provide approximately 75% of the energy that your brain requires. The balance of the energy will come from glycerol, which also is released from your body's fat reserves—and from glucose synthesized in the liver from protein. As long as there is high-quality fat and protein in the diet, your brain will always have plenty of fuel. [166]

This is what happens when we miss a meal or while we are sleeping. Normally, with the presence of insulin diminished (between meals and while we sleep) our bodies feed off our stored fat. As the night passes and insulin's presence recedes, more stored fat is released from our fat cells and our livers increase their production of ketones, the by-product of burning fat for energy. After a few days of this, we enter the state of "ketosis" (when the liver's stores of glycogen are depleted) and our brains and bodies are using ketones for fuel. This same phenomenon occurs on a low-carb diet. Far from starving, researchers report that the brain actually operates more efficiently on ketones compared with glucose. [167]

Incidentally, the preferred energy source for the heart is ketones. Studies show there is a 28% greater efficiency of the heart when ketones are used as a fuel source.[168]

Taubes points out that humans existed in a state of mild ketosis (elevated level of ketones in the body) for 99.9% of human history, long before the modern carbohydrate existed. [169] Indeed, we evolved on a diet almost wholly composed of fat and protein—with a tiny bit of plant matter (roots, berries, and leaves). Today, this eating approach has been recreated as the Paleolithic Diet, a dietary approach that is gaining popularity. But, there are some real concerns with this diet, including the vital vitamins and minerals you miss out on by not eating foods such as grains and dairy. If your primary goals are control of your blood pressure, blood sugar and insulin, along with weight loss, you will achieve better and healthier results by eating in accord with *The 30-Day Blood Pressure Cure Plan* in Part Two of this book, beginning on page 175.

HOW HEALTHY ARE YOUR ARTERIES?

Today, there are a variety of excellent diagnostic tests that can help determine the health of your arteries and your risk of heart attack or stroke. Here are the essentials:

Testing for inflammation. C-Reactive Protein (CRP) is a blood marker for inflammation. Along with triglyceride levels, CRP is far more reliable in predicting your risk of heart disease than cholesterol levels, because it indicates the extent of inflammation in your body in general and your arteries in particular. CRP is usually not included in standard lipid panel tests, so be sure to request it the next time you have your cholesterol levels tested. Be sure to specify the "high-sensitivity" CRP blood test, as the test most commonly administered does not register background levels of inflammation. If your CRP is elevated, your doctor may suggest aspirin therapy or other medication. Chapters Twelve and Thirteen suggest specific foods and supplements that have been shown to effectively reduce inflammation levels.

Agatston calcium score. This test (named after Arthur Agatston, MD, Dr. Heilbron's friend and associate from the South Beach Diet) measures the amount of calcified plaque in your arteries and thus the amount of "hardening" that has occurred. As you will recall, hypertension can result from hardened arteries (arteriosclerosis). To check for the buildup of calcium in plaque on the walls of the arteries of the heart (coronary arteries), this test uses a special X-ray device called computed tomography (CT), which takes pictures of the arteries in thin sections to identify the locations and concentrations of calcified plaque. This test allows the physician to check for coronary artery disease (CAD) in its early stages and to determine how severe it is.

The higher your score, the more plaque you have in the arteries of your heart. This increases your chance of having a heart attack. If you have a high Agatston calcium score, you may need more tests to further investigate the condition. One such test, called coronary catheterization, allows doctors to look directly into your arteries. Agatston calcium scoring is not done as part of a routine screening and may not be covered by all health insurance plans but it is relatively inexpensive (about $99). Don't be too concerned about cholesterol and other indirect markers, but we recommend that you check your Agatston calcium score to know if you are at risk.

Testing your glucose and insulin levels. Chronically elevated blood glucose promotes glycation, as well as other aging processes and degenerative diseases. The higher the blood sugar, the greater the chance that destructive reactions between proteins, fats, and sugars will take place. The process can eventually lead to the deterioration of cellular function. Since insulin resistance often occurs with hypertension, you'll want to be sure to be checked, so you can either rule this out or get appropriate medical treatment. Several tests can measure your glucose and insulin levels, either directly or indirectly, including C-peptide, glucose, glucose tolerance test (GTT), and hemoglobin A1C. Each of these four tests can be beneficial. Ask your doctor which ones are right for you.

Many people don't realize that they can display a normal glucose level (less than 126) and still have elevated levels of insulin in their blood. This will give you almost the same risk of coronary artery disease as someone with full-blown diabetes. [170]

TESTING FOR YOUR RISK OF HEART ATTACK

As mentioned earlier, you should think of hypertension as a symptom of trouble, and not solely a medical condition that needs to be controlled. Ultimately, what you really should care about is the overall health of your cardiovascular system and your risk of heart attack or stroke. The reason for controlling hypertension, either with drugs or natural treatments, is to lower this risk. Having elevated blood pressure should make you more than a little curious about your odds of having a heart attack in the near future. These two tests will give you the most reliable answers.

HDL cholesterol. The majority of doctors still consider elevated LDL (what we have come to call "the bad cholesterol") the most trusted predictor of heart attack risk. It is not. Other factors are far more predictive, including the size of those LDL particles. A more serious danger is low HDL cholesterol (otherwise known as the "good cholesterol"). People with low HDL (less than 40 for men and below 50 for women) [171] are at far greater risk of having a heart attack than those with a high total cholesterol or elevated LDL cholesterol. [172] For women, HDL is so accurate at predicting future heart disease that it is, effectively, the only predictor of risk that matters. In fact, when researchers look for genes that predispose men or women to living an exceedingly lengthy life—longer than 95 or 100 years—one of the few genes that stands out is a gene for a naturally high HDL cholesterol level. However, also note that very high HDL (over 70 and especially over 100) is a very strong marker of toxicity.

97

You should be aware, then, that the sugars and sweeteners added to processed foods spell trouble for our arteries and our hearts. A study published in a recent issue of the *Journal of the American Medical Association* found that the more added sugars we consume, the more our HDL or "good" cholesterol goes down. For this reason, the American Heart Association recently recommended limiting added sugar intake to no more than 5% of our total calories, which comes out to roughly 100 calories per day for women and 150 calories per day for men. [173]

But the AHA's advice doesn't go far enough. It isn't just sugar that lowers HDL, but refined carbohydrates (bread, pastries, breakfast cereals, chips, and cookies) as well. [174] See the "Top 10 Worst 'Fast Carb' Foods" on page 92, as a reminder of the foods you should avoid.

Triglycerides. A high triglyceride level is another serious risk factor for heart disease, although many doctors remain far more concerned with a patient's cholesterol levels. Triglycerides are simply fats stored in fat cells and the liver if we eat too many sweets and refined carbohydrates. Triglycerides also build up in the blood as the result of metabolic disorders and obesity. The higher their level, the greater the risk for heart attack.

Elevated triglycerides (above 150) are also a major risk factor for heart disease, Type 2 diabetes, and metabolic syndrome. On the other hand, low triglyceride levels are a hallmark of excellent health and coincide with elevated levels of protective HDL. In a 40-year study conducted by researchers at the University of Hawaii, scientists found that low triglyceride levels at middle age best predicted "exceptional survival"—defined as living until age 85 without suffering from a major disease.

Metabolic syndrome. Remember our discussion of this serious condition back on page 7? People with metabolic syndrome are up to 400% more likely to have a heart attack or stroke compared with the general population. [175,176] Metabolic syndrome is defined as having any three of these symptoms simultaneously: Elevated triglycerides, low HDL cholesterol, accumulated abdominal fat, and high blood sugar and insulin levels.

Currently, having any three of these symptoms of metabolic syndrome is the most reliable predictor of an impending heart attack, although many doctors fail to connect the dots and continue to treat each symptom separately. If you suspect you have metabolic syndrome, we strongly urge you to bring this to your doctor's attention right away. And if your physician has not recognized the problem on his own, we also recommend that you find another doctor.

SHOCKING SECRET ABOUT TOM HANKS' DIABETES

Actor Tom Hanks has joined the growing list of celebrities who have been diagnosed with Type 2 diabetes or pre-diabetes. During a recent appearance on the Late Show with David Letterman to promote his new film *Captain Phillips*, Hanks casually announced that his physician finally moved him from a pre-diabetic diagnosis to Type 2.

In his own words, Hanks told Letterman: "I went to the doctor and he said, 'You know those high blood sugar numbers you've been dealing with since you were 36? Well, you've graduated. You've got Type 2 diabetes, young man.'"

NO WONDER TYPE 2 DIABETES IS A GLOBAL EPIDEMIC!

What is so shocking about Tom Hanks' diagnosis is that his doctor allowed his blood glucose levels to linger at pre-diabetic levels for more than 20 years! Given what we know about the dangers of chronically elevated glucose levels, this action (or rather, inaction) by Tom Hanks' doctor should qualify as medical malpractice. By his doctor's own words, Tom Hanks' blood glucose levels hovered between 100 mg/dL and 125 mg/dL for more than two decades. This is truly "bad medicine"!

THAT MUCH GLUCOSE IS TOXIC TO THE BODY

High levels of glucose in the bloodstream have a damaging effect on arteries, tissues, organs, and the metabolism—and accelerate the rate at which your body and brain age. Elevated glucose levels are highly inflammatory. This inflammation "burns" delicate artery linings and sets the stage for heart attack, high blood pressure, and stroke—not to mention cancer, dementia and Alzheimer's disease, and kidney failure.

Moreover, through a process called glucotoxicity, high glucose levels begin to destroy the beta cells in the pancreas that are responsible for producing the hormone insulin. When this happens, your body is effectively being "poisoned by sugar." This further hastens the development of Type 2 and, ultimately, Type 1 diabetes. By that point you have become dependent on insulin injections for life.

In a nutshell, greater inflammation means faster aging, more disease, and a shorter life span.

TOM HANKS' DOCTOR SHOULD HAVE REALIZED THIS DANGER

More than a decade ago, the DECODE study of 22,000 people found significant risk of heart disease and diabetic complications starting at glucose levels of 95 mg/dl. As it happens, these levels are considered perfectly "normal" by the American Diabetes Association (ADA) and almost all doctors because they are well below the official cutoff for pre-diabetes and Type 2 diabetes.[177]

Another important study discovered that the risk of heart attack rises with any increase in average blood sugar—even for those who do not have diabetes.[178]

The most recent research shows that glucose begins to damage the body at levels above 85 mg/dL[179]—and that the risk of cardiovascular disease climbs significantly from this point. [180]

All of these studies were highly publicized. Every doctor—regardless of his specialty—should be aware of them.

DOCTORS ARE WRONG ABOUT "HEALTHY" BLOOD GLUCOSE LEVELS

If Tom Hanks' personal physician didn't realize the harm being done, you can imagine how out of touch your doctor might be. But don't blame your doctor. The official guidelines distributed to all physicians by the ADA state that a person officially has Type 2 diabetes when his/her fasting glucose level is 126 mg/dL—and pre-diabetes when the level is above 100 mg/dL. But these definitions are arbitrary and dangerous. Why? Because these cutoff levels ignore the proven damage done to the body that begins at much lower levels of blood glucose. Even worse…

TOO MANY DOCTORS TREAT PRE-DIABETES AS "NO BIG DEAL"

Tom Hanks' physician is a perfect example. Because the ADA doesn't endorse a program of diet and lifestyle improvements for people with pre-diabetes, most doctors simply wait until a patient's blood glucose crosses the official type 2 threshold before beginning any treatment. In almost all cases this means multiple drugs. A small percentage of physicians may mutter something about "losing some weight" and "come back in six months"—but they rarely (if ever) provide pre-diabetes patients with any specifics.

This casual attitude of doctors about pre-diabetes naturally carries over to the patient and the public at large. And given the previously mentioned studies confirming the serious harm done at "pre-diabetic" levels of blood glucose, this furthers the case of medical malpractice against them. Because, in reality…

"PRE-DIABETES" IS A KILLER!

Many people with pre-diabetes never get Type 2—yet they are at serious risk for cardiovascular disease, life-threatening health problems, and death just the same.

- A study performed at Crittenton Hospital Medical Center in Detroit showed that 36% of people with pre-diabetes already had coronary artery disease—similar to the 42% with Type 2 diabetes. [181]

- In addition, most people with pre-diabetes already show signs of retinopathy (eye damage), nephropathy (kidney damage) and neuropathy (nerve damage), all of which are common complications of diabetes.[182]

- This risk is confirmed by yet another study which found that nearly two-thirds of all patients admitted to the emergency room with heart attacks were found to have had pre-diabetes or undiagnosed diabetes. [183]

- Another important study found that the risk of heart attack increases with any increase in average blood sugar, even for those who don't have diabetes.[184]

PRE-DIABETES IS ACTUALLY STAGE 1 DIABETES

Popular diabetes blogger Riva Greenberg put it succinctly in her *Huffington Post* article entitled "Pre-Diabetes: The Lie That's Killing Us:" "Pre-diabetes doesn't exist. And the lie we tell that it does, does incredible harm. It stops the nearly 80 million Americans who have it from making the lifestyle changes necessary to prevent advanced type 2 diabetes. Pre-diabetes is, in truth, Stage 1 diabetes."

Doctors are making a serious mistake about blood glucose levels and heart disease. While they continue to determine your risk for a heart attack or stroke based on your cholesterol level (which, by the way, has never been proven), a more reliable gauge is clearly your blood glucose level.

HERE'S HOW TO PROTECT YOURSELF:

Our current healthcare system is badly broken, so I advise you not to place too much faith in it. Please do not relax your guard if your physician or healthcare provider assures you that your glucose level is "perfectly normal" or that you "only have pre-diabetes." Instead, consider this a red alert wake-up call that should boot you into immediate action. Unless your glucose levels are consistently below 85 mg/dL, you should be vigilant and proactive by strictly limiting (or completely avoiding) the consumption of sugar, sweets and sweeteners, and simple carbohydrates. If you are uncertain about how to do this, Jim created an easy-to-follow, step-by step plan in his bestselling book, *The 30-Day Diabetes Cure* (www.30daydiabetescure.com).

THE BEST WAYS TO MONITOR YOUR OWN HEALTH

Next to your blood pressure readings, your blood glucose levels are the most important indicators of your health and your chances of experiencing serious illness. While doctors continue to blame cholesterol for heart disease, the real foe is elevated blood glucose and the harmful inflammation and diseases that it causes. You should be keeping close track of these two vital factors daily after age 40—regardless of whether or not you have Type 2 diabetes and/or high blood pressure. Of course, regularly monitoring these two factors is absolutely essential if you have a diagnosis of either condition.

CHAPTER TEN

DOES HIGH CHOLESTEROL REALLY CAUSE HEART DISEASE?

So much for the dietary fat "theory" of heart disease. Even more dubious is the idea that elevated cholesterol causes heart disease. Doctors have never been able to explain why more than half of all heart attack victims have cholesterol levels in the normal range. Or why the French, who have the highest cholesterol in Europe (average measurement around 250), also have the lowest incidence of heart disease—and only half the incidence of heart attack as here in the US. It is a well-known medical fact, proven by the famous Framingham Heart Study, that there are as many heart attacks in people with cholesterol levels under 200 as there are in those whose levels are 300 and over. [185]

THE BIRTH OF "THE CHOLESTEROL MYTH"

How did the cholesterol theory of heart disease get its start? Through a colossal error that never should have occurred. It appears that when researchers autopsied the arteries of deceased heart attack victims, they discovered cholesterol in artery plaques and jumped to conclusions. Incredibly, they assumed that because cholesterol was present, it was somehow the cause of heart disease. This has to be one of the biggest research blunders ever made. Then, they further assumed that if they could reduce the presence of artery plaques—by using drugs to suppress the liver's production of cholesterol—they could reduce the risk of heart attack. Thus, the "cholesterol theory" of heart disease was born.

But this was a massive mistake. Medical researchers should have realized that the immune system uses cholesterol and other blood fats to patch the tiny tears in artery walls caused by inflammation and excessive blood pressure. The more artery damage there is, the more cholesterol is produced so it can be used for this repair. Blaming cholesterol for heart disease makes as much sense as blaming the firefighters for the blazes to which they respond.

Now you can understand why taking a statin drug to lower your cholesterol is so absurd. Cholesterol is not the cause of heart disease; inflammation is. And the diet and lifestyle factors that cause it. While statins have demonstrated a very modest ability to prevent a second or third episode in male patients who have already suffered a heart attack, this is not due to a lowering of cholesterol. Instead, this protection is attributed to a mild anti-inflammatory effect produced by statins—an effect that can be achieved by any number of natural inflammation-fighting agents, including fish oil.

Statins provide little to no protection for otherwise healthy individuals exhibiting elevated cholesterol. If your cardiologist is pressuring you, as Jim's was, to use statin therapy to lower your cholesterol and thereby lower your risk of heart attack, we suggest you find a doctor who is up on the latest research. The greatest benefit that statin drugs provide is to make their manufacturers rich. How these companies managed to convince the medical community and the American public that 60 million of us needed to be on these drugs remains one of the greatest unsolved medical mysteries of our time.

HOW A HEART ATTACK OR STROKE HAPPENS

Even under normal conditions, arteries suffer a lot of wear and tear and are constantly being repaired. In a healthy body, this repair is usually triggered by temporary inflammation; so the rise in cholesterol levels subsides once the repair has been made. However, when inflammation is chronic, say in a smoker, a person with hypertension or someone with a poor diet, the problem becomes systemic and constant.

This is what happens with atherosclerosis. Plaques are forever forming, rupturing, re-repairing, and hardening over with calcium, which narrows arteries and can further raise blood pressure. In an unhealthy body, artery damage is not fully repaired and leads instead to chronic inflammation and damage caused by free radical molecules. In response, the body manufactures more cholesterol, which is rushed to the scene, becomes oxidized, and forms additional plaques.

A vicious cycle is now underway. When one of these plaques ruptures, it creates a blood clot which can dislodge and block one of the tiny capillaries downstream, depriving the heart or brain of oxygen. This blockage can result in a heart attack or stroke.

Oxidized cholesterol is the real danger in heart disease. Cholesterol is harmless in its un-oxidized state, but once it becomes oxidized (a state similar to rancid cooking oil), it spews free radical molecules which destroy healthy tissue and trigger the inflammation response. [186] This is why some people with normal cholesterol levels have heart attacks, while others with high cholesterol levels do not. The difference lies in the amount of chronic inflammation in their bodies and whether or not their cholesterol is being *oxidized*. It doesn't really matter whether your total cholesterol is high or low.

THE OVERLOOKED EXPLANATION FOR THE FRENCH PARADOX

Our modern diet and lifestyle are the leading cause of this inflammation. As we've seen previously, diets high in sugar, refined carbohydrates, and the insulin they generate are extremely inflammatory. Easily oxidized oils, such as polyunsaturated vegetable oils, along with trans-fats, are also major contributors to heart disease and greatly increase both inflammation and oxidation.

104

You'll recall that the French have higher cholesterol levels than we do in the US, yet they have a significantly lower rate of heart disease. Their average blood pressure also is higher than ours and they are notorious smokers. So why do they have 50% *fewer* heart attacks than we do? Researchers refer to this conundrum as the "French Paradox," and it has bewildered scientists for decades.

The answer seems to be that, while French cholesterol numbers are higher, their cholesterol remains un-oxidized, and therefore harmless. Experts have speculated that this may be due to the large amount of antioxidants in their diet. The French, like most people of the Mediterranean, consume far more fresh vegetables, fruits, olive oil, garlic, and fish than Americans. Their custom of drinking red wine with meals also may be an important factor. While it's true that antioxidants are important, almost no one has considered the obvious: That this "mysterious" protection is a result of the saturated fat in the French diet. Dr. Dean Ornish also noted that the French take time to eat (no drive thru for them) and usually share meals with friends and family.

Numerous studies[187] have shown that populations consuming the lowest amounts of fat have the highest rates of heart disease and cancers—and vice-versa. Looking purely at the statistics, it is apparent that dietary fat—and saturated fat in particular—exerts a protective effect on human health. We realize this is contrary to what doctors have been telling us for decades, but these studies do not lie. This is the 800-pound gorilla that the medical community wishes would go away, and so it continues to ignore these studies. Doctors' anti-fat bias is so strongly held that they have gone to great lengths over the past 40 years to skew the facts and obfuscate their conclusions.

Personally, we're sticking with the science and have no intention of giving up the protection that good quality fat provides—and this includes saturated fats. Meat, eggs, full-fat dairy products, including organic yogurt and cheese, are part of our diets. This decision is not just based on numerous medical studies, but also on history. Humans (*Homo sapiens*) evolved on animal fat and protein for more than 500,000 years. Heart disease, cancer, and diabetes did not start showing up until refined carbohydrates and vegetable oils became part of the modern diet. Coincidence? We don't think so.

ANTIOXIDANTS ARE IMPORTANT, TOO

Of course, the antioxidant-rich fruits, veggies, and red wine in the Mediterranean diet provide protection against cardiovascular problems and cancer, too. Antioxidants are a class of vitamins/nutrients that neutralize free radicals and the inflammation they cause. Volumes of evidence show that increasing consumption of antioxidant foods and supplements reduces your chances of getting atherosclerosis. (We'll discuss these in more detail in chapters Twelve and Thirteen.)

Red grapes are especially high in antioxidant flavonoids (also called bioflavonoids), which are a class of antioxidants that work synergistically with vitamin C. They are found in abundance in many fruits and vegetables—especially grapes, apples, citrus, onions, tomatoes, squash, eggplant, parsley, berries, and green tea. Research shows that consuming more of these foods substantially retards the development of atherosclerosis and cardiovascular disease.

Typical of Mediterranean peoples, the French also consume garlic and olive oil quite liberally. Garlic prevents the oxidation of cholesterol and reduces plaque accumulation in the arteries. Studies show that people who consume a lot of olive oil have 20% higher levels of oleic acid in their cholesterol, making it more resistant to oxidation. Other phenol compounds in olive oil add to its antioxidant value (the better quality the olive oil, the more phenols there will be).[188]

Since each antioxidant plays a somewhat different role in fighting inflammation, a wide range of antioxidant foods and supplements in your diet will reap the greatest rewards. Dr. Linus Pauling, the father of orthomolecular medicine and a multiple Nobel Prize winner, considered atherosclerosis to be a vitamin C deficiency disease. Pauling believed that vitamin C is one of our most important antioxidants and found it crucial for the production of collagen, which is needed to build and repair artery walls. Dr. Heilbron takes 12,000 to 20,000 mg of vitamin C daily. At age 49 his Agatston Calcium Score is zero, which is very rare.

Vitamin E is another antioxidant that is crucial for heart health. Studies show that low levels of vitamin E are a reliable predictor of CVD mortality. Beta-carotene, vitamin D, lipoic acid, selenium, and zinc are all important antioxidants to include. We'll discuss each of these in more detail in Chapter Thirteen.

"PYRAMID POWER" GONE WRONG

Back in the 1990s, putting together a healthful diet seemed easy. All you had to do was follow the US Department of Agriculture's new food guide pyramid, and you would lower your risk for heart disease, cancer, and a long list of other health problems supposedly caused by dietary fat.[189]

At the base of the pyramid—its foundation—was carbohydrates…lots and lots of carbohydrates. In other words: Fill your plate with potatoes, pasta, bread, rice, and corn, along with vegetables and fruit.

At the peak of the structure were fats and oils. The implication was that you should basically avoid them. Mind you, the *type* of fat or oil never entered the conversation. All fats were considered bad. If you had to eat meat, butter, and cheese, better to keep consumption down to a bare minimum.

The Pyramid was convincing. It was created, after all, by the venerable—and supposedly trustworthy—USDA. Nearly everyone, from moms to family doctors, bought into the idea that fats were evil.

Of course, we now know they were wrong. "The National Institutes of Health (NIH) spent several hundred million dollars trying to demonstrate a connection between eating fat and getting heart disease," writes Gary Taubes in a 2002 *New York Times* article entitled "What If It's All Been A Big Fat Lie?" "...and despite what we might think," Taubes writes: "...it [the NIH] failed [to prove its case]." He's referring to five major studies that could find no such link between fats and heart disease. "They failed to demonstrate...that eating less fat had any health benefits."

Nevertheless, the NIH continued campaigning for its cause. Like all crusades based on a false belief, this one led to some spectacularly wrong-headed ideas. such as that consuming fat is a major cause of weight gain and obesity. That notion flew in the face of common sense. As every farmer knows, you fatten a pig or steer by feeding it corn, which is low in fat and extraordinarily rich in carbs. Yet, doctors at the time were telling people to consume all the cornflakes they wanted, so long as the milk they used was fat-free.

Looking back, the results now seem all too predictable. Corporations made fortunes selling low-fat, high-carb products. Americans got heavier. And the rates of chronic illnesses such as heart disease and diabetes began to spike. That is because carbs cause broad swings in blood glucose and insulin levels, which drive hunger and cause overeating and body fat accumulation. Cutting nearly all fat from the diet, including the beneficial ones, has two unhealthy effects: It lowers HDL (the protective type of cholesterol), and it raises triglycerides (blood fats that help cause heart attacks).

Surprisingly, the risk for other diseases, primarily cancer, did not go down either. Scientists had always believed that a high-fat diet led to breast and colon tumors. But several large studies demonstrated that lowering total fat intake, in fact, had no effect on these diseases.

A huge study launched in 1993, The Women's Health Initiative (WHI) Dietary Modification Trial, bore this out. With funding from the National Heart, Lung and Blood Institute (NHLBI), researchers recruited 50,000 women between the ages of 50 and 79. Of these, 19,541 were randomly assigned to follow a low-fat diet. Their goal was to lower their fat intake from almost 38% of calories to 20%. They were helped in this effort by a series of individual and group counseling sessions. Another 29,294 women were randomly assigned to continue their usual diets and were given just generic diet-related educational materials.

After eight years, the researchers looked at how many women in each group had developed breast cancer or colorectal cancer. Researchers also tallied up heart attacks, strokes, and other forms of heart disease. And they looked at things like weight gain or loss, cholesterol levels, and other measures of health.

The results, published in the *Journal of the American Medical Association*, showed no benefits derived from a low-fat diet. Women assigned to this eating strategy did not appear to gain protection against breast cancer, colorectal cancer, or cardiovascular disease. And after eight years, their weights were generally the same as those of women following their usual diets.

That's not to say, of course, that dietary changes in fat consumption can not change your health for the better. In fact, a switch to healthful fat sources can produce significant beneficial effects.

YOUR BODY NEEDS AN OIL CHANGE

In 1995, Dr. Michel de Lorgeril and researchers from the French National Center for Health Research initiated the Lyon Diet Heart Study to look deeper into whether a Mediterranean-style diet could improve the health and survival of people already stricken with heart disease and damaged by heart attack, compared with a group that ate the AHA-approved, heart-healthy, low-fat diet called the "prudent diet."

The Mediterranean diet is hardly what you would call "low-fat." In fact, 30% to 40% of its calories come from fat, mostly from olive oil, butter, fish, and nuts. What makes this unique is not the amount, but the *type of fat* it contains—none of the fat is trans-fat or polyunsaturated fat from vegetable oils.

Originally scheduled to last for five years, the study was abruptly halted after only two years, for "ethical" reasons. Participants in the Mediterranean diet group experienced a 70% reduction in deaths from a second heart attack and a 61% lower rate of cancer compared with the "prudent diet" group.

"The results were spectacular and of unexpected magnitude," reported one of the lead researchers. "The protective effects of the diet began to occur within two months of observation." Benefits this dramatic had not been seen with any other diet, drug, or medical procedure. Indeed, the results were so impressive that they were promptly published in three of the world's most prestigious medical journals: *The American Journal of Clinical Nutrition, The Lancet* and the *Journal of the American College of Cardiology.*[190], [191] (Ironically, the *New England Journal of Medicine* would not publish the study results, some say, because of its dogmatic belief in LDL cholesterol and fat as the dietary cause of heart disease.)[192]

More recent research shows that the Mediterranean diet also reduces the risk of Alzheimer's disease and Parkinson's disease.

CHAPTER ELEVEN

HOW TO START REVERSING YOUR HYPERTENSION

The good news about high blood pressure is that you don't have to use drugs to treat it. There are plenty of simple ways to help heal yourself and get back on track to living a healthy life.

The very first steps you must take are to increase your consumption of heart-healthy foods, and cease consuming those foods and beverages that adversely affect your blood pressure. We refer to these as the Hypertension Harming Foods because they either contribute to elevating your blood pressure to dangerously high levels, or they add to the inflammation load in your body. Often these foods and beverages do both.

We recommend that you begin reducing your consumption of these unhealthful foods and beverages (or completely eliminate them) and replace them with the Hypertension Healing Superfoods we list and describe in Chapter Twelve. As a result of replacing harmful foods with Superfoods, your health will improve, your blood sugar metabolism will rebalance, and your blood pressure should greatly improve.

Your consumption of the following foods, food products, and beverages should be reduced or eliminated as soon as possible. Make sure you read food labels carefully to be sure you aren't unknowingly consuming these detrimental substances:

Sweeteners, including sugar, high fructose corn syrup (HFCS), agave syrup, brown sugar, molasses, corn syrup, artificial sweeteners (Splenda, NutraSweet, Sweet' N Low), and all sugar alcohols, such as sorbitol, malitol, and erythritol.

You may use stevia in place of other sweeteners, unless you don't care for its bitter aftertaste. Small amounts of honey may also be used, unless you have diabetes, pre-diabetes, or other blood sugar issues.

Soda pop, both regular and "diet" soft drinks, fruit juices, sports drinks, energy drinks, and sweetened teas.

Sweets, including candy, energy bars, granola bars, sugary desserts, ice cream or sorbet of any kind. Be particularly vigilant about eliminating all foods and beverages containing high fructose corn syrup (HFCS).

Sweetened dairy products and flavored yogurts.

Bread and baked goods. Eliminate any foods containing refined wheat, including white flour, rice flour, or soy flour. These include muffins, bagels, rolls, pastries, cookies, donuts, waffles, and pancakes.

Refined grain products, including prepared breakfast cereals, sweetened granola, chips, crackers, pasta (even those labeled "whole grain"), and all processed snack foods.

Fast food, including burgers, hot dogs, French fries, fried chicken, and the usual fare.

All deep-fried foods.

Margarine and foods containing hydrogenated or partially hydrogenated oils. This includes most snack foods and processed cheeses (such as Velveeta or American slices).

Refined vegetable oils, including corn, safflower, sunflower, soybean, peanut, and canola.

All highly processed meats, cold cuts, sausages, and jerky containing nitrates and chemical preservatives.

Ketchup, sweet condiments, creamy salad dressings, and relishes (because they usually contain sugar or HFCS).

Avoid all beers and ales (they contain barley malt and dextrose). If you must drink alcohol, limit yourself to one glass per day of wine or spirits. Avoid cocktails made with soda pop or juice-mixers.

IMPORTANT SHOPPING TIPS AND REMINDERS

Beware of food products labeled as "fat-free," "lite," "diet," and "Great for Low-Carb Diets." These often contain sweeteners, sodium, and other chemicals that are harmful to your body.

Avoid prepared deli foods containing hidden sugars and starches (for example, potato salad, coleslaw, and baked beans).

Check labels of liquid medications, cough syrups, cough drops, and other over-the-counter medications that may contain sugar.

Check salad dressings carefully. Many contain sweeteners, such as HFCS.

"Gosh! This doesn't leave me much to eat."

At first glance, you may be thinking that these healthy guidelines may seem like harsh dietary restrictions.

However, if you look a little closer, you'll see that many of the "foods" we are encouraging you to avoid aren't really foods at all, but rather factory and lab-created food-like substances.

Will choosing these Hypertension Healing Superfoods require some changes for you? Probably. But the long-term benefits are wonderfully worth the short-term effort it takes to choose to be healthy. Especially when you consider the very serious health dangers and complications you're facing with uncontrolled hypertension—or the nasty side effects you'll have to endure on drug therapy.

Besides, you really do have a wide selection of delicious, healthful foods and beverages that can improve your blood pressure, as you'll see in Chapter Twelve.

Your diet is the single most important factor that determines your health, for better or worse. Indeed, poor diet is one of the main causes of high blood pressure in the first place. Time and again, we've seen dramatic improvements in peoples' blood pressure when they restrict or reduce their consumption of those highly processed and artificial foods and beverages.

But why do people crave and over-consume those harmful "foods" in the first place?

A BRIEF HISTORY OF EATING

It may surprise you to learn that our primitive, reptilian brains are genetically and biologically programmed to "seek and eat" high-calorie, fatty foods. You see, the brain's urge to binge on sweet, fatty, calorie-rich foods developed in the days when our ancestors were hunter-gatherers. Eating as many calories as possible, whenever possible, enabled our ancestors to store excess calories as fat so they could survive lean times. Consuming high-fat food whenever it was available was a survival strategy that worked well for the human race for 2.4 million years.

Today, that same strategy is killing people. Fat and sugary calories are cheap and abundant today, so our genetic programming is backfiring by making us fat and sick. We are operating in a modern world with ancient appetites.

This is because our brains have not evolved fast enough to keep pace with our food environment. Prior to about 10,000 years ago, when agriculture developed, the human diet was restricted to the animals we could hunt or find and the wild plants we could gather. This is very different from today when we are literally surrounded by tens of thousands of food products and cheap calories. [193]

All that hunting and gathering was also hard work. Our ancestors expended a tremendous number of calories acquiring their food. When they were successful in locating a food supply, they gorged upon it because food preservation and storage techniques had not been perfected.

Foods that were calorie-dense, such as carbohydrates and fats, were the most prized—and animal protein (red meat, fowl, and fish) was the most common and important food that hunter-gatherers ate. They also consumed wild fruit and berries, roots, grasses, seeds, and nuts. This was the diet that sustained the human race since its appearance on the planet.

This is how our preference for sweets and fats developed. Hunter-gatherers came to recognize that foods with the highest concentrations of calories either tasted "sweet," as did wild berries and fruits, or were "fatty," like the organs of animals, which were usually consumed on the spot at a kill. Over time, our ancestors came to attach feelings of pleasure to these foods as they stimulated the reward center in the brain. This is why eating a scoop of ice cream, a hunk of chocolate, or a slice of cheesecake feels so delightful today. They contain both sensations of sweet and fat.

WHY IT FEELS SO GOOD TO BE LAZY

Another important component of our brain's programming is the conservation of energy. Just as sweets and fatty foods taste good to us today, it generally feels good to relax on the couch and do nothing. This stimulates the same reward centers—and has its primal origins in a time when conserving energy was also an important survival mechanism. Early human life was arduous, and those hunter-gatherers who were well-rested were usually the ones who could outrun a hungry predator, defeat an attacking enemy, or keep hunting until they found game. This is why relaxation feels so pleasurable to us in modern times, even if we have a 9-to-5 desk job.

With the advent of agriculture about 10,000 years ago—and the era of industrialization that followed it—the human diet and lifestyle changed dramatically. Carbohydrates, in the form of bread and grains (and later sugar), became the predominant source of calories. For the first time in human history, we could relax and even sleep undisturbed because our food supply was assured.

Today, 60% of our calories come from refined carbohydrates—foods that our ancestors never ate, including cereal grains, sugary drinks, baked goods, chips, snacks, and processed foods.[194] Yet, the primitive brain is still driven to gorge on these abundant and easily obtained calories, even though our modern bodies and metabolism suffer from this excessive consumption and inadequate physical activity. Diet- and lifestyle-related diseases such as hypertension, obesity, Type 2 diabetes, heart disease, stroke, and various cancers are sickening us and striking us down in record numbers.

HOW EXCESS BLOOD SUGAR AND INSULIN ARE KILLING US

When you consume sugar and refined carbohydrates, they break down almost instantly into simple sugar (glucose) and quickly enter the bloodstream. Immediately, blood sugar levels rise. To control this rise in glucose, the body releases the hormone insulin, which opens cells so the sugar can enter and be metabolized as fuel. As sugar exits the bloodstream, healthy levels are restored, and insulin retreats.

But when sugar and simple carbohydrate foods are continuously consumed, the body must produce and release increasing amounts of insulin. Over time, the cells become resistant to insulin and still greater amounts are required. This is the condition known as insulin resistance, the precursor to Type 2 diabetes.

Insulin resistance causes the body to accumulate belly fat, raises blood pressure, produces blood fats called triglycerides, increases cholesterol levels, triggers widespread inflammation throughout the body, damages brain cells, causes depression and fatigue, blunts the sex drive, impairs circulation (especially to the capillaries of the eyes and limbs), and feeds tumor growth.

Left unchecked, the result can be heart attack or stroke, cancer, Alzheimer's disease, kidney failure, and death. These are the very "plagues" of modern civilization that kill and cripple millions every year.

It would seem ironic if it weren't so tragic: The same consumption impulses and programming that led to our survival through millions of years of evolution now threaten our decline and demise.

WE MUST BREAK WITH OUR GENETIC PROGRAMMING
BEFORE IT DESTROYS US

These twin impulses, to gorge on calories and conserve energy, remain strongly programmed in our modern brains. Yet if we are to escape their unfortunate consequences, individually and collectively, we have some important choices to make, choices that our environment always made for us in the past. It was difficult to over-consume in ancient times because calories were too scarce. In addition, we couldn't take it easy as we do today because there was just too much to do in order to survive.

For the first time in human evolution, we must confront and defy our ancient programming if we are to enjoy good health and a long life. If we don't change our behaviors, our genetically driven impulses will be our undoing.

In truth, the killer diseases of our time are *behavioral* problems, not true medical conditions. As such, we must address and correct them with behavioral changes instead of relying on pharmaceutical solutions to save us. This is why, with regard to hypertension, changes in your diet and lifestyle can be the best "medicine" at your disposal.

You can—with awareness, determination, and practice—learn to control those primitive parts of your brain, effectively "rewiring" your brain by making better food and lifestyle choices. Making the decision to eliminate the Hypertension Harming Foods from your diet is an important first step. In the next chapter you'll learn how to replace them with the Hypertension Healing Superfoods. For now, here are the three most important changes you can make today to make a quick transition to a healing lifestyle:

1. Eliminate soda pop, soft drinks, fruit drinks, and artificial sweeteners—the leading source of empty calories in the modern diet. This one action will produce a dramatic improvement on your blood pressure, your blood sugar, and your weight. Soda pop is full of HFCS, which damages your liver.

In an international study published in *Hypertension: Journal of the American Heart Association,* researchers found a direct link between high blood pressure and consumption of sweetened beverages. Subjects who drank sugar-sweetened beverages daily had significantly higher systolic and diastolic blood pressure on average than those who avoided the sweet drinks. People who consumed the highest quantities of high-fructose corn syrup (the most common sweetener used by the soft drink industry) had the highest blood pressure levels. Indeed, the more sugar that study participants consumed, the higher their blood pressure spiked upward.

Fruit juices aren't much better for you because they are loaded with sugar, too, and will spike blood glucose. And diet beverages containing artificial sweeteners may be the worst of the lot. There's extensive evidence linking artificial sweeteners such as aspartame to health problems ranging from brain tumors to fatty liver disease.

In the aforementioned study, the INTERMAP researchers discovered that those who drank *diet soda* were fatter than those who consumed regular sodas. [195] This is because diet drinks fool your body into thinking it is ingesting sugar, which creates the same insulin spike and cravings as regular sugar.

In a separate Japanese study, researchers followed 39,786 middle-aged men and women for 18 years between 1990 and 2008. They tracked soft drink consumption via self-administered questionnaires. Results showed that stroke risk was *significantly* higher for people who drank soft drinks every day, compared with those who drank them rarely or never. This association was especially pronounced among female subjects suffering from ischemic stroke. Stroke is the third leading cause of death in the US and is the leading cause of serious, long-term disability. Meanwhile, nearly *half* of all Americans drink one or more glasses of soda pop every day.

What does all this mean to you? Stick with water, coffee, and green tea, which contains plant compounds that are good for your health.

2. Eat a high-quality breakfast. Why are you always hearing that breakfast is the most important meal of the day? *Because it is.* Breakfast jump-starts your metabolism and gets your energy going—provided you eat protein for breakfast. Breakfasts consisting of fast carbs such as breakfast cereal, a bagel, and OJ will immediately break down into glucose and spike your blood sugar and insulin. Then, once your bloodstream is cleared, your body and brain start screaming for more glucose. How? By making you feel drowsy, unable to focus, and hungry again (otherwise known as the "mid-morning slump").

This will not happen when you build your breakfast around protein (such as eggs, nitrate–free bacon or steel-cut oats—in the latter have about 7 grams of protein per one cup cooked), healthy fat (as in eggs, avocado, butter, and full-fat yogurt) and slow carbs (such as berries, black beans, or the veggies in an omelet). A protein-based breakfast (ideally, one that includes 15-18 grams of protein) will perk you up mentally without spiking your blood sugar and insulin levels. This way, glucose will be slowly released into your bloodstream for a steady energy supply. The fat in your morning meal will keep your hunger satisfied until lunchtime. Best of all, your carb cravings will diminish or vanish. You will lose weight without "trying," because insulin, the body's fat storage hormone, will remain in the shadows.

3. Take a 30-minute walk every day. The great thing about physical activity is that it is the spark that gets your body's metabolism going. This isn't about exercise or trying to lose weight. Instead, it's realizing that your body and brain just work better when you're physically active. Blood glucose gets burned off, your cells use insulin more efficiently (so you need less of it), more oxygen gets into your bloodstream and to your organs, and your mood and self-confidence perk up.

USE YOUR WILLPOWER TO REIN IN YOUR DNA

Physical activity is another trait we share with our hunter-gatherer ancestors. They were constantly in motion and therefore in peak physical condition. Scientists tell us that after periods of physical activity, brain chemicals called endorphins kick in to create a sense of euphoria and well-being.

These three simple practices—eliminating sugary drinks, eating a protein-rich breakfast, and walking at least 30 minutes a day—are the foundation upon which you can build your entire hypertension-reversing lifestyle.

Psychologists have found that it generally takes about 21 to 28 days to replace a bad habit with a good one. This is why most drug and alcohol recovery programs last about one month. This also is why we designed *The 30-Day Blood Pressure Cure Plan* for you, which follows in Part Two of this book.

While you will need to exert some effort and regular practice in the beginning, these practices will become natural after a short time. They will become ingrained habits that you will find yourself performing automatically and unconsciously. In short, you'll be rewiring your brain to create healthy blood pressure and good health for yourself.

Imagine. No longer must you cave in to the urges that seduce your primitive reptilian brain. Instead, you will exert conscious control over your caveman cravings—and actually start *enjoying* the state of healthfulness. In the process, instead of being a slave to your impulses, you will be cultivating real personal power and the freedom to make choices that truly matter.

In this way, healing your hypertension can actually heal your entire life. It will heal our world, too. Because, as your family, friends, and co-workers notice your marvelous transformation, they'll be inspired to heal and improve themselves, too.

You see, you really *can* change the world.

Remember: Nothing succeeds like success. Once you begin to experience the fruits of your labors (more energy, positive moods, appreciation for your life, more meaningful relationships—in addition to your slimmer waistline and lower blood pressure), you will just naturally want to "keep getting better."

After you get pretty good at the three basic practices described above (eliminating sugary drinks, eating a protein-rich breakfast, and walking at least 30 minutes a day), you may want to consider the following as possible next steps…

TAKE OFF SOME POUNDS

That's right, "lose weight." Extra fat on your body means your heart has to pump harder to push your blood through your arteries. And that's not good.

Why? Because eventually your heart (which is a muscle, after all) will get tired and wear out. Doctors call this condition "congenital heart failure"—and it is not a pretty way to go. So give your heart a break and lose a little weight.

In fact, when it comes to preventing hypertension, losing weight may even be more important than exercising. A study recently published in the *American Heart Journal* found that healthful weight was a greater determinant of lower blood pressure than being physically fit. The results were from the Cooper Center Longitudinal Study, which evaluated the health of more than 35,000 patients over a 20-year period. [196]

Losing weight is shockingly easy once you stop following the conventional bad advice about what to eat (carbs and low-fat foods, for example). There are several eating plans out there crafted to help you both shed pounds (some are faster than others) *and* lower your blood pressure.

In Appendix C, we've described the popular eating plans that will produce sustainable results, both for your weight and your blood pressure.

CLIMB OFF THE COUCH

After diet, the most potent weapon against high blood pressure is regular physical activity. Like all muscles, the heart becomes stronger as a result of exercise. In turn, this means it has to work less to pump blood through the body. A lesser-known benefit of working up a sweat is that it stimulates the body to produce nitric oxide, which activates chemical pathways that relax and open blood vessels, allowing blood to flow through them with more ease. Researchers at Emory University School of Medicine found that the nitric oxide produced during exercise protects the heart from injury. [197]

Whether you walk, run, swim, dance, clean your house, or do yard work, 30 minutes of vigorous physical activity a day is excellent medicine for high blood pressure. The secret is to start off slowly. Make sure to warm up for at least five to 10 minutes, and measure your heart rate periodically once you begin working out, aiming for a rate that is 65% to 85% of your maximum.

(*Note:* To calculate your maximum heart rate, subtract your age from 220. If you are 50, your maximum heart rate is 170, so your target heart rate would be between 110 to 145 beats per minute.)

If you are out of shape, you don't have to start off with 30 minutes of exercise right off the bat. Begin with 10 to 15 minutes—even that short amount of time can have a clear positive impact. Then gradually, work your way up. Over time, you might find yourself able to walk or run for longer than you think is possible for you to do. According to a *New York Times* article, moderate exercise may be better than intense aerobic activity for those with high blood pressure. One study showed that jogging two miles a day does such a great job alleviating hypertension that patients were able to completely come off their medication. [198]

The article went on to say that the slower-paced activities of yoga and tai chi may do just as well at lowering blood pressure as moderate activity. (See more about the stress-reducing effects of these two activities under the "Chill Out" section in Chapter Fourteen.) It doesn't take much effort for exercise to have an effect. However, be sure to consult a physician before you start your exercise program.

TAKE A WALK—OR FOUR

According to researchers at Indiana University, three or four short, brisk walks throughout the day can be more beneficial to people watching their blood pressure than one continuous bout of exercise.

"The biggest problem for most people is they don't have the time," said Janet P. Wallace, professor in the Department of Kinesiology at the IU School of Health, Physical Education and Recreation. "You might think, 'I don't have the time to go to the gym or work out for 40 minutes, but I might have the time to do 10 minutes here, 10 minutes here and another 10 minutes here.' Four 10-minute walks would be ideal."

Wallace's study compared the effect of accumulated exercise versus continuous physical activity on people with pre-hypertension—an elevated blood pressure level that typically progresses to hypertension or high blood pressure.

The randomized crossover study involved a group of men and women diagnosed with pre-hypertension. The subjects walked on a treadmill continuously for 40 minutes one day, and on another day, four times for 10 minutes over the course of 3.5 hours. On average, their systolic blood pressure dropped 5.4 to 5.6 mm Hg and their diastolic blood pressure dropped 3.2 mmHg. The drop is significant because a reduction of 5 mmHg in systolic blood pressure has been reported to substantially reduce mortality and to reduce the incidence of stroke and coronary heart disease.

The study found that these blood pressure readings decreased by the same amount whether the study participants utilized continuous exercise or broke their exercise down in multiple shorter sessions. Interestingly, the beneficial effects lasted longer (around 11 hours) in the group who took four 10-minute walks, compared with seven hours for the group that walked continuously for 40 minutes.

"We had no idea the short bouts would be better [for blood pressure]," Wallace said. Most previous studies recommend long, continuous exercise sessions as being more effective for overall health. Wallace's findings were published in the *Journal of Hypertension.*

PHYSICAL ACTIVITY HELPS REDUCE BLOOD PRESSURE

Findings from another study confirm that physical activity reduces blood pressure in patients with high blood pressure, even if they are already taking medications to address this problem.

As reported in the *Clinical Journal of Sports Medicine,* Dr. Domenico Di Raimondo and colleagues from Universita Degli Studi Di Palermo in Italy assessed the effects of a fast-walking program on a group of patients with high blood pressure.

To be eligible for the study, subjects needed to have systolic blood pressures between 140 and 159 and diastolic readings between 90 and 99 mmHg. All of the subjects were taking medications for their high blood pressure. None had limited mobility and none was obese.

Three times a week, under the guidance of an experienced physiotherapist, the participants engaged in fast-walking sessions. After six weeks, the average systolic blood pressure fell from 143.1 to 135.5 mmHg, the report indicates. At the same time, the average diastolic pressure dropped from 91.1 to 84.8 mmHg. No gender-based differences were found.

The authors concluded that these results support exercise training as an important part of the treatment for individuals with mild elevations in blood pressure.

TO EXERCISE OR NOT TO EXERCISE?

If you have high blood pressure, that is the question.

For people with normal BP, exercise causes a healthy increase in blood flow to the muscles. One recent study from the University of Texas, however, showed that in people with hypertension, intense exercise actually *constricts* blood vessels, decreases blood flow, and raises blood pressure even higher. [199]

This doesn't mean you should give up regular physical activity. You can still do gentle types of exercise, such as yoga, tai chi, qigong, brisk walking, or easy bicycling. Heavy weight lifting, however, may not be a good choice for you.

There's a simple, easy way to determine if you should put a limit on the intensity of your exercise. Just check your blood pressure immediately after you work out. If it approaches 220/120, your intensity is too high.

Be sure to discuss your findings with your doctor. He or she may be able to suggest other exercise options.

CHAPTER TWELVE

THE BLOOD PRESSURE-HEALING FOODS

We've already discussed how the right foods and diet are an essential part of lowering blood pressure. Besides eliminating fast carbs and improving the ratio of carbohydrates to protein to fats, there are specific foods that are particularly good at fighting high blood pressure. Many of the foods listed here are high in potassium, which keeps sodium levels in balance. As you may remember from our earlier discussion in Chapter Five, it's not sodium *consumption,* but rather sodium *retention* that affects blood pressure. If you eat it and excrete it, there's no problem. If you eat it and keep it, it causes fluid retention, which in turn drives up blood pressure. Potassium causes you to excrete sodium.

Many of these healing foods also contain magnesium. Magnesium relaxes arterial walls, allowing blood to pass through easily. Some of these healing foods also contain fiber and phytochemicals (plant-derived chemicals) such as flavonoids, which protect the integrity of arterial walls.

Tulane University researchers investigated the data from 25 randomized, controlled trials involving more than 1,400 adults. They found that study participants who ate between seven and 19 grams of fiber per day for at least eight weeks enjoyed a reduction in blood pressure.[200]

BEST FRUITS AND VEGGIES FOR BETTER BLOOD PRESSURE

Apples. Besides being a great source of fiber, apples, along with onions and wine, contain the blood-vessel-dilating plant chemical quercetin. But this important nutrient is in the skin of the fruit, so keep that skin in the game! Apples are also a great source of potassium. One large apple has only about 115 calories, yet provides about 240 mg of potassium. Additionally, apples contain hypertension-healing pectin, a natural fiber that can help clear the blood of toxins and cholesterol. Over time, the effect of apples on blood pressure is impressive.

In one small study, researchers gave healthy adults a Red or Golden Delicious apple to eat every day for four weeks. A second group took capsules containing mixed apple polyphenols—antioxidants found in apples. A third group was given a daily placebo. At the end of the trial, the apple eaters had lowered their LDL cholesterol levels by 40%. The results for those taking the polyphenols capsules were similar, though the capsules were not quite as effective as eating apples themselves.[201]

Another study from the Netherlands analyzed the data of men who ate an apple a day plus a small amount of onions (also rich in quercetin) and tea, which contains flavonoids. Apples, onions, and tea may make for an odd meal, but the men who consumed them were one-third less likely to experience a heart attack then those who did not eat these flavonoid-rich foods.

Here's a great snack idea: Create a relish by sautéeing sliced apples and cooked onions, and serve it alongside baked pork chops or chicken. You can even add cabbage to the mix and make a slaw!

Bananas. This portable fruit is a fabulous source of potassium, magnesium, and fiber, all of which are fantastic allies for reducing blood pressure. The FDA has even allowed the banana industry to make claims that the fruit lowers blood pressure. And a recent study published in the *New England Journal of Medicine* found that eating bananas as part of your regular diet can cut your risk of stroke by a whopping 40%. [202]   However, bananas contain a lot of natural fruit sugar, so eat them in moderation.

If it seems like your bananas are always overripe before you get a chance to eat them all, extend their shelf life by keeping them in the refrigerator, where they will stay firmer longer, or slice them and store the frozen slices in the freezer to add to yogurt or smoothies. Conversely, you can speed the ripening of green bananas by keeping them in a paper bag on your kitchen counter.

THE TOP 10 POTASSIUM-RICH FOODS

1. Swiss chard	6. Tomatoes
2. Crimini mushrooms	7. Collard greens
3. Spinach	8. Squash (both summer and winter varieties)
4. Celery	9. Cantaloupe
5. Broccoli	10. Green beans

Beans, legumes, and whole grains. Fiber plays an important role in controlling blood pressure. Beans, legumes, and whole grains contain heart-healthy fiber that can help reduce the risk of heart attack and flush plaque from your body. In addition to soluble fiber, beans also provide calcium, iron, and vitamin B. Whole grains are also a good source of B vitamins, selenium and magnesium. The fiber, vitamins, and minerals in beans and whole grains can also help with satiety and weight management.

Blueberries. If you eat enough blueberries, your tongue will turn blue and you may reduce your risk of developing high blood pressure. *Anthocyanins,* the same compound responsible for dyeing your tongue, are a kind of flavonoid that have been shown to be particularly beneficial in lowering blood pressure. Anthocyanins are found mainly in fruits and vegetables such as blueberries, raspberries, cranberries, strawberries, black currants, blood oranges, and eggplant. An analysis of data collected over a 14-year period from 156,957 health professionals reveals that those participants over the age of 60 who ate more than one serving of blueberries per week were 10% less likely to develop high blood pressure. Because a large amount of these beneficial flavonoids are present in an average serving of blueberries, getting the beneficial effects of anthocyanins through dietary means is relatively easy.[203]

Broccoli. According to a new laboratory study published in the *American Journal of Hypertension,* broccoli may be near the top of the list of anti-hypertensive foods. Broccoli contains a compound called sulforaphane that significantly improves not only blood pressure, but kidney function as well.[204] This beneficial substance is also present in other cruciferous vegetables such as Brussels sprouts, cabbage, cauliflower, horseradish, and arugula.

Cardamom. Cardamom is a spice frequently used in East Indian and Middle Eastern cuisine. Not only does it add flavor to curries and chai, it's also great for your heart. *The Indian Journal of Biochemistry and Biophysics* reported the findings of one study showing that just 3 grams of cardamom a day effectively lowered blood pressure. In that study, 20 people who were newly diagnosed with hypertension were given 3 grams of cardamom daily for 90 days. The study showed that cardamom improved antioxidant levels and helped break down blood clots without altering blood fibrinogen or lipid levels. As an added bonus, after three months on the cardamom regimen, all the study participants reported experiencing increasing feelings of well-being.

Spice Up Your Health. The following herbs and spices have been shown to have a beneficial effect on blood pressure. Stock up on these healing spices, and add them generously to salads, smoothies, and meals:

- Cardamom
- Cayenne
- Celery seed
- Cinnamon

- Garlic
- Ginger
- Oregano
- Parsley

Celery and parsley. Celery and parsley are both considered diuretics. They lessen blood volume by helping the body eliminate water. Diuretics can be dangerous in that they can cause your body to release necessary nutrients along with extra fluid, but both celery and parsley contain potassium, so the body stays nourished with an important electrolyte even while it is eliminating excess water.

Celery seed isn't well known among Western herbalists, but Ayurvedic practitioners have been using it to treat water retention, arthritis, and certain diseases of the liver and spleen for thousands of years. It's one of many foods on our healing food list that contains antioxidants that protect cells from free radical damage.[205]

In addition to the benefits of celery seeds, the celery plant contains several compounds that work like blood pressure medications without the corresponding side effects. Celery, celery extract, and celery oil all contain a compound called *apigenin*, which causes the smooth muscles of blood vessels to relax, thereby decreasing the pressure the blood exerts as it flows through the body. Celery also contains substances that act like calcium-channel blockers, indirectly dilating blood vessels and reducing the blood levels of BP-elevating hormones called *catecholamines.*

In traditional Chinese medicine, celery is a time-honored treatment for high blood pressure. Several modern studies show that people who eat more celery experience significant drops in blood pressure. Celery contains a chemical compound called *apigenin,* which dilates blood vessels and reduces the circulatory force of the bloodstream. Another chemical in celery, *3-n-butylphtalide*, not only relaxes arteries but also reduces levels of adrenaline and other hormones that cause blood pressure to rise. University of Chicago researchers found that animals given 3-n-butylphtalide had a 12-point drop in blood pressure. Extrapolated to humans, these results would be enough to shift a patient with mild hypertension into the safe zone.[206]

Some doctors hesitate to recommend celery because they've heard its high in sodium. They forget that a three-ounce serving of celery has more than 340 mg of potassium, which can neutralize the sodium's pressure-raising effects. We advise patients to have no more than four or five stalks of celery a day—and to check their blood pressure regularly just to be safe. In most cases, they notice that their pressure goes down. [207]

A relative of celery, parsley (its name comes from the Greek word meaning "rock celery"), has been used as a culinary herb for a couple of thousand years. The root is often prescribed by herbalists for its many therapeutic benefits, which include vasodilation, or improving the elastic flexibility of blood vessels. The leaves are packed with vitamin C, vitamin A, iron, and potassium. So the next time you see this humble decoration on your dinner plate, don't overlook it. It is actually a storehouse of vital nutrients. Eating parsley will help freshen your breath, too. [208]

Cheese, from raw milk. Getting enough calcium can make it easier to keep your blood pressure down. Research data points to adequate calcium intake as a contributing factor in hypertension control. Cheeses made from hormone-free raw milk are a tasty way to add more calcium to your diet. (For more calcium benefits, read "Milk" on page 130).

Cinnamon. Who would have thought that being healthy could taste so good? *The Center for Applied Health Sciences* in Ohio conducted a study of 22 subjects, half of whom were given a 250mg of water-soluble cinnamon daily, while the other half were given a placebo. It was discovered that those who drank cinnamon had a 13% to 23% increase in antioxidants connected with lowering blood sugar levels. Cinnamon sprinkled on hot oatmeal or a baked apple is a treat—and good medicine. Research shows that cinnamon can reduce both insulin levels and blood pressure, so use the sweet-smelling spice liberally.

CHOCOLATE POWER FOR YOUR BLOOD PRESSURE!

Good news, chocolate lovers. Chocolate may help lower blood pressure. Let's be clear here. Gorging on bonbons or candy bars is most definitely not good for your health. However, a little bit of extra dark chocolate every day may have some minor health benefits.

In a meta-analysis of 20 short-term studies, scientists concluded that the high cocoa content in dark chocolate can lower blood pressure by two to three points. This may not sound like much, but even one point matters. The report, published by Cochrane Collaborations, emphasizes that the benefits are received only when the chocolate has a high cocoa content. [209] Moderation is also key. Chocolate contains a lot of calories, so more is not better. The report recommends chocolate lovers keep their consumption under three ounces.

The research was inspired by the indigenous people of Central America's San Blas Islands.These folks consume a lot of cocoa, and yet they generally have normal blood pressure. This led scientists to investigate the effects of cocoa on blood pressure.

Cocoa contains flavanols, antioxidants that assist the cardiovascular system. These antioxidants provoke the body to produce nitric oxide. Nitric oxide causes blood vessels to relax, allowing blood to flow more freely. Researchers made it clear that the positive effects dark chocolate had on blood pressure were small and that no long-term studies have been done.

It is the cocoa, not the candy made from it, that provides the benefit; The higher the cocoa content in your chocolate, the better. We recommend a cocoa content of at least 70%. Dark chocolate has a higher cocoa content than semi-sweet or milk choco-late.

You can skip the sugar, fat, and calories added in processing chocolate and get your antioxidants from other healthier sources. If it's the chocolate taste you crave, try using unsweetened cocoa powder, which provides the same benefits and is packed with essential minerals. Apples, apricots, beans, and blackberries also contain similar flavanols; plus they have fiber, vitamins, and minerals not found in any chocolate bar.

Chocolate is not health food. However, if you are a chocolate lover, you can enjoy a small square of extra dark organic chocolate daily without ruining your health or your waistline. And it may even help lower your blood pressure by a few points.

FAMOUS FERMENTED FOODS

Fermented foods benefit digestion and therefore support the immune system. Specifically, fermented foods have been shown to support the beneficial bacteria in our digestive tract. When our digestion is functioning like a well-oiled machine and we are absorbing all the nutrients we need, our immune system tends to be happy, and thus more able to wage war against disease and illness.

Here are some of the best fermented foods to help your digestive system operate at its best:

Apple cider vinegar. You may be familiar with its strengths as a natural antiseptic and antibiotic—but did you also know that apple cider vinegar can be used to help lower blood pressure? [210, 211] You can add the vinegar to your salads or just stir two tablespoons into a glass of water and drink it down. As an added benefit, apple cider vinegar may also help to lower your blood sugar over time.

Kimchi (kimchee). This pungent Korean food is made with cabbage and often with white radishes. It can be eaten fresh or fermented. The most popular version is pickled, and with good reason. It turns out that the fermented version has a more positive impact on health. [212] Kimchi is an acquired taste. It is fermented and seasoned with hot chili and garlic and sometimes ginger. A small study at Aju University in Korea found that fermented kimchi helped lower blood pressure and cholesterol. Some people tame and cool their kimchi by mixing it with yogurt.

Yogurt. Speaking of yogurt, researchers at Tufts University reported that a study of 2,197 adults showed a slightly reduced incidence of hypertension among those who ate an average of one serving (a cup) of low-fat yogurt every three days. [213]

Although blood pressure generally increased with age, systolic pressure generally rose less among the yogurt eaters. One caution: Commercially prepared, flavored, low-fat yogurt can contain a lot of added sugar; so your best bet is to buy plain (no sugar added) Greek yogurt and sweeten with fruits or berries. To assure your yogurt is of the highest quality, we recommend that you make your own.

THE BEST YOGURT ON EARTH AT HALF THE PRICE—OR LESS!

Yogurt is so versatile. Yogurt is a heart-healthy food. [214]   It's also delicious. Another reason to keep a steady supply of yogurt on hand is its versatility. Use it in place of sour cream in tacos and burritos or instead of mayonnaise in spreads for sandwiches or wraps. Use plain or combine with pureed cottage cheese to replace ricotta in eggplant lasagna. Squeeze in a little lemon or lime juice to make a cream sauce with fresh herbs to go over grilled fish or chicken.

Getting started: Although you can buy specialty yogurt-makers, there's no need to clutter your kitchen with more appliances. I've found that using either a thermos bottle or a small beverage cooler is the cheapest and easiest way to achieve sure success with no fuss. To get started, you'll need:

- 1 quart organic whole or low-fat milk or consider dairy alternatives such as coconut or almond milk.

- yogurt starter (see below)

- cooking thermometer—available at most grocery stores

- 2-quart sauce pan

- 2 quart jars with lids

- bath towel

- Thermos bottle or a small picnic cooler

- optional: organic powdered milk (to use as a thickening agent if the yogurt is too thin) consider dairy alternatives such as coconut or almond milk.

JIM HEALTHY'S HOMEMADE YOGURT RECIPE

Be sure to plan ahead with this recipe. Though preparation of the cultured milk mixture takes only about 10 minutes, an additional 4–8 hours are needed for the yogurt to thicken. During this period no further tinkering is required, though the yogurt will need to be transferred to a refrigerator as soon as it has thickened.

First, be sure your pots and utensils are very clean and free of all soap residue. Next, you'll need a "starter" of the right bacteria cultures to get the yogurt going. My favorite yogurt starter is Probiotic Acidophilus by American Health, located at most health-food stores. One tablespoon of the acidophilus starter is all you need.

I also tried the Yogourmet starter, priced at $8 for a package of three starters. This product was totally acceptable. It has milk powder and three strains of bacteria. The end result was a nice thick and tangy yogurt that was a little firmer than the other types.

The cheapest starter of all (under $1) is a cup of whole plain organic yogurt with "live active cultures." Look for specific bacteria that fight inflammation, such as the *Lactobacillus* strains and *Propionibacterium.* You'll only have to purchase a starter once because your own homemade yogurt will provide you with a continuous supply. Just remember not to eat it all! One cup will provide all the cultures you need for the next batch.

Instructions:

1. Heat ¾-quart of organic, non-bGH milk in a saucepan to 170-180 degrees.
2. Turn off the heat and let the milk cool to 108–112 degrees.
3. Add the starter of your choice and stir.
4. Pour this cultured milk mixture into a thermos or a quart jar (see instructions below).
5. Let sit 4–8 hours, or until thickened. Do not bump, move or otherwise disturb!
6. After it has thickened, store your finished yogurt in the refrigerator.

The Thermos method. This is the easiest method by far. Once the starter has been added to the milk, pour it into a wide-mouth, quart-size Thermos bottle. Cap it, wrap the thermos in a thick kitchen towel, and set it in a warm place. When the yogurt has thickened (4–8 hours), transfer it to a glass jar and store in the fridge.

The cooler method. After adding the starter to the warm milk, pour the mixture into a quart jar and set it in the cooler. Fill a second quart jar with boiling water, and nestle it right up against the yogurt. Cap the jars, cover them with towels and close the cooler. When the yogurt has thickened (4–8 hours), put it in the fridge.

This method works well for bigger batches. For a double batch, mix two quarts of milk and two cups of starter and pour the mixture into two glass quart jars. Fill two more quart jars with boiling water and nestle them in the cooler, right next to the yogurt jars. Top with a towel, and close the cooler.

For the insatiably curious. I can never follow instructions unless I know *why* I am supposed to do something a certain way. For those stricken with a similar affliction, here's the explanation:

Heating the milk to just below boiling kills off any "bad" bacteria that might interfere with the good bugs.

Cooling the milk to 108–112 degrees brings the temperature into a range that will help the good bacteria multiply. Any warmer, and you'll destroy the friendly bugs. Any cooler and they'll be shivering so much they won't procreate.

I say "do not disturb" because any rocking of the container interferes with the bacteria setting up and thickening the milk. So position the container in a place that's easy to access. Avoid jostling it while checking for progress.

Yummy yogurt! My tests found that this simple method results in yogurt with a tangy, complex flavor. This yogurt has a slightly tart bite and is creamier than store-bought brands, but still sturdy enough when making a sauce or dip. Adding the acidophilus gives it a sharper taste, while adding powdered milk mellows the tang and thickens the yogurt. Experiment with different batches until you get the texture just as you like it. Once you have created a yogurt you prefer, you can use one cup of it to start your next batch. After a few tries, you'll easily master the art of yogurt-making.

To make a richer, thicker Greek yogurt. Pour the yogurt into a muslin cloth hanging over a bowl. A probiotic-rich liquid will drain off. Do not waste it! Drink it—or add it to juices or smoothies. Scrape the Greek yogurt from the cloth after two hours and refrigerate.

Yogurt will keep for at least a week in the fridge. Remember to reserve one cup of your last batch to start your next batch. Your starter culture will last several months if kept sealed in a refrigerator. Consume at least one cup of yogurt daily and resupply your stash every few days so you don't run out.

I like to eat yogurt every morning. I start with a bowl of fresh berries (strawberries, blueberries, blackberries, and raspberries), mix in a cup of yogurt, sprinkle generously with ground flaxseed and a dash of cinnamon. This keeps me going strong. In addition to helping me control my weight and keep my blood pressure down, the berries contain natural pain-relieving compounds and anti-inflammatory and joint-healing properties that soothe my arthritis. (I describe my personal drug-free arthritis program described in the book coauthored with Stephen Sinatra, MD, *Arthritis Interrupted*, www.arthritishealing book.com.)

Garlic. This robust aromatic may not be the greatest for your breath, but your cardiovascular system loves it. Garlic is one of the most extensively studied healing foods. It consistently has been found to reduce both systolic and diastolic pressure, as well as the risk of blood clots in the arteries. Garlic contains *allicin,* a substance with antibacterial, antioxidant, lipid-lowering, and anti-hypertension properties. Full of antioxidants, garlic's heart benefits are many.

As a vasodilator, it relaxes arterial walls and reduces blood clots. In a pilot study at Clinical Research Center of New Orleans, patients with severe hypertension were given a garlic preparation containing 1.3% allicin. Sitting blood pressure fell with a significant decrease in diastolic blood pressure only five to 14 hours after the dose. [215]

Scientists at the German Centre for Cardiovascular Pharmacology wanted to measure the effects of garlic on hardening of the arteries. They selected 200 middle-aged men and divided them into two groups. One group was given 300 mg of garlic extract daily for two years—the equivalent of one to two fresh cloves—while the second group got none. At the end of the two-year period, the men in the garlic group had significantly more flexible blood vessels.

When researchers conducted a review of studies on garlic, they found that it significantly reduced both systolic and diastolic blood pressure numbers. That is one great heart-healthy clove! But take note: garlic's main components, such as allicin, are most potent when raw. [216, 217]

We aren't asking you to chew on raw garlic cloves. Use your food processor or blender to puree raw garlic cloves and add the pureed garlic to pesto, mix with Greek yogurt for a healthy dip, or add to salads or chilled soups. Jarred and frozen garlic work just as well. Garlic may also be taken in the form of a supplement.

Ginger. You can add an antihypertensive kick to your stir fries and salads with ginger, which is so good for lowering blood pressure. However, please be aware that ginger can interact with some drugs and cause unwanted side effects. These include blood-thinners such as *phenprocoumon* and *warfarin* (Coumadin); many diabetes drugs, such as *glimepiride* (Amaryl), *glyburide* (DiaBeta, Glynase PresTab, Micronase), *insulin*, *metformin* (Glucophage), *pioglitazone* (Actos), *rosiglitazone* (Avandia); and a class of anti-hypertensive medications called calcium channel blockers, including *nifedipine* (Adalat, Procardia), *verapamil* (Calan, Isoptin, Verelan), *diltiazem* (Cardizem), *isradipine* (DynaCirc), *felodipine* (Plendil), and *amlodipine* (Norvasc).[218]

Ginger works by stimulating the sweat glands and the circulatory system. Blood goes outward toward the extremities, and this action lowers blood pressure. Ginger also slows down platelet aggregation, which means that, like garlic, it reduces blood clots.

Try ginger wrapped up in sushi or juiced with carrots and apples. In some dishes, it's especially good when mixed with other blood-pressure friendly ingredients such as garlic and hot peppers. Add raw ginger slices or ginger tea bags to cool filtered water to make a delicious ginger drink.

Grapefruit. This familiar citrus fruit supplies vitamin C, pectin, folic acid, and lycopene, which help prevent symptoms of arterial plaque. Grapefruit helps flush LDL cholesterol from arteries and lessen high blood pressure problems.

Milk. While we encourage choosing whole organic milk over skim milk for its healthy fats, milk in general can provide dramatic hypertension benefits. A two-year study of 6,000 people published in the *American Journal of Clinical Nutrition* found that people who drank skim milk had 50% less hypertension than those who drank less. Scientists credit milk's calcium with helping to counteract the pressure-raising effects of sodium. But for blood-pressure control, any milk seems to help. Dr. John Laragh, who studied hypertension at Weill-Cornell Medical College, found that patients with mild hypertension, defined as a diastolic reading between 90 and 104 (the bottom number of your reading), showed significant improvement just by drinking more milk. [219]

Another study, this one conducted at the National Heart, Lung and Blood Institute, looked at the dietary habits and blood pressure of 8,000 adult males. The researchers discovered that men who drank about two cups of milk a day were 100% less likely to develop hypertension than those men who didn't drink as much. That's a fantastic finding and it confirms other reports, including research from the famous Framingham Heart Study, which found that people who get the most calcium are the least likely to develop high blood pressure. Another study done in Spain demonstrated that both men and women who consume more dairy products have a 50% lower risk of hypertension. [220]

The recommended daily intake of calcium depends on your age and sex: Women need more calcium than men, and the recommended amounts increase. Everyone should get at least 750 mg of calcium daily and up to 1,500 mg may be ideal for post menopausal women, but only women should drink this much. But men shouldn't overdo it. Studies show that adult males who consume excess calcium, over 2,000 mg/day, may increase their risk of prostate cancer. [221]

Millions of Americans are deficient in calcium because they are lactose intolerant and are unable to digest cow's milk. For them, soy milk is a good alternative because most brands today are fortified with calcium. Soy also contains *genistein*, a chemical compound that increases levels of nitric oxide, the gas that dilates blood vessels to help lower blood pressure. Research shows that animals on a soy-based diet tend to have lower blood pressure than those on a regular diet and soy is thought to have similar effects in humans. A recent study of men and women with mild-to-moderate hypertension found that those who drank soy milk had a decrease in systolic blood pressure of about 18 points, and a drop in diastolic pressure of about 15 points. Drink soymilk regularly—about one glass a day—to take advantage of its benefits.

Nuts. Nuts are a versatile, high-protein food. Ounce for ounce, nuts contain nearly twice as much protein as lean meat and, unlike many protein sources, nuts don't require refrigeration. Although they are high in calories, they are also high in fiber, vitamins, minerals, and antioxidants. Nuts are a wonderful source of healthful monounsaturated fat, and they won't spike your blood sugar. Their portability and versatility make nuts a great snack food. You can eat them as is, add them to stir-fries, sprinkle them on your salad, and mix them with yogurt and berries. Purée them in your food processor and make your own nut butter to spread on celery or carrots. Just remember they are high in calories, so you don't want to "go nuts" with nuts. Just a few will do.

One of the most important benefits nuts provide is in aiding heart health. In a Harvard University study, nuts were shown to reduce the risk of developing cardiovascular disease and Type 2 diabetes. The study involved 83,000 women. The women who frequently ate walnuts, almonds, peanuts, pecans, cashews, pistachios, Brazil nuts, hazelnuts, pine nuts, or macadamia nuts were 27% less likely to develop diabetes than women who rarely ate nuts. That's because nuts help control glucose levels and can improve the body's insulin response. As an added benefit, the women who ate nuts also tended to lose body fat. Data from four large studies revealed that those who ate nuts at least four times a week lowered their risk of coronary heart disease by an astonishing 37%. These findings were reported by the Physician's Study, the Adventist Health Study, the Nurses' Health Study and the Iowa Women's Study.

Even nut butters had a beneficial effect. Those who ate at least two tablespoons of peanut butter five times a week reduced their risk of cardiovascular disease and Type 2 diabetes by 20%—pretty impressive, right? Before you reach for that jar of peanut butter, remember the study showed a greater benefit from eating whole nuts than from nut butter.

To increase the benefit, make your own fresh nut butter. If you prefer to buy your nut butter ready-made, choose natural nut butters with no additives and store them in the refrigerator.

- **Almonds.** According to a study published in the *Journal of Nutrition*,[222] the high antioxidant content in almonds (they are rich in vitamin E) can also assist those with chronically elevated insulin and glucose levels. Almonds are low on the Glycemic Index (GI), and they help neutralize free radicals and control blood sugar.[223] A study published in the medical journal *Metabolism* reported that almonds also have the ability to lower the total GI of any meal in which they are included.

- The *International Journal of Obesity and Related Metabolic Disorders* published a study indicating that almonds can assist in weight loss, which can help lower blood pressure. In that six-month study, those who ate almonds as part of a low-calorie diet reduced their weight by more than 10%. Moreover, 96% of the participants who had Type 1 diabetes were able to reduce their medications. In a clinical trial in Spain, researchers found that those who ate nuts at least twice a week were far less likely to gain weight than those who did not eat nuts. That study had 8,865 adult participants and the data showed that those who ate nuts were 31% less likely to pack on the pounds.

- **Walnuts.** Here are four key discoveries researchers have made in studies involving walnuts:

1. *Diabetes Care* published a study reporting a 10% reduction in LDL cholesterol was linked to eating walnuts. Study participants also demonstrated a significant increase in the ratio of HDL to total cholesterol.

2. According to a study published in the *British Journal of Nutrition,* walnuts, as well as pecans and chestnuts, are exceptionally high in antioxidants. Eating antioxidant-rich nuts also lowers your risk for coronary heart disease, which often results from having insulin resistance and diabetes.

3. The research journal *Phytochemistry* identified 16 different beneficial antioxidant polyphenols in walnuts.

4. Researchers in Spain reported that just a quarter cup of walnuts can provide over 90% of your daily requirement of omega-3s. In that study, adults who ate walnuts lowered their LDL cholesterol by between 6.4% and 10%.

Peanuts. Not technically a nut, the peanut (a legume) is a similarly great source of antioxidants. They are also high in resveratrol, vitamin E, and that same healthy fat (oleic acid) found in olive oil. Resveratrol is the "anti-aging" antioxidant compound that is found in red grapes and red wine. A study published in the *Journal of Agricultural and Food Chemistry* revealed that resveratrol created a significant increase in blood flow to the brain, and that it helped reduce the risk of stroke by as much as 30%. [224] Cool beans! As long as you have no allergies to them, peanuts are a healthy addition to your diet.

Olive oil. Not only is olive oil good for you, it's also very healing—especially for hypertension. A number of studies show that consuming olive oil can significantly reduce both systolic and diastolic blood pressure. In fact, these studies indicate that most people can lower their blood pressure just by consuming more olive oil, even if they don't make other dietary changes.

In one clinical trial, researchers at the University of Barcelona, Spain, recruited men from Germany, Denmark, and Finland—countries where olive oil is not commonly used—and had the men add about one-and-a-half tablespoons to their daily diets. By the end of the study, the men saw reductions in their systolic blood pressure of about 3%.

While it's still not clear exactly how olive oil lowers blood pressure, researchers think it may be due to the large amount of polyphenols it contains. These high-powered antioxidant compounds help protect arterial linings and promote better circulation by keeping them free of plaque buildup. [225]

In a study conducted on the importance of olive oil, Dr. L. Aldo Ferrara, Associate Professor at the Frederico II University of Naples in Italy, discovered that daily consumption of 40 grams of olive oil reduced the dosage of blood pressure medication in hypertensive patients by about 50%. The *polyphenols* in extra-virgin olive oil are credited with the significant reduction of blood pressure. [226]

Olives. Olives are a significant part of the Mediterranean diet, recognized to be one of the healthiest diets in the world. And where does all that healthy olive oil come from? From olives, of course. Slice them up and add to salads and wraps. Mince them and add to hummus and yogurt dips. Or simply snack on them whole.

Onions. They may make you cry, but onions are worth the weep if only for one tiny compound—*quercetin.* Onions are rich in quercetin, a type of flavonoid (a compound found in plants and vegetables that is high in antioxidants) with potent artery-opening effects. You don't have to live in the Mediterranean to reap these rewards. An important study done in the Netherlands examined men who ate an apple a day, small amounts of onions and drank tea—three foods that are high in flavonoids. The men experienced one-third fewer heart attacks than those who didn't consume the same quercetin-rich diet. [227]

In a more recent clinical trial, researchers at the University of Utah studied a group of adults with hypertension, giving them either a placebo or quercetin every day. The patients receiving the quercetin experienced reductions in blood pressure of 7 mmHg (systolic) and 5 mmHg (diastolic) compared with the placebo group. Researchers speculated that the quercetin may reduce the body's production of a blood vessel constricting protein called angiotensin II. Results of this important study were published in the *Journal of Nutrition.* [228]

Oranges. The juicy fruit from the sunshine state is packed with vitamins, minerals and phytochemicals perfect for fending off heart disease and keeping blood pressure low.

Oranges contain potassium, folate, calcium, magnesium, and Vitamin C. The latter protects arteries from the effects of cell-damaging free radicals. Research published in the *American Journal of Clinical Nutrition* indicates that drinking orange juice daily may greatly lower the blood pressure of slightly overweight men.[229] Orange juice, however, is high in natural sugars. So rather than drinking orange juice, we recommend you eat your oranges and receive the full benefit of all the nutrients and fiber contained in the whole fruit. Both lemons and oranges contain fruit pectin and potassium. Both of these compounds help protect the body from arterial plaque buildup and aid in the regulation of blood pressure.

Papaya. This fleshy, melon-like fruit is perfect for potassium-rich smoothies with a tropical feel. As we've discussed, this mineral counteracts the effects of sodium and, in so doing, helps keep blood pressure in a normal range. An older study from 2000, published in *Phytotherapy Research,* demonstrated that a form of papaya extract may help lower blood pressure.[230]

Pears. The mellow fruit is full of potassium and fiber and even some quercetin. Like apples, most of the nutrients are in the skin. So, wash your pears well, and eat the skins.

Plantains. A staple food in much of Africa and the Caribbean, plantains are a cross between a banana and potato. The plantain looks like a banana, but is larger and has a thicker skin, with the starchy texture of a potato. Chock full of potassium, you can bake, mash, fry, or boil them. But they aren't too palatable raw.

Potatoes. The humble potato has been much maligned and gastronomically abused. If they are not drowned in hot grease or smothered in margarine, potatoes eaten in moderation can actually help fight against hypertension. The earthy food is loaded with vitamins, phytochemicals and minerals. Potatoes do have a high Glycemic Index (GI) rating, but they are most definitely not "bad" for you.

The problem with potatoes lies in both the way they are cooked and the way they are served. The average potato contains only about 110 calories. It is what we add to our potato that causes problems.

Eating a large baked potato every once in a while can help knock out hypertension because it is rich in potassium, a mineral "that acts like a super-hero" when it comes to blood pressure function. In one clinical study, people with hypertension who ate more potassium-rich foods, including potatoes, saw their blood pressure levels decline so much that they were able to reduce their doses of blood-pressure medicine. And this benefit applies to sweet potatoes, too. They also contain a hefty wallop of potassium to keep your blood pressure normal and your heart beating in a regular rhythm.

In a review of 33 studies examining the effect of potassium on blood pressure, researchers found that people who get at least 2,340 mg of potassium daily—from foods, supplements, or both—lowered their risk of hypertension by 25%. And people who had the highest blood pressures benefited the most.[231]

Again, hang on to that skin! More than 60% of the potassium resides very close to the skin and will be removed if you peel your potatoes. Also, potatoes pack a huge carbohydrate punch. So eat potatoes in moderation and balance a potato-containing meal with a healthy source of protein. Too many potatoes eaten at one sitting can lead to raised insulin levels, and over time this can cause insulin resistance, which as we explained earlier is something you want to prevent.[232]

Colored potatoes pack more of a nutritional punch than white ones, with purple potatoes coming in as the nutritional champions. Potatoes are high in hypertension, fighting magnesium and potassium. They also contain phenols, zinc, iron phosphorus, B vitamins, vitamin C, and carotenoids. Carotenoids are the plant pigments found in most richly colored vegetables. Carotenoids support our metabolic processes, and most have important antioxidant activity. Our bodies require these phytochemicals but do not manufacture them. We must get them by eating colorful plant foods.

Joe Vinson, PhD, is a chemistry professor at the University of Scranton in Pennsylvania. He has been studying the humble spud and is intent on bringing its nutritional power to light. Did you know, for example, that a single raw potato can provide 25% of the body's requirement of vitamin C? Professor Vinson's studies even revealed that potatoes, when eaten properly, do not cause weight gain.

Working with a test group of people who were hypertensive and overweight, Dr. Vinson set out to study the effects of purple potatoes on their conditions. Study participants ate six to eight purple potatoes with skins, twice a day, for an entire month. At the end of the month, they had an average reduction of 3.5 points in systolic pressure and 4.3 points in diastolic pressure. Equally interesting was the fact that in spite of consuming an admittedly large volume of potatoes, test subjects did not gain any weight or note any other ill health effects.

We're not recommending you eat that many potatoes, but it is interesting to note that there was no weight gain for those who did.

Dr. Vinson hypothesizes that potatoes can be effective tools in managing hypertension. It seems potatoes contain phytochemicals that work like ACE-inhibitors, without the negative side effects of drugs. The professor warns that cooking potatoes at high temperatures and frying potatoes destroys these precious nutrients.

Seafood. We have known for a long time that the omega-3 fatty acids in fish are good for cardiovascular health. Mackerel, along with salmon and sardines, are among the richest sources of it. Now it appears that mackerel is also one of the best foods for normalizing blood pressure. In a study at Berlin's Central Institute for Cardiovascular Research, researchers divided hypertensive men into two groups. Both groups ate a standard Western type diet, but one group also consumed two daily servings of canned mackerel, or about 14 ounces. They followed this diet for two weeks, and then cut back to three servings of mackerel a week for eight months. While they ate the mackerel, their blood pressure dropped by 7%. That is enough of a reduction to take most people with mildly elevated blood pressure out of danger.

We are certainly not suggesting that you eat mackerel twice a day, but this study suggests that any of these omega-3 fish can help bring your numbers down.

Mackerel isn't the only fish that lowers blood pressure. Peptides, which naturally occur in bonito tuna and sardines, also reduce hypertension by inhibiting the *angiotensin-converting enzyme* (ACE) that constricts blood vessels. By the way, this is exactly the way ACE-inhibitor drugs work—and these fish peptides block ACE better than any naturally occurring substance known. Five separate clinical studies have demonstrated that the peptides in bonito and sardines perform just as well as many anti hypertensive prescription drugs. And the blood-pressure reduction in these studies was significant, usually dropping people with borderline hypertension into the normal range.

A meta-analysis of numerous studies examining fish oil's effect on blood pressure found that eating omega-3 rich fish three times per week is as effective at reducing high blood pressure as taking mega-doses of fish-oil supplements. Omega-3s reduce blood pressure by softening and improving the flexibility of artery walls.[233]

We addressed the many splendored health benefits of omega-3s in Chapter Eight. Both wild-caught salmon and clams are rich in sterols and omega-3 oils. Salmon is high in calcium and mono-unsaturated fat, two nutrients that reduce the risk of heart attack and help prevent arterial plaque buildup. Clams are also strong allies in the fight against arterial plaques. These are good sources of protein and helpful foods to eat when you are serious about managing your blood pressure.

Sesame oil. Commonly used in Asian countries, sesame oil (toasted or untoasted) is another smart choice. Several animal studies have shown that sesame oil reduces blood pressure, as well as the arterial damage caused by hypertension. A human clinical trial confirmed this effect. Hypertensive patients taking a calcium-channel blocker medicine were given seven teaspoons of sesame oil daily for two months and not only saw their blood pressure reduced, but they also experienced a decrease in triglycerides and LDL (the "bad" cholesterol), while their good HDL cholesterol went up.[234]

Soy nuts and edamame. Soy is a favorite protein source for vegetarians. Soy proteins help dilate blood vessels, which improves circulation and helps to lower blood pressure. As an added bonus, soy also helps stabilize blood sugar.

In a study involving 60 women, soy was found to contribute to a significant drop in blood pressure. The women were asked to eat two different diets, staying on each one for a period of eight weeks. Both diets were low-fat and high-carbohydrate and both diets contained the same ratio of fats to proteins.

The difference came in the source of protein. In one of the diets, the participants ate a half-cup of unsalted soy nuts a day. And the result? Regardless of their starting blood pressure, all of the women who were hypertensive experienced a notable drop in blood pressure readings. And nearly 80% of the women with normal blood pressure also experienced a drop in both systolic and diastolic numbers.

In a similar Chinese study with a test group of 300 people, one group ate wheat protein and another ate soy protein. The soy eaters with hypertension dropped their numbers by an average 4 points systolic and 3 points diastolic. The proteins in soy help dilate blood vessels, which lowers blood pressure. Soy also contains a compound called *genistein* that promotes the production of nitric oxide, another chemical that allows the arterial walls to relax. Now that you know the benefits of soy, enjoy some yummy edamame! [235]

Spinach. Popeye was right about the nutritional power of this leafy green veggie! Spinach contains antioxidants and is also rich in folate (vitamin B-9), both of which help arteries stay strong. A 2005 study published in the *Journal of the American Medical Association* showed that women who ate at least 1,000 micrograms of folate daily decreased their risk of hypertension by 20% to 45%.

People suffering with hypertension often have high levels of homocysteine, an amino acid that contributes to the buildup of plaque along arterial walls. Folate, especially when taken with vitamins B-6 and B-12, helps reduce levels of homocysteine. [236]

Another study discovered that an enzyme in spinach acts exactly like ACE-inhibitor drugs to lower blood pressure by blocking the enzyme that constricts and tightens blood vessels. When laboratory animals with hypertension were fed spinach, it significantly dropped their blood pressure within two to four hours. [237]

But wait, there's more. Spinach also contains certain amino acids called peptides, which act as a kind of natural ACE inhibitor. [238]

One more thing—a no-brainer that probably took researchers much work and thousands of dollars to figure out: Pick spinach (and other veggies) with leaves that are very dark and beautiful. Science has shown that the prettier the leaves are to the eye, the higher the concentration of vitamin C.

While you're in the produce section sourcing spinach, also look for dandelion leaves, which contain potassium, a natural diuretic. They taste great in salads, wilted, or in green smoothies.

Tomatoes. Ever wonder what gives tomatoes their fiery red hue? It is lycopene, a type of antioxidant called a carotenoid, which helps lower blood pressure. Tomatoes are the best food source for lycopene.

In a study published in the *American Heart Journal,* tomato extract lowered blood pressure in people who had mild hypertension. Every day for eight weeks, 31 subjects were given 250 mg of tomato extract; each capsule contained 15 mg of lycopene, the amount you would find in three-ounces of tomato sauce. The results: Both systolic and diastolic numbers went down the most dramatically during the last two weeks.

Tomatoes also contain several other heart-healthy substances, including *gamma-aminobutyric acid* (GABA). So go ahead and have some marinara sauce on your spaghetti squash. [239]

Lycopene may also lower the risk of stroke. Researchers at the University of Eastern Finland found that men who had higher concentrations of lycopene had significantly lower risks of having a stroke.

Researcher Jouni Karppi, PhD, and colleagues, studied over 1,000 Finnish men ages 42 to 61 in the longitudinal Kuopio Ischemic Heart Disease Risk Factor study. The researchers measured serum concentrations of various carotenoids, including lycopene, alpha-carotene, beta-carotene, alpha-tocopherol, and retinol. After adjustment for potential confounders, greater serum concentrations of lycopene—but none of the other carotenoids—were associated with a lower stroke risk.

Researchers found the relationships remained significant after adjustment for age, examination year, body mass index, systolic blood pressure, smoking, serum LDL cholesterol, diabetes, and history of stroke.

"One possible reason that lycopene might decrease the risk of stroke more than other antioxidants …may be the consequence of antioxidant activity," they wrote. "Lycopene is a potent antioxidant and the most effective quencher of singlet oxygen, and it was reported to be more effective than beta-carotene in cell protection against hydrogen peroxide and nitrogen dioxide radicals."

Lycopene also serves other functions. It reduces inflammation, blocks cholesterol synthesis, boosts immune function, and inhibits platelet aggregation and thrombosis.

"This study supports the recommendation of eating [more] servings of fruits and vegetables a day," said Nancy Copperman, MS, RD, director of public health initiatives at the North Shore-Long Island Jewish Health System in Great Neck, NY.

"Foods such as tomatoes, guava, watermelon, and grapefruit are good sources of lycopene," she said in a statement. "When a tomato is cooked, the heat processing actually increases the levels of cis-lycopene, which is easily absorbed by the body."

Watermelon. Watermelon has been shown to naturally lower blood pressure. A study at Florida State University followed nine subjects for six weeks. Four men and five menopausal women ingested six grams daily of an extract of watermelon (equivalent to about two pounds of watermelon). All nine of the subjects were pre-hypertensive and all were between the ages of 51 and 57.

In the test, participants were given watermelon extract. The amino acids in watermelon extract are broken down in the body by enzymes, creating nitric oxide. Although nitric oxide is a pollutant in the external world, in our bodies, it is a vital messaging molecule and plays an important role in keeping our blood vessels supple and regulating our blood pressure.

One could take the amino acid L-arginine by itself, but we do not recommend that. Taken in that form, it can cause nausea, gastrointestinal upset, and diarrhea.

Watermelon has none of these side effects. And if you eat your watermelon instead of taking extract, you will receive even more nutritional benefits. Watermelon contains potassium, fiber, vitamins A, B6 and C, and lycopene—a helpful antioxidant once thought to be found only in tomatoes.

After six weeks of watermelon extract, all study participants showed increased aortic blood flow and lowered blood pressure.

"We are the first to document improved aortic hemodynamics in pre-hypertensive but otherwise healthy middle-aged men and women receiving therapeutic doses of watermelon," said FSU assistant professor Arturo Figueroa, MD, PhD. "These findings suggest that this 'functional food' has a vasodilatory effect, and one that may prevent pre-hypertension from progressing to full-blown hypertension, a major risk factor for heart attacks and strokes."

The results of this study, which appeared in the *American Journal of Hypertension*, may pave the way for an L-citrulline supplement to be used in treating pre-hypertension and hypertension. A watermelon extract may prevent the onset of hypertension altogether.

The benefits of watermelon don't end there though. A study conducted in 2008 by Texas A&M's Fruit and Vegetable Improvement Center suggests that this summertime thirst quencher may also increase libido by relaxing blood vessels and increasing blood flow to other areas of the body.

GET INTO THE WHOLE GRAIN GROOVE

One of the best things you can do for healing hypertension is to replace simple, processed carbohydrates, such as white bread and pasta, with whole grains, such as brown rice, oats, millet and quinoa (these last two are technically seeds, though commonly classified as grains) millet, and oats. Whole grains pack more fiber, which research proves helps lower blood pressure.

How? Your body can't digest insoluble fiber—the kind you get in grain husks. By some process not yet fully understood, the fiber in whole grains slows digestion and absorption, which also keeps insulin from rising too quickly. All of this helps keep blood sugar levels stable, and balanced blood sugar levels lead to stable blood pressure. In addition to fiber, many whole grains contain magnesium, which relaxes blood vessels and also helps to keep blood pressure down.

Whole grains have more nutrients because they are far less processed and retain the husk around their kernels. In the same way that many fruits and vegetables carry a large percentage of their nutrients in their skins, the husk around the rice grain contains the fiber and magnesium that helps lower blood pressure. Eliminating this husk gives white rice its paper-pale hue, and strips the rice of many essential nutrients.

Many people have an undiagnosed sensitivity to gluten. Gluten is present even in whole grain wheat, so we recommend you investigate gluten-free whole grains like amaranth, millet, quinoa, rice, sorghum, and teff.

Another caveat: Although the body doesn't digest the fiber in grain husk, it will eventually break the husk down and digest the kernel inside. That kernel is almost pure carbohydrate. So go easy on grain consumption. Even if you are eating healthful whole grains, if you eat too much, you'll overwhelm the protective effects of its fiber with insulin-raising carbs.

THE "911 EMERGENCY DIET"

If your blood pressure is high and you need to bring it down quickly but don't want to use medications, let rice come to your rescue. A diet of steamed brown rice, fruit and vegetables, known as the Kempner Rice Diet, reduces blood pressure by at least 20 points in a matter of days. This is an old trick used by commercial airline pilots who routinely are checked for hypertension but are not allowed to take medications to bring it down. This rice diet really produces fast results. [240]

While the diet is restrictive—no other foods are allowed, including oils, sweeteners, spices, alcohol, caffeinated beverages, meat, and dairy products—the rapid results are worth it. Eating such a bland diet like this cannot hold most people's interest for longer than a few weeks. But once you get your hypertension under control, you can shift over to a more varied Hypertension Healing Diet which can offer you plenty of flavor and variety, while keeping your blood pressure in the safety zone more permanently.

THE TOP 10 MAGNESIUM-RICH FOODS

Magnesium is essential for hundreds of different chemical reactions in the body, including maintaining your energy level, helping you relax, and sustaining the health of your heart and blood vessels. To reap its many benefits, stock your cupboards and refrigerator with these foods.

1. Swiss chard
2. Spinach
3. Pumpkin seeds
4. Broccoli
5. Basil
6. Cucumbers
7. Flaxseeds
8. Gingers
9. Sunflower seeds
10. Wild salmon

BEVERAGES FOR BETTER BLOOD PRESSURE

It is not just what you eat that matters. What you drink will also have a profound effect on your blood pressure.

Beet juice. Want an effective fix that lasts? While we don't usually encourage people to think about magic pills for health issues such as high blood pressure, beet juice is an exception. Researchers at Queen Mary's William Harvey Research Institute in London found that beet juice not only lowers blood pressure, but it does so quickly—within three hours of drinking just over a cupful. And the effects last for 24 hours. It is thought that the nitrates in beetroot contribute to its blood pressure-lowering effects.

A study by the London School of Medicine and Dentistry found that volunteers who drink just 16 ounces of beet juice daily experienced reductions in blood pressure of more than 10 points—and their pressure remained lower over 24 hours.[241] The researchers explained that the beets and other green leafy vegetables are converted into nitric oxide, a gas that opens arteries wider so blood flows with less pressure. "There have been some very large studies showing that when people were put on a fruit-and-vegetable diet—particularly green leafy vegetables—that their cardiovascular function and cardiovascular health improved," says Dr. Amrita Ahluwalia, senior author of the study. In the past, doctors have credited the antioxidants in beets and other vegetables for their cardio-protective effects. Now it seems that nitric oxide is the real hero.

One of the easiest ways to get plenty of these anti-hypertensive vegetables into your diet is by drinking fresh vegetable juice. (For Jim's favorite recipe, see "Jim Healthy's Blood Pressure Lowering Juice" on the next page.) Some commercial vegetable juices also are quite effective. According to a study published in the *Journal of the American Medical Association* in 2001, V8 juice lowers blood pressure significantly. [242]

JIM HEALTHY'S BLOOD PRESSURE-LOWERING JUICE

Here's a yummy blood pressure-lowering tip from Jim: One of my favorite beverages is this super-healing fresh veggie juice, which I drink every day at lunchtime when I am not traveling. It is packed with phytonutrients, vitamins, minerals, and inflammation-fighting compounds that lower cholesterol and blood pressure, clean my arteries, boost my brain-power, sharpen my vision and memory, and even ease my joint pain.

It took me a while to get the mix right, so feel free to adjust the recipe until it suits your taste buds. If you don't already own a good-quality juicer, you'll need one, but it's one of the best investments you can make in your health. One of the best manufacturers of reliable juicers is Breville (www.brevilleusa.com)—it's the brand I use.

All of the produce listed below should be organically grown.

Makes one 8–10 oz. serving

Ingredients

   2 stalks of celery

   4 or 5 sprigs of parsley

   1 stalk of kale

   1 stalk of Swiss chard

   ½ red beet and a few of the greens

   Small bunch of spinach

   ½–1 sweet apple

   Plug of fresh ginger (about the size of your thumb)

   5–8 carrots

The beet, apple, and carrots will sweeten the bitter taste of the greens, so you may want to use more of these until you get used to the flavor.

Since I drink this almost every day, my wife and I have found a clever way to slash the prep and clean-up time by making a one-month supply (about five gallons). Every 30 days or so we juice about three gallons and freeze it in 8-oz plastic ice tea bottles. The whole operation takes the two of us about two hours from start to finish. Then, every morning I remove a bottle from the freezer and by lunchtime it's thawed and ready. If I am going to be away, I take a frozen bottle on the road.

The Kuna Indians of the San Blas Islands of Panama have a diet high in salt, yet as a group, they have normal blood pressure. Norman K. Hollenberg, MD, professor of medicine at Brigham and Women's Hospital and Harvard Medical School, investigated the Kuna Indians to see if he could discover the secrets of their cardiovascular health. Hollenberg found that although they ate a diet rich in salt, they also consumed a drink made with locally grown cocoa at nearly every meal. Furthering his studies, Dr. Hollenberg then monitored the health of indigenous Kuna people who had moved to the city. Those who had moved to the city began to consume commercially ground cocoa. As they did, their blood pressure reading began to rise.

Hollenberg's research was published in the December 2003 issue of the *Journal of Hypertension.* In presenting his findings, he revealed that a second study indicated that natural cocoa, rich in flavanoids, also helped increase circulation to the brain and the extremities.

In that second study, 27 healthy people, aged 18 to 72, consumed a daily cocoa beverage that contained 900 milligrams of flavanols. After just five days, researchers measured "significant improvement" in both blood flow and in the function of the endothelial cells that line blood vessels.

The take-away from Dr. Hollenberg's research is that consuming natural cocoa with high-flavonol content can be good for your health. The studies show that cocoa's flavanols help regulate the body's ability to synthesize biologic nitric oxide, and improve vasodialation and blood flow. The flavanols in cocoa may also help keep platelets from clustering on the walls of blood vessels.

According to Dr. Harold H. Schmitz, executive director of the Mars Center for Cocoa Health Science, one problem in conducting the studies stems from differences in types and amounts of flavanols in commercially available chocolate and cocoa. The products are affected by the way the raw materials are handled and processed and by the variety of the cacao.

According to Carl L. Keen, PhD, chairman of the nutrition department at UC Davis, cocoa has a similar effect to baby aspirin on the body, and may be a good alternative for people who cannot tolerate the aspirin.

Says Dr. Schmitz: "Most chocolate that is currently available is delightful and delicious, but not necessarily good for you. We hope that in a year or two, it is possible to change that."

Dr. Hollenberg warned that chocolates, like vitamins and other substances, have to be tailored to the individual because "good isn't always good; it depends on who you are."

Coconut water. These days most health food stores and supermarkets carry coconut water, which is the fluid found inside coconuts. Coconut water is not the same as coconut milk which is made from the meat of this delicious fruit. Coconut water has long been used as a source of nutrition during famines, and it is so bio-compatible that it can be safely injected into the human blood stream. In a 2005 article in the *West Indian Medical Journal,* researchers reported on the effectiveness of coconut water and another tropical drink, mauby, for reducing hypertension. Mauby is made from the bark of the buckhorn tree and is popular in the Caribbean.

For this study, 28 subjects were divided into four groups. One group received water, while the others received mauby, coconut water or a combination of the two. After two weeks, results showed 71% of the coconut water, group had a significant reduction in their systolic blood pressure, compared with a decrease of 40% of the mauby group and 43% for the group that drank the mixture of mauby and coconut water. Similarly, 29% of the coconut group saw significant declines in their diastolic pressure, as did 40% and 57% of the other two treatment groups.

Coconut water's high potassium content may explain its effectiveness in lowering blood pressure. Increased potassium intake helps reduce blood pressure as it balances out the sodium that promotes hypertension.

Green tea. In Asia, the healing potential of antioxidant-rich green tea has been celebrated for thousands of years. One study of 1,507 Chinese people found that participants who consumed from one-half to five cups of green tea daily for a minimum of a year lowered their risk of developing high blood pressure by a whopping 46%, compared with those who consumed less than that; and drinking more than five cups lowered risk by 65%. [243]

Some researchers think that green tea's exceptional blood-pressure lowering capacity comes from its ability to act like an ACE-inhibitor (see Appendix A on page 307 for more information on ACE inhibitors). ACE stands for *angiotensin-converting enzyme*. Angiotensin is a chemical in the body that causes arteries to constrict, so inhibiting its effect is a good thing.

JIM HEALTHY'S HYPERTENSION PUNCH

This easy, inexpensive beverage combines four Hypertension Healing ingredients. It's yummy and refreshing and I sip on it when working out in the gym or when hiking outdoors. It keeps me hydrated and packs a four-way benefit for my blood pressure. Plus I love the way it tastes.

Makes 1 gallon

Ingredients

   3 ½ quarts of decaffeinated green tea

   2–3 cups of unsweetened pomegranate juice

   6–8 tablespoons of hibiscus leaves (wrapped in tithing cheesecloth)

   Sliced ginger root to taste

Instructions:

Put all ingredients in a one-gallon glass jar with a screw-on lid. Place in the sun to brew for two to three hours and then chill. Drink throughout the day.

Hibiscus tea. It seems appropriate that a flower that lowers blood pressure levels would hail from the land of warm breezes and ocean surf. Hibiscus is native to Hawaii, and recent research reveals that it indeed brings the relaxing ambiance of a Hawaiian beach to your arteries.

Hibiscus (*Hibiscus sabdariffa*) is a well-respected traditional remedy for high blood pressure in many countries around the world, so researchers decided to clinically measure its validity on hypertensive patients. The participants stopped taking their high blood pressure medication for one week prior to the study and drank a cup of hibiscus tea one hour before having their blood pressure taken, which was done three times throughout the 15-day study. After 12 days, the subjects who drank the hibiscus tea experienced an average 11.7% drop in systolic blood pressure and a 10.7% drop in diastolic blood pressure from their initial readings. For someone with a blood pressure of around 160/115, this would be a reduction to roughly 145/95, which is so impressive that the results of the study were reported in the *Journal of Ethnopharmacology.*[244]

In another study, hibiscus tea worked almost as well as medication for bringing down blood pressure. Seventy-five people were divided into two groups. One group drank 16 ounces of hibiscus tea a day while a second group took 25 mg of the drug captopril twice a day. Nearly 80% of the hibiscus tea drinkers saw a reduction of at least 10 points in diastolic blood pressure, compared with 84% of the drug users. A subsequent study with a larger participant pool had similar results. [245]

In yet another study, researchers divided 193 participants into two groups. One received hibiscus extract containing a total of 250 mg of anthocyanins (the flavonoid that gives hibiscus its hypertension-healing power) and the other received 10 mg of the drug lisinopril daily. After just four weeks, participants taking hibiscus saw a reduction of an average of 16 points in systolic pressure and 12 points diastolic pressure. [246]

While the hibiscus tea produces reductions rather quickly, they may not be long-lasting for all people; so it is wise to drink the tea on a regular basis (we recommend two cups daily). The tea is brewed from the flowers and fruit of the plant, using a teaspoon or less per cup. Sweeten to taste. Never discontinue any medication without speaking to your doctor first. Hibiscus tea is available commercially as Red Zinger Tea.

H₂0 for a happier heart. Most Americans do not drink enough water. In fact, up to 75% of the population may be chronically dehydrated without even being aware of it. Since our bodies are mainly composed of water, if we don't give it a steady supply of its primary juice, there will be consequences. Arterial walls need to be well-hydrated in order to stay flexible and allow blood to flow through them with ease. If your arteries aren't well-hydrated, they become more rigid and blood pressure will increase. Another problem with chronic dehydration is a decreased metabolism, which can result in weight gain.

A wise guideline for staying hydrated is to drink at least eight 8-oz glasses of water a day. Make sure to use a quality filter to assure you're nourishing your cells with clean, pure water. You don't have to buy an expensive filter, but we enthusiastically encourage you to make this investment in your family's health. With all of the water that we hope your family will be consuming, you are going to need a reliable unit. The one we like best is the Katadyn Combi Water Filter, with an attachment for your tap. It has a ceramic element that filters more than 13,000 gallons of drinking water before requiring replacement. This filter removes both bacteria and toxic chemicals from your water. [247] While you may pay a little more for this water filter, it is worth it. The Katadyn Combi filters water to .2 microns, which is as safe as you can get. Be sure to use a glass bottle, glass-lined thermos, or stainless steel bottle to carry your drinking water with you. Waterwise Systems also sells water distillers that are very good. In addition, the Rettin Company makes a good filter/ionizer that also gets our "thumbs up." (We suggest getting a filter for your shower too, because the chlorine in heated tap water is especially toxic.)

To be extra good to your health, drink mineral-enriched water. You can make your own at home (see recipe in the box that follows). The magnesium content will help your arteries stay relaxed.

One easy way to determine if you are taking in enough fluids is to watch your urine. If it's dark yellow, you need more liquids; if it's pale yellow or clear, you are doing just fine.

MAKE YOUR OWN MINERAL WATER

You can make your own mineral water with all-natural Himalayan crystal rock salt, which contains 84 essential minerals. [248] You can purchase it online at www.source naturals.com.

Here's what you'll need:

- Clean 8-oz glass jar

- Natural spring water or filtered tap water

- Himalayan crystal rock salt

Instructions:

Pour a thin layer of rock salt over the bottom of the jar. Add natural spring water to a depth of two inches above the salt. Put a lid on the jar and let the mixture sit over night. If there's no salt visible in the solution in the morning, add more. Continue this process until some salt remains un-dissolved. Add 1 tsp of the salt solution to 8 ounces of filtered drinking water. Store the remaining salt solution in the refrigerator.

CHAPTER THIRTEEN

SUPPLEMENTS FOR HEALTHIER BLOOD PRESSURE

It would be wonderful if we could get all the nutrients we need to fight hypertension simply by eating a wide variety of fresh, whole foods. Unfortunately, it doesn't seem that we can. Decades of modern farming methods—mechanized tilling, chemical fertilizers, and mono-cropping—have left soils depleted of nutrients (unless they have been maintained organically). And if nutrients are missing from the soil, they will also be missing from the plant foods grown in that soil.

Even if it were possible to eat a perfect diet, however, our bodies still could not fully metabolize all the nutrition we take in. The production of digestive enzymes slows and weakens with age. If you cannot fully digest your meals, then you cannot get complete nutritive benefit from them. Additionally, many illnesses require extra nutrition, far beyond what even the best ordinary diet can offer.

For all these reasons, nutritional supplements can be critical for good health, in general, and for lowering blood pressure, in particular. Following is a list of vitamins, minerals, and herbs that will help you treat your high blood pressure.

ANTIOXIDANTS LOWER STROKE RISK BY 60%

Antioxidant vitamins are your allies in reversing hypertension and protecting yourself from the debilitating effects of cardiovascular disease and stroke. Sometimes, people can become cavalier or fatalistic about their high blood pressure. "When I die, I die," they might say. But what if you don't die? What if you suffer for years in a body that will no longer obey your wishes?

Stroke is a very real threat for those with hypertension. It is a leading cause of disability and death in the US, and yet according to the National Stroke Association, up to 80% of all strokes are preventable. [249]

When a blood clot blocks an artery, or a blood vessel in the brain is severely damaged, blood flow to the brain is blocked. Brain cells in that area begin to die and the patient is left with brain damage. We call this a stroke. Depending on the area of the brain affected, a person could lose memory, their ability to speak or move or relate socially. Sounds pretty horrible, doesn't it?

The good news is that antioxidants can lower your risk of stroke by 60%! Yes, the same antioxidants that lower your blood pressure also lower your risk of having a stroke. A study

148

published in the *Journal of Nutrition* found that keeping your antioxidant levels high keeps your stroke risk low. Simply taking vitamin C enabled study participants to lower their risk by 40%.

The journal *Nature* published a study that addresses the underlying physical cause of hypertension. Researchers made great strides identifying and treating the root cause of the problem, rather than just addressing the symptoms. It all has to do with a protein called angiotensinogen. Among other things, this essential protein helps control blood pressure. Unfortunately, it is easily damaged by free radicals. [250]

Free radicals assault the angiotensinogen, damaging the vascular system, raising blood pressure, and putting you at greater risk for stroke and other problems.

Antioxidants help protect your body, including the delicate endothelial lining of blood vessels, from free radicals. In this study, researchers found that increasing antioxidant intake via natural foods and supplements lowered blood pressure and stroke risk. The greatest results were achieved when other mitigating factors, such as stress and overweight, were also addressed.

Following is a list of vitamins, minerals, and herbs that will help you treat your high blood pressure:

Alpha-Lipoic Acid (ALA). A multifaceted antioxidant, ALA defeats damaging free radicals. Recent research published in the *Annals of the New York Academy of Science* shows how it works: Cells are busy little centers of energy production, thanks to mitochondria— the powerhouse of the cell. But not all the work of this critical cell structure is positive, because as mitochondria are churning out energy, they are also producing cell-damaging free radicals.

Enter ALA. This antioxidant forms a barrier around the mitochondria that protects it from free radicals. This is great news for your high blood pressure.

Besides lowering blood pressure, ALA has an impressive laundry list of other health benefits, including deterring atherosclerosis, improving insulin sensitivity for people with Type 2 diabetes, controlling obesity, and improving mental clarity. [251]

Mitochondria are the energy power plants in each cell. Like external power plants they generate some undesirable "pollution" as they do their job. Energy production in our bodies can create large numbers of free radicals. These free radicals contribute to premature aging, hypertension, insulin resistance, and other diseases. Mitochondria are especially vulnerable to damage from free radicals.

In a study published in the *Annals of the New York Academy of Science*, researchers detailed how lipoic acid prevents damage to cellular mitochondria by providing a sort of antioxidant shield to the cellular structure. In addition to known antioxidant heroes like raw vegetables and fruits and other natural foods, R-lipoic acid was shown to be a strong defender of cells. Protect your internal power plants with healthy nutrition and lipoic acid.

Calcium. You're probably used to opening up a magazine and seeing a celebrity with a white mustache inquiring, "Got milk?" If you've got hypertension, your answer should be, "Yes."

Drinking milk and consuming other dairy products may help keep your blood pressure down because calcium, like potassium and magnesium, helps to relax the walls of the arteries. A study in Puerto Rico found that men who did not drink milk were twice as likely to develop high blood pressure as were their peers who drank more than a quart of the white stuff a day.

It is not clear how much dairy you need to help your blood pressure, but it has been shown that dietary calcium (not calcium supplements) may help your blood pressure, too. A report published in the *Journal of Human Hypertension* found that a daily calcium intake equivalent to 1,000 mg of calcium could decrease blood pressure. [252] Green vegetables such as kale, broccoli and spinach, as well as nuts and seeds, are good non-dairy sources of dietary calcium.

PUT DOWN THOSE CALCIUM SUPPLEMENTS!

Get your calcium from food, not pills. That's the latest medical advice. Too much of a good thing may be just that: too much. That's the conclusion of a prospective, longitudinal, population-based study of Swedish women looking at calcium intake and cardiovascular mortality. [253]

In the study, high rates of calcium intake were associated with higher all-cause and cardiovascular death rates (except stroke), as reported in an article published online in the February 13, 2013, issue of the *British Medical Journal.*

The Swedish research is the latest in a series of worrisome studies linking calcium intake and cardiovascular events. (A National Institutes of Health study showed that a high intake of supplemental calcium increased the risk of cardiovascular disease death in men, but not women.)

The Swedish researchers found that the highest intakes of calcium (more than 1,400 mg/day) were associated with higher all-cause risk of death, after adjustment for age, total energy, vitamin D and calcium-supplement intake, and other dietary, physical and demographic factors, compared with intakes of 600-1000 mg/day.

The lead researcher, Karl Michaëlsson, MD, PhD, said the association of calcium intake with all-cause and cardiovascular mortality "was especially strong if a high dietary intake of calcium was combined with calcium supplements."

Women with the highest intake of calcium (more than 1,400 mg/day) who used supplement tablets had a 2.5-times higher risk of all-cause death than women with similar total intakes not taking a supplement. "My present recommendation," Dr. Michaëlsson said, "is to avoid calcium-supplement use, if you have a normal varied diet."

This advice was echoed by John Cleland, MD (Hull York Medical School, Kingston-upon-Hull, UK), who said that calcium tablets "have not been shown to reduce fracture rates or improve any other patient outcome that I know of." He recommended that people stop taking calcium supplements "until efficacy/safety is shown," and this advice "should definitely include those taking them for osteoporosis." [254]

Chlorella. This green algae is considered to be one of the most powerful superfoods known to man. Chlorella contains vast amounts of chlorophyll within its cell walls. The cell walls of chlorella are tough and indigestible, so many chlorella producers break the cell walls before selling the product. Broken cell chlorella releases the nutrients inside the cell walls so the human body can use them. Besides being possibly the richest source of chlorophyll on Earth, chlorella is also very high in plant protein. Chlorella contains 58 grams of protein per 100 grams of weight. By comparison, beef and chicken have 24 to 28 grams of protein per 100 grams of weight. Besides reducing hypertension, chlorella is a pain reliever, reduces hypertension, enhances the immune system, and chelates heavy metals.

In another clinical study, patients with hypertension were given 10g chlorella tablets and 100 mL of chlorella extract for two months. Patients were taken off all blood pressure medications and then treated with chlorella. One-fourth of the patients saw a decrease in blood pressure after taking chlorella for two months. The other three-fourths did not see a rise in blood pressure, despite being taken off their blood pressure medication.

Coleus Forskohlii. Used in the Ayurvedic tradition for thousands of years to treat heart-related illnesses, Coleus Forskohlii is gaining attention from Western health practitioners for its ability to reduce blood pressure. As an added bonus, the herb assists in the breakdown of stored fat cells, helping you lose weight and lessening the burden on the heart.

Cordyceps. This type of mushroom is a powerful Chinese herb that not only reduces blood pressure and heart rate, but also increases blood supply to arteries and heart. Take cordyceps in tablet or capsule form.

CoQ10. Co-enzyme Q10 (CoQ10) is a humble enzyme with an important role: kick-starting mitochondria, the energy-producing element of cells. Not only does CoQ10 energize mitochondria, it is a powerful antioxidant that helps arteries manage blood flow. Both of these functions may be why it's so superb for heart health. Check this out: Taking CoQ10 as a supplement has been found to lower both systolic and diastolic blood pressure by a significant amount in people suffering from hypertension. In one study, daily 100 mg doses of CoQ10 given to hypertensives for 10 weeks resulted in a 10% reduction in blood pressure.

The body makes its own reserves of CoQ10, but as you age, the levels seriously decrease. Moreover, it's hard to get enough through diet alone; many foods contain CoQ10, but in minimal amounts. So taking a supplement is necessary.

Evening primrose oil. Extracted from the seeds of the bold yellow evening primrose flower, this oil contains alpha-lipoic acid which, as mentioned earlier, is a free-radical fighting antioxidant that has proven effective in lowering blood pressure. Taking evening primrose oil can shave off as much as 10 points from systolic and diastolic numbers. [255]

Garlic. This popular kitchen herb is also a well-known heart health remedy and tonic. Now, a recent Australian medical study adds to its impressive cardiovascular benefits. The research showed that subjects who took two capsules (480 mg) of aged garlic extract experienced significant drops in systolic blood pressure, averaging around 12 mmHg. To put this improvement into perspective, every 10 mmHg drop in blood pressure can cut cardiovascular risk by as much as 40%.

Aged garlic extract, which contains standardized amounts of the antioxidant *s-allylcysteine,* is far more potent than its culinary counterpart. But using garlic in the preparation of your meals (ideally raw) is still a wise way to combat high blood pressure. [256]

Grape seed extract. Dressed in red, green or purple, grapes—the fruit itself, leaves, sap, and wine—have been used for centuries for many medicinal purposes.

Recently, studies have revealed what may be the key to their healing power—antioxidants. Grape seed extract is chock full of antioxidants. They protect blood vessels from damage by free radicals and help lower blood pressure.

In a 2009 study, researchers gave grape seed extract to subjects who had metabolic syndrome (a combination of health problems that includes high blood pressure, high cholesterol, and insulin resistance) for four weeks. The results? Lower blood pressure—both systolic and diastolic. [254] Grape seed extract may also improve control of insulin levels in those suffering from diabetes, and this, of course, also helps to protect blood vessels from buildup of plaque and other obstructions. The extract is available in capsules, tablets, and liquid. [258, 259]

Hawthorn. A symbol of hope in ancient Greece, Hawthorn is packed with free-radical-fighting flavonoids, particularly anthocyanidins and proanthocyanidins. (It's the flavonoids that give Hawthorn its red color.) Hawthorn improves blood flow by dilating arteries, increasing flexibility in blood vessels, and reducing blood volume. It is kind of a natural ACE-inhibitor and may also strengthen heart muscles and positively influence the balance between water and salt in the body.

Hawthorn has long been used to treat hypertension, and with good reason. In a study done in the UK, patients with Type 2 diabetes and high blood pressure were divided into two groups. One group received pharmaceutical blood pressure medications, and the other group took 1,200 mg of hawthorn extract daily. After four months, those taking hawthorn showed a lower average diastolic reading.

The herb can be taken in capsules, liquid and solid extracts, and tinctures. There are also teas on the market containing hawthorn berry. [260] The results are not immediate. Once you start taking hawthorn, you may have to wait from two to four weeks to see blood pressure lower. [261]

L-arginine. Remember how we discussed that nitric oxide helps blood vessels dilate (a good thing for lowering blood pressure)? Well, here is a substance that promotes the production of that wonderful vasodilator, L-arginine. It is an amino acid that, when taken in supplement form, has been shown to decrease blood pressure. L-arginine can be found in the body and also can be ingested via poultry, fish, and dairy products. [262]

L-carnitine. This is also an amino acid, but this one functions in the process of metabolizing fat. Taking L-carnitine increases energy by providing more fat to the muscles, and this indirectly helps blood pressure.

Magnesium. Magnesium lowers blood pressure by relaxing the arterial muscles, which helps blood to circulate with greater ease. Those who don't get enough magnesium are putting themselves at risk for hypertension and heart disease. Luckily, foods that are high in magnesium are also often rich in potassium and dietary fiber as well; so you don't have to work too hard to get several hypertension-healing boosts at once.

You should be able to get enough magnesium in your diet by eating green powerhouses such as spinach and other green vegetables; nuts such as almonds and cashews, legumes such as soybeans and lentils; and whole, unrefined grains. Want to drink your magnesium? Milk is a good source, as is mineral water.

If you are taking a diuretic or other anti-hypertensive drug, you might be losing the mineral through your urine and may need to supplement. Ask your doctor.

Omega-3s. Research reveals that omega-3s can help lower blood pressure, as well as help tame atherosclerosis by keeping plaque from building up on arterial walls.

An examination of 17 studies found that taking three or more grams of fish oil daily might bring down high blood pressure. (There is a risk of bleeding at levels higher than 3 grams a day, so consult with your physician if you decide to try this supplement.)

Good sources of omega-3s include walnuts, chia and flax seeds, soybeans, navy and kidney beans, Pacific wild-caught, cold water fish, winter squash, and olive oil. You can also find omega-3s in algae and krill, and in some plants and nut oils. [263, 264]

Potassium. This common mineral possesses the ability to dilate (open) arteries and helps the body excrete excess sodium. Both these traits help potassium lower blood pressure. The typical American, however, consumes only a third of the potassium our ancestors ate. Organically grown natural foods are a good source of potassium, but you have to eat them, in order to receive the benefits.

Potassium deficiency is a significant factor in hypertension. Researchers publishing in the *Archives of Internal Medicine* found that the imbalance of potassium to sodium in the diet drives up blood pressure. Studying data from 21 countries, it was found that only 20% to 30% of the adult population maintained normal blood pressure readings. Meanwhile, potassium intake was below the recommended daily allowance of 4.7 grams.

According to the authors of the study: "An effective way of increasing potassium intake is to follow the guidelines for healthy nutrition more closely, including a higher consumption of vegetables and fruit. In addition, the use of mineral salts in processed foods—by which sodium is partly replaced by potassium—would contribute to an improved intake of both sodium and potassium." (Mineral salts are the natural, unprocessed salts, such as Himalayan salt and Celtic Sea Salt, which we told you about in Chapter Seven.)

The study concluded that people could lower their blood pressure by eating a diet rich in avocados, carrots, spinach and other greens, tomatoes, and other vegetables, and by reducing or even eliminating the consumption of processed foods.

Research shows that you don't have to take a supplement to get enough potassium to help lower your blood pressure. [265] You can make yourself a sunshine-colored fruit salad with bananas, papaya, and cantaloupe, or chomp on some carrots or celery; enjoy a turkey sandwich, or make yourself a nourishing plate of beans and squash with a side of leafy greens. [266]

Vitamin B-complex. Your standard B-complex supplement is made up of eight separate vitamins and three related substances: vitamin B1 (thiamine), B2 (riboflavin), B3 (niacin), B6 (pyridoxine), B12 (cobalamin), B9 (folic acid), B5 (pantothenic), B7 (biotin), choline, inositol, and para-aminobenzoic acid. B-complex is kind of a wonder supplement, doing everything from nourishing skin and hair to relieving fatigue. But most importantly, it helps the body manage anxiety and stress—and a relaxed body means lower blood pressure. [267]

Vitamin C. Many folks reach for this vitamin as the first line of defense when they're feeling under the weather. But did you know that vitamin C can also help lower blood pressure? It is not clear why, but it may be that vitamin C is an antioxidant that fights free radicals, rogue molecules that bind with oxygen and destroy cells. Researchers at Boston University School of Medicine found that one large dose of 2,000 mg, followed by daily doses of 500 mg of vitamin C over one month, resulted in lower blood pressure.

The average systolic pressure of the participants taking vitamin C decreased from 155 mm Hg to 142 mm Hg and the mean pressure decreased from 110 to 100 mm Hg. [268]

In another study, researchers at the Johns Hopkins University School of medicine found that taking 500 mg of vitamin C daily dropped blood pressure in those with hypertension by about five points. While that may not sound like a lot, it does mean a lower risk of cardiovascular events and stroke. Vitamin C improves the endothelial function of artery walls, restoring elasticity and helping repair micro-tears in the vessels. Vitamin C also acts as a mild diuretic, which also helps lower blood pressure.

Edgar (Pete) Miller, MD, PhD, lead author of the study, summed up the study this way, "Our research suggests a modest blood pressure lowering effect with vitamin C supplementation." Dr. Miller noted that taking in more than the recommended daily requirement effectively lowers blood pressure enough to lower risk of a heart attack or stroke.

If you would rather get your vitamin C from your diet than from a supplement, then eat citrus fruits, spice up your meals with red chili peppers, fill up with thick-leaved greens such as kale and collards, and go pick some strawberries. Other foods that pack some vitamin C are sweet peppers, parsley, turnip greens, broccoli, Brussels sprouts, watercress, cauliflower, and cabbage. Both of us like to flavor the drinking water we carry with us with a vitamin C product called Emergen-C (www.emergenc.com). For higher dosing we like BioEnRgyC formulated by Garry F. Gordon, MD, DO. We take between 12,000 mg to 20,000 mg daily.

CHAPTER FOURTEEN

ALTERNATIVE HEALING TECHNIQUES

In addition to a nutritious diet, adequate exercise and powerful supplements, alternative healing techniques can also help bring your blood pressure down to healthful levels. Here are some you might want to try.

Restful sleep. When we sleep, our bodies and minds rest, regenerate and heal. During deep sleep, blood pressure drops up to 20 points, arterial walls relax and the immune system is strengthened. Brain function and mood are both greatly improved with sleep. Sleep helps to reduce the levels of stress and inflammation in your body. High levels of "inflammatory markers" are linked to heart disease and strokes. During sleep, respiration, heart rate, blood pressure, and the body's level of stress hormones are all lowered. Sleep also helps to slow the aging effects of stress.

Achieving restful sleep begins with creating a bedroom environment and a nighttime routine that supports sleep. Remove all electronics from the bedroom. Use low-level lighting. As much as possible, maintain a consistent bedtime. To give yourself the best chance of a restful sleep, avoid caffeine for at least six hours before bedtime, aerobic exercise for at least two hours before bedtime, television news, and negative conversations. Add meditation or deep breathing and gratitude to your evening routine. Studies have shown that counting your blessings can make you happier and improves both your health and your sleep. [269]

POOR SLEEP LINKED TO RESISTANT HYPERTENSION

Poor sleep makes hypertension worse. That's the conclusion of research presented at the American Heart Association's Blood Pressure Research 2012 Scientific Session, showing that sleep plays an important role in regulating high blood pressure. In fact, poor sleep quality *doubled* the risk of developing drug-resistant hypertension in women.

Researchers, led by Dr. Rosa Maria Bruno, found a link between poor sleep quality and resistant hypertension. Her research noted marked differences in the patterns among women and men. "In women, poor sleep quality was strongly related to anxiety, depression, and resistant hypertension," Dr. Bruno explains, "but this was not the case for men."

"In women, we found that poor sleep quality was associated with a fivefold increase in the probability of having resistant hypertension," Dr. Bruno noted. "I would say that treating insomnia may improve resistant hypertension, although we need further data…on this."

Her conclusion? "We believe that insomnia is making hypertension worse."

Evidence from other sources adds strength to this hypothesis. Interrupted sleep increases cortisol levels and stimulates the nervous system. Both of these factors are directly related to elevated blood pressure readings.

The takeaway from this is to do all you can to relax more and improve the quality of your sleep. Here are some proven tips that can help…

Stick it to hypertension with acupuncture. There is a reason acupuncture has been used for thousands of years to treat heart-related issues in Chinese medicine: It works. In one study, the blood pressure levels of 160 hypertensives dropped significantly after they received 22 30-minute acupuncture treatments over a period of six weeks. If you feel a little wary of being stuck by needles—do not be. Acupuncture is painless, and many people find it downright relaxing. [270]

Chill out. If you're tired of looking at all the bottles of drugs you're taking for your high blood pressure, there may be a different kind of medication you want to take—a chill pill! One of the most enjoyable prescriptions for high blood pressure is to relax. If you find it difficult to calm yourself (and most likely many with high blood pressure do), there are effective, pleasurable techniques to relieve stress (see Day 26 of the 30-Day Plan, p.285).

Meditate. If you think you have to smell like sandalwood and wear Birkenstocks to try out meditation, think again. Meditation is nothing more than training your mind to focus your thoughts. This allows the body to become relaxed and balanced.

If you prefer a no-frills version of meditation, try this: Pay attention to your breathing. Just sit quietly, with perhaps some soothing music playing, breathe normally and focus your attention on your breath. When you notice your attention leave your breath, simply bring it back. Do that for 20 minutes and see how you feel. If focusing on your breath does not work for you, you can choose an image or flower or a word such as *breathe* or *relax*. But the basic technique stays the same: When you notice your attention lapsing, gently bring it back. Dr. Heilbron credits Kriya yoga and meditation as the most important contributions to his spiritual development.

Use your imagination. When some people meditate, they use a method called creative visualization. Even Olympic athletes use this method to help them create the outcome they desire. In fact, a cardiologist named John Kennedy, MD, created a special technique for heart patients that combines breathing with guided imagery. It is explained in his book entitled *The 15-Minute Heart Cure,* and his patients have seen results with it in as little as two weeks.

Simply move. If the idea of sitting still makes you feel even more stressed, think of more action-oriented ways to calm your mind, the so-called "moving meditations," including *tai chi, qi gong,* and yoga.

We can thank China for *tai-chi* and *qi gong,* which have been used for centuries in that country as forms of gentle exercise that calm the mind as they relax the body. Both were developed as martial art forms before being implemented as exercise forms, and both use a combination of focusing breath and mind to regulate the body.

Tai chi and *qi gong* involve doing a series of very slow, flowing, almost dance-like movements that help you feel what *tai chi* and *qi gong* practitioners call *qi* (pronounced "chee") or subtle energy in your body. In *tai chi,* the movements are more complex and choreographed, while *qi gong* features simpler movements.

What exactly is *qi*? Qi is the invisible-to-the-eye life force of all things. If you put your palms together closely without actually allowing them to touch, you may feel an energy in the space in between your hands. If you do, you are sensing *qi*.

In Chinese medicine, cultivating *qi* helps heal the body. Whether you sense *qi* or not, *tai chi* and *qi gong* get results. A large review of 22 studies on tai chi, sponsored by the National Center for Complementary and Alternative Medicine, found that performing *tai chi* regularly lowers blood pressure. [271] In some studies, it has even proven itself to be just as effective as aerobic exercise for mitigating hypertension. *Tai chi's* healing effects has made it pretty popular. According to a 2007 National Health Interview Survey, approximately 2.3 million adults in the US had performed tai chi in the previous year. So if you decide to give tai chi a try, you'll be in good company.

Qi gong is also a winner for those struggling with high blood pressure. A 30-year study followed the progress of two groups of hypertensive patients. All of them had been given blood pressure medication, but half also practiced *qi gong*. Those who did not practice *qi gong* were twice as likely to suffer a stroke or die from stroke, as those who were doing the simple *qi gong* exercises.

In addition, *qi gong* practitioners were able to cut back on their hypertension drugs—30% even eliminated them completely—whereas those who did not practice *qi gong* had to increase the dosage of blood pressure medication over time. You don't have to practice *qi gong* for decades to see results. Another study found that the positive, blood pressure-lowering effects of *qi gong* were experienced after just 10 weeks. [272]

Yoga. This is another increasingly popular way to reduce stress, and your blood pressure. And no, you don't have to be a human rubber band to do it. More than 13 million Americans use this form of exercise from India to stretch, strengthen, and generally calm down.

Yoga uses physical postures (in Sanskrit, *asanas*) and breathing exercises (*pranayama*) to achieve a harmonious relationship between body and mind, thus living up to its name yoga, which means "union" in Sanskrit. There are many varieties of *yoga*, including *kriya, bikram, vinyasa, ashtanga,* and *hatha*. Most Americans practice hatha. [273] There are different skill levels as well, from easy beginner to difficult advanced. If you are a newbie and you want to see if yoga's stress-relieving poses will work for you, check out a restorative or gentle yoga class. There are even classes called "Round Body Yoga" that are especially geared toward people who are overweight.

LOWER YOUR BLOOD PRESSURE WITH YOGA

The American Heart Association (AHA) cites stress management, weight management and exercise as proven strategies to prevent high blood pressure. Well, yoga does all three! Yoga is known to lower blood pressure, promote stress reduction, improve physical strength and flexibility, and assist in weight management.

In fact, yoga has been used for thousands of years to treat concerns like high blood pressure (HBP), a condition the University of Maryland Medical Center (UMMC) calls "the silent killer." *Yoga Journal* recommends certain yoga poses as therapeutic for high blood pressure. Well-known poses like Downward Facing Dog and Easy Pose are beneficial, but so are lesser-known exercises like the Big Toe Pose and Seated Forward Bend. You can find photographs of these poses at www.yogajournal.com or you can search the Internet. Here's how to perform these beneficial poses:

Big Toe Pose. Stand with feet together. Inhale through the nose. Exhale through the nose and bend forward at the waist, keeping the back straight. Grab the big toes and gently pull down.

Seated Forward Bend. Sit with legs straight and pressed together. Exhale through the nose and bend forward at the hips. Keep the back straight and reach for the toes.

MedIndia.net, a website managed by the MedIndia Network for Health, also recommends Camel Pose and the Knee Squeeze as being effective for high blood pressure:

Camel Pose. Kneel on the floor. Exhale and arch the back, reaching back for the ankles. Tilt the head and look at the ceiling. Hips remain in line with the knees.

Knee Squeeze. Lie face up on the floor with the legs straight. Exhale, bend one knee and hug it into the chest. Keep the other leg straight. Switch legs.

WARNING: AVOID THESE YOGA POSES

According to *Yoga Journal*, people with high blood pressure need to be careful with inversion poses such as standing on your head. This position increases pressure inside the blood vessels of the neck and head. However, starting with mild inversions and gradually increasing the degree of inversion over time may strengthen the blood vessels and could be beneficial in the long run. Just start out slow, and take it easy.

GADGETS THAT DE-PRESSURIZE YOU

In addition to exercising and meditating, there are also some smart new technologies that can help you reduce high blood pressure.

HeartMath. Founded by Doc Childre, HeartMath is a biofeedback modality based on over 20 years of published research and clinical studies that have demonstrated the critical link between emotions, heart function, and cognitive performance. These studies have been published in numerous peer-reviewed journals such as *American Journal of Cardiology, Stress Medicine, Preventive Cardiology, and Journal of the American College of Cardiology.*

The modality is used to reduce stress, improve performance and experience a more balanced life. It helps to cultivate a deep sense of inner calm and a life filled with increased energy and confidence and overall wellness. HeartMath uses a three-step process that can reduce blood pressure by up to 20% instantly. It now has a convenient iPhone app version. For more information, visit www.heartmath.org

Get into the Zona. A small, hand held electronic device, Zona, helps you perform isometric exercises with your hands to lower your blood pressure. Approved by the FDA, Zona relaxes the autonomic nervous system, which is responsible for the fight-or-flight response, and stimulates the parasympathetic nervous system, which is responsible for relaxation.

Relaxing and stimulating the two different nervous systems in this way has been tied to proper blood vessel dilation. The isometric exercises that Zona facilitates may also result in the body producing nitric oxide, which, as mentioned earlier, is known to help blood vessels open and relax. Learn more about Zona at www.zona.com.

Use a wrist cuff. Advances in blood pressure monitoring are happening all the time. The new type of cuff worn on the wrist may allow for a more accurate blood pressure reading.

British researchers from the University of Leicester, working with a health technology manufacturer in Singapore, HealthSTATS, have created a blood pressure cuff that measures blood pressure in the largest artery in the body, the aorta. The aorta is closer to the heart and the brain than those arteries in the arm, and researchers working on the project maintain that measuring the blood pressure from the aorta makes for a more accurate reading.*

It's well known that blood pressure from the aorta is *lower* than that measured in arteries in the arm. So, if your blood pressure is on the cusp of what is defined as hypertension, it could be that measured with the proper device, your blood pressure is less severe than you or your doctor believes.

Whatever type of device you use, self-monitoring is a terrific way to help you feel on top of your numbers, and take greater responsibility for your health. You will be able to tell your doctor

*http://www2.le.ac.uk/news/blog/2011-archive/february/blood-pressure

what your blood pressure levels are when you take them in your own environment, where you are at ease. Having your blood pressure taken in a medical office can make your numbers higher than usual because of "white coat hypertension," which we discussed earlier.

Also, monitoring your blood pressure at home lets you know how well your treatment strategies are working. As you try out new diet changes, exercises, and supplements, you can see for yourself how effective they are. And lastly, reading your own blood pressure means fewer trips to the doctor's office to have him or her do it for you—and that means less damage to your wallet. [274]

iHealth. You can now use your laptop for blood pressure monitoring! The iHealth Blood Pressure Dock works in tandem with an arm cuff and an app for your iOS-compatible device, such as iPhone, iPad, or iPod Touch. Dynamic, easy-to-read graphics illustrate the testing process while it is taking place, and help you chart your blood pressure measurements. You can even e-mail your healthcare provider or family members your daily results and history, helping your healthcare treatment to be that much more tailor-made for you.

CHAPTER FIFTEEN

DETOXIFY YOUR BODY
AND YOUR HOME

We couldn't end this section of the book without a discussion of toxins. As you read in Chapter Six, there is a direct relationship between the accumulation of heavy metals in the body and cardiovascular diseases, including hypertension. Environmental toxins have become a serious threat to human health and are now linked to numerous medical conditions. Indeed, there is much evidence linking these substances to ill health in general. This chapter should help you protect yourself and your family from this growing menace.

Persistent organic pollutants (POPs) are everywhere. These environmental toxins accumulate in body tissues, stressing the heart, liver, lungs, and kidneys as the body tries to eliminate them… causing cell mutations (which can become cancer)…disrupting the endocrine system (that includes all hormones, blood sugar metabolism, and the reproductive system)…and depressing the immune system, which leaves you vulnerable to infections and disease. POPs are in our water, air, and household cleaners. They are present in body care products such as shampoo and lotion. They are also in our foods and the materials used in processing and packaging what we eat.

WHAT ARE POPS?

The EPA defines POPs as "toxic chemicals that adversely affect human health and the global environment. Because they can be transported by wind and water, most POPs generated in one country can and do affect people and wildlife far from where they are used and released. They persist for long periods in the environment and can accumulate and pass from one species to the next through the food chain." [275] Here are some specific POPs and where they "pop up" in your daily life:

- **Antibiotics and growth hormones.** These are routinely added to the grains eaten by factory feedlot animals. They lodge in the animals' fat and are transferred to your body when you eat these meats. Whatever toxins your body is able to eliminate end up in your neighborhood wastewater system, which is recycled into tap water. The balance is absorbed into your body's fatty tissue. The more body fat you have, the more "opportunities" you have to accumulate these substances.

- **Pesticides and fungicides** are routinely sprayed on non-organic crops and absorbed by the plants themselves. [276] These have long been linked to the development of various cancers.

163

- **Genetically modified (GMO) crops**, are human-designed plants that have had their very DNA tinkered with. There are no long-term studies showing whether these crops are safe for animals or humans who eat them.

- **Meats and vegetables packaged in plastic and Styrofoam,** PVC (polyvinyl chloride), bisphenol A (BPA), and styrene. All of these are known human toxins. In addition, BPA is also linked to a higher incidence of diabetes. Some commercial food cans are lined with BPA and hard plastic water bottles may be made with it.

- **Dioxins and furans** are produced during industrial processes such as bleaching wood pulp to make paper and from burning trash, including medical and municipal waste. They are also found in wood preservatives and garden and agricultural herbicides. Nearly 90% of human exposure comes from eating animals (or dairy products) in whose tissues these chemicals have accumulated. [277]

- **Heavy metals**—including lead, mercury, arsenic, cadmium, and a host of other heavy metal toxins—are present in the environment and can disrupt our cells' abilities to create and use energy. Lead is ubiquitous in water, air, and food. Mercury is heavily absorbed from vaccines and seafood such as tuna and other large fish. Arsenic is present in foods treated with pesticides. Cadmium is generated by cigarette smoke.

IN YOUR HOUSE AND IN YOUR BODY

The tremendous amount of plastic used in our food supply is simply incalculable—and some of its residue ends up in our bodies. Think of all those salad bar containers, milk jugs, yogurt tubs, and bags of nuts and veggies you may use. Add to that plastic spatulas, rubber scrapers, cups, and plates, all of which come into contact with heat via cooking or dishwasher.

Cleaning products are another source of toxic exposure. They contain dangerous chemicals such as formaldehyde, trisodium phosphate, hydrofluoric acid, and others labeled as "irritants." Shampoos are made with *sodium laureth sulphate*, a suspected carcinogen linked to kidney and liver damage. Parabens are known hormone disrupters, yet they remain in deodorants, cosmetics, and hair dyes. Hormone disrupting *phthalates*—found in hair spray, nail polish, and products containing "fragrance"—are banned in Europe because of their link to birth defects and cancer, yet they remain largely unregulated in the US. [278]

In 2008, Jane Houlihan, the director of research for the Environmental Working Group, told a US House subcommittee that personal care products, including shampoo and cosmetics, are "the single largest source of risky chemicals that Americans are exposed to." Houlihan told the subcommittee: "Companies are free to use almost any ingredient they choose in personal care products, with no proof of safety required." [279]

HOW TO PROTECT YOURSELF FROM TOXINS

It's impossible to prevent your body from being contaminated by these environmental toxins. Even the Inuit Eskimos of Greenland, who generate no real pollution at all, display unacceptably high levels of man-made toxins that are produced in distant industrial countries. It is astonishing how far these toxins can travel to end up in the fat of the whale, seal and polar bear meat that make up the traditional Inuit diet.

While it is impossible to escape today's toxic chemicals, you can reduce your exposure by changing your purchasing, cooking, and food storage habits. More importantly, you can help your body's elimination system rid your bloodstream and fatty tissues of toxins that have accumulated over time. Happily, your liver is your body's "toxin filter." It helps disarm toxins and sends them to the kidneys for further processing so that they can be excreted via urine. (Yet another reason to keep your kidney function healthy.) Your colon also is involved in this detoxification process. Its mucous membrane keeps harmful bacteria and other toxins from entering your body, and the beneficial bacteria in your large intestine removes toxic wastes from the food you eat.

Here's the best news of all: You can begin detoxing your body on Day 1 of *The 30-Day Blood Pressure Cure Plan*. Here's how:

- By eliminating processed foods and factory meats, you are removing a major source of toxic chemicals from your daily life.

- Loading up on vegetables, fruits, and fiber-rich foods provides extraordinary support to your digestive system (including your liver) in clearing toxins from your body.

- Our focus on high-fiber foods works in your favor, since fiber binds to wastes and moves them out of your body.

- Daily exercise and physical activity begin stimulating your respiratory system, your heart and lungs, and are natural detoxifiers.

- As you begin to lose weight by eliminating sugar and other refined carbohydrates, you will be shedding the fat that stores toxins.

HOW PURE IS YOUR DRINKING WATER?

We couldn't survive very long without water, and yet our supply is swimming with toxins. Health officials continually remind us that tap water is safe, but this is far from true. If you don't already have one, you should get a good-quality water filter right away. Consider these facts:

- In 2009, a comprehensive survey of US drinking water identified widespread levels of pharmaceuticals and "hormonally active" chemicals all across America. The Southern

Nevada Water authority tested tap water from 19 US locations and found the most common residues included atenolol, a beta-blocker used to treat heart disease, antidepressant drugs used by people with bipolar disorder, estrogen hormones, the tranquilizer *meprobamate*, an epilepsy anticonvulsant, plus numerous antibiotics. [280]

- A 2010 *Chicago Tribune* story looked at the health-destroying effects of the herbicide atrazine, the most common chemical found in US streams and rivers. [281, 282] Researchers at Indiana University discovered an increase in nine different types of birth defects in infants whose mothers were pregnant during the spring planting season (April through July), when atrazine is sprayed on farmland.

Because of its harmful effects, this chemical is banned in Europe. But in the US, farmers, golf course owners, and homeowners still use this dangerous weed killer. Atrazine is a *feminizing endocrine disruptor*—a chemical that disrupts human hormones. According to new research, it is more dangerous at lower concentrations than once believed.

Atrazine ultimately ends up in our drinking water. Residents of corn-growing states have the worst contaminations, with up to 50% of them exposed to atrazine in drinking water, in that levels spike to 10 times the legal limit during planting season. Even at concentrations that meet federal standards, atrazine is linked to low birth weight, birth defects, and menstrual problems. Independent researchers are finding that children's reproductive and nervous systems suffer disproportionately from exposure. Wildlife also suffers: Male frogs reared in an atrazine environment turned into females and were able to breed with males.

For more on purifying your drinking water, see page 172.

DO YOU NEED A SPECIAL DETOX PLAN?

Detoxification diets are all the rage in some corners, but do you need one? Let us remind you that our book contains one of the best there is. Just follow *The 30-Day Blood Pressure Cure Plan* (found in Part 2, page 175) and your body will begin to detox naturally.

We don't recommend special detox "cleansing" diets and fasting regimens because they can dramatically disturb your metabolism—and may even do long-term damage. Your body needs a steady source of nutrients that are sorely lacking in fad diets, so avoid these quick fixes. We recommend that you reject any dietary protocol that could overstress your body's metabolism. [283] Here's what you can and should do to reduce your body's toxic load instead:

HELP YOUR LIVER DO A BETTER JOB

Your liver is your body's filter for toxins. It is an amazing toxin clearinghouse. All blood leaving your stomach and intestines heads first to the liver, which metabolizes nutrients and sends them off to where they are needed. At the same time, the liver breaks down chemicals as it cleanses your blood of toxins such as alcohol and any other chemicals you've ingested, absorbed, or inhaled.

A healthy liver is highly efficient, filtering up to two liters of blood every minute. [284] It also screens out pathogenic bacteria from the bloodstream, thus helping you resist infection and sickness. The bile your liver secretes helps break down fats in the blood so they can be absorbed for nourishment or stored for energy later. Your liver also produces good HDL cholesterol needed to carry fats through the body for the creation of hormones and to keep the walls of your cells strong and impermeable.

Cholesterol is the building block for all your hormones. If a doctor or someone tells you your cholesterol is high and tries to start you on a statin drug, please have him or her check your hormones first, including cortisol, estrogen, progesterone, testosterone, and DHEA. Cholesterol is the building block for all of these. Thyroid also regulates cholesterol production. So get your hormones checked before you tinker with your cholesterol. Your real problem could be an easily corrected hormonal imbalance. (For a more in-depth understanding of cholesterol, see Dr. Heilbron's YouTube presentation, "Cholesterol High? Ask Why!" at http://www.youtube.com/watch?v=35TObk1_60w.)

Below are some other practical detoxification tips. For more information and suggestions about detoxing, see Day 26 in the 30-Day Plan (p.285).

Be extra kind to your liver. Given its important role in cleaning up your body's toxic load, you should avoid damaging it with harmful foods and substances (such as POPs, HFCS and PUFA oils) or keep it busy with one task (such as clearing out excess alcohol). Otherwise, it can't be available when you need it to filter other environmental toxins.

Beat the yeast. Having any kind of yeast infection overtaxes your body. The standard medical solution is antibiotic treatment, but there is a reliable alternative. Caproyl is a liquid antifungal made from liquid caprylic acid and mixed into a high-quality, non-GMO, first-pressed, solvent-free oil base. In a study at Japan's Niigata University School of Medicine, caproyl was found to be extremely effective in fighting yeast infections and other systemic infections. Researchers concluded: "The fungicidal effect of caprylic acid on *Candida albicans* was exceedingly powerful…Caprylic acid exhibits remarkable fungistatic and fungicidal properties." Caproyl can be purchased at your local health food store or online.

Perfect your elimination. Your body is marvelously designed to clear out all the toxins to which it is exposed. The liver, the kidneys, and the intestines all eliminate waste. When you observe domestic animals, you can see that every time they eat, they eliminate. We humans should be the same. Having several bowel movements throughout the day pushes toxins out of your body before they can contaminate you.

We recommend beginning your day with a morning tablespoon of Caproyl, a teaspoon of psyllium seed powder, a tablespoon of liquid bentonite (a clay made of hydrated aluminum silicate that contains minerals such as calcium, magnesium and iron), and one-third teaspoon of Multidophilus (a probiotic) mixed into eight ounces of water. This protocol opens up your bowels, liver, and kidneys. This will help keep your bowel movements regular. (Without regular bowel movements, the body reabsorbs the toxins into the gut and can create an overgrowth of *Candida* bacteria.)

HERBAL DETOX HELPERS

Chemical pollutants, exhaustion, poor eating habits, and chronic allergies can cause your liver to go sluggish. [285] Once this occurs, it is fine to use herbs to coax the detox process along. People have been using healing herbs for thousands of years. Remember, though, that as your liver gets assistance from herbs in clearing the junk from your body, the toxins themselves will move through your bloodstream on their way out the door. This can cause temporary fatigue, a little malaise, nausea, or even a mild skin rash. (These are common symptoms when detoxification is occurring.) Start gently on low doses of detox herbs so you don't have any extreme reactions. Here are some of our favorite liver-supporting herbs:

Milk thistle. Also known as *silymarin*, this plant remedy has been used for more than 2,000 years [286] to protect the liver from damage and help it regenerate healthy cells. Multiple studies show that milk thistle is effective in protecting the liver from environmental toxins, including long-term alcohol use, plus the damage caused by pharmaceutical and over-the-counter drugs. Milk thistle's magic lies in the seeds that hold its active ingredient, *flavonolignans*, which actually alter cell membranes so that only tiny amounts of toxins can enter liver cells. It also stimulates protein synthesis for regeneration and repair of liver cells. In addition, these seeds contain essential fatty acids that serve as anti-inflammatory compounds in the liver.

Professional herbalists and alternative practitioners often recommend milk thistle as an herbal tincture for liver cleansing and healing—but you can also benefit from the capsule form. By stimulating the flow of bile through the liver, digestion and elimination are both improved.

Visit a naturopath, clinical herbalist or natural pharmacy for guidance on taking milk thistle. Generally, tinctures and extracts sold in natural foods stores can be taken by the dropper, added to a small amount of warm water. Start with one dropper once or twice a day and gradually increase it to two or three until you experience results. Milk thistle is often combined with licorice or dandelion, which also support liver health.

Burdock. This is another thistle herb used to cleanse the blood by helping your kidneys filter out impurities. We like to use a tincture of burdock along with milk thistle to ensure that toxins released from the liver don't hang around in your bloodstream very long.

Turmeric. Called the "king of spices," this Ayurvedic herb has long been used for liver cleansing. Its active ingredient is *curcumin,* a potent anti-inflammatory and antioxidant. Remember that your liver produces bile to move out toxins. Turmeric speeds the flow of bile and its toxic load. If you don't want to purchase supplements, just locate some organic turmeric and start sprinkling it on everything from eggs to chili. While it is boosting your liver function, you also will be boosting brain power. A study published by the *American Journal of Epidemiology* looked at the link between curry consumption (curry is made with turmeric) and brain function in older Asian adults. The researchers found that those who ate the most turmeric had the lowest rates of cognitive decline. [287]

There's even more good news if you're concerned about Alzheimer's disease. According to the *Journal of Neuroscience Research,* curcumin actually inhibits amyloid proteins from forming in the brain. These proteins are a hallmark of Alzheimer's. [288] Turmeric also helps to reduce the inflammation associated with arthritis. Other research shows that it helps prevent infections and cancer, so shake it on your food liberally.

HEAVY METAL-REMOVERS

Heavy metal toxins such as mercury and lead have been implicated in cardiovascular disease. Dr. Heilbron has observed patients with elevated lead and mercury levels who, after chelation therapy with EDTA and DMSA (discussed below), displayed dramatic improvements in their lipid profiles. Here are some other effective detoxification helpers:

Cilantro. Also called Chinese parsley or coriander, cilantro (*Coriandrum sativum*) has been shown to help prevent lead from being absorbed by the body. A solution made with cilantro also helped remove mercury from the body in laboratory animal studies.

Chlorella. This green algae has demonstrated the ability to take up toxic metals in its environment, thus decreasing reabsorption of heavy metals excreted into the gut from the liver-biliary system. Chlorella's influence is even stronger when used in conjunction with garlic and cilantro. Researchers observed a dramatic reduction of 66.03% in blood lead levels in laboratory animals receiving chlorella extract while being exposed to lead.

Garlic. It has been demonstrated by researchers to be beneficial in the management of heavy metal toxicity. Garlic was especially effective in dealing with lead, cadmium, and mercury.

Alpha Lipoic Acid (ALA). Mostly known for its attribute as a powerful antioxidant, ALA also possesses the ability to directly chelate heavy metals—especially mercury, arsenic, cadmium, and copper.

YOUR SKIN RELEASES TOXINS, TOO

Your body's largest organ is your skin—and it is the frontline defender and detoxifier. Just as skin absorbs toxins, it also purges them, releasing toxins in perspiration and body oils via sweat glands and oil glands. Each sweat gland acts like a tiny kidney, sweating out heavy metals such as mercury and oil-based toxins like petroleum products, which occur in many cosmetics. In keeping with the idea of a gentle detox, avoid extremes such as extended stays in any hot environment, such as steam baths and saunas. Sweat out toxins in short spurts, while keeping your cool by following these tips:

- Work up a sweat by exerting yourself with vigorous exercise regularly to stimulate perspiration and detoxing.

- Sweat in a sauna, steam room, or hot tub to open up pores and warm your body. This helps mobilize toxins to exit your body via the skin. Just a few minutes in any of these, with lots of fresh cool water afterward to replenish your liquid reserves, can be remarkably effective in releasing toxins through the skin.

- Drink a liberal amount of fresh water throughout the day to support normal perspiration, which also eliminates unfriendly chemicals.

Washing: How you bathe is very important. Be certain to systematically clean every part of your body. Use only natural, organic, non-perfumed soaps. Give yourself a little massage into the muscles while you're at it.

Massage: Speaking of massage, this is an excellent way to relax your muscles, remove tension, and improve circulation. Massage has multiple health benefits. One popular masseuse we know now claims that we store "emotional issues in the tissues." Massage can help you release toxic patterns from the muscles and your body.

CHELATION THERAPY

Since 1953, EDTA-chelation has been approved by the FDA to remove toxic heavy metals such as lead, mercury, cadmium, and arsenic from the bloodstream. Lowering the levels of these toxins will allow your liver to more effectively remove other toxins as well.

Toxins block the ability of your cells to function correctly. When cells can't function correctly or stop producing certain chemicals, illness can occur. This, in turn, initiates a decrease in hormone production, triggers inflammatory problems such as arthritis, stimulates allergies and plaque buildup, and causes a decrease in brain function with memory loss and "brain-fog." The removal of toxins will help your cells to work better and improve your health in general.

One of the main reported benefits of chelation therapy is the improvement—and some say the *reversal*—of cardiovascular disease. While there have been tens of thousands of anecdotally reported case histories of cardiovascular benefit, chelation therapy has never had an "official" double-blind study proving its effectiveness. This changed with the November 4, 2012, release of a 10-year, $30 million nationwide study sponsored by the National Institutes of Health (NIH) called TACT (the Trial to Assess Chelation Therapy). (Dr. Heilbron was one of the TACT investigators for Mount Sinai Hospital in Miami, Florida.)

CHELATION PROVEN TO WORK

According to the results of the TACT study, chelation therapy is indeed effective at improving cardiovascular disease and preventing heart attacks. Take a look:

Chelation Therapy Results:

Overall improvement with vitamins	26%
Overall improvement	18%
Death reduced	7%
Heart attacks reduced	23%
Hospitalizations reduced	28%
Diabetes cardiac complications reduced	39%
Surgeries reduced	19%
Strokes reduced	23%

Chelation is usually administered intravenously (IV) over a three-hour period or through a daily oral program. Dr. Heilbron offers both IV and oral chelation therapy at his clinic in Santa Fe, New Mexico. Most patients do 10 to 20 IV treatments initially, usually by getting one or two treatments per week, followed by monthly IV maintenance therapy. In between IVs, patients continue their therapy by taking daily oral chelation pills and high-quality daily multivitamins with minerals to replenish and support the process. Patients are closely monitored during this process. Kidney function is checked regularly, and the Metal Toxins Test is repeated every six months.

The American College for Advancement in Medicine (ACAM) provides a list of physicians with intensive training in the use of EDTA chelation therapy. Ask your doctor if she/he has been trained by ACAM. For further information and to obtain a Physician Referral to a Complementary, Alternative and Integrative Medicine (CAIM) physician that is affiliated to ACAM, please visit www.acam.org.

11 WAYS TO DETOX YOUR SURROUNDINGS

We recognize that making big shifts in your lifestyle can be challenging and tough to implement all at once. That's why *The 30-Day Blood Pressure Cure Plan,* which begins on page 175, gives you plenty of time to acclimate to new ideas, foods, and habits. Making small incremental daily changes is a much easier and more sustainable way to change your life. It is the same with detoxing your environment and your body. You won't do it in a single day, but you *can* start today by taking steps that will clear your kitchen, bathroom, and cosmetics shelf of products that make it harder to heal your hypertension. Here are some helpful tips:

Get a water filter. Stop buying bottled water—it's bad for your budget and all those plastic bottles represent an environmental disaster. Instead, as we recommended earlier, buy a high-quality water filter to remove pesticides, pharmaceuticals, and other impurities from your drinking water. You don't have to buy an expensive filter, but we enthusiastically encourage you to make this investment in your family's health. We recommend that you drink 64 ounces of pure water every day, so you are going to need a reliable unit. The one we like best is the Katadyn Combi Water Filter, with an attachment for your tap. It has a ceramic element that filters more than 13,000 gallons of drinking water before requiring replacement. This filter removes both bacteria and toxic chemicals from your water. [289] While you may pay a little more for this water filter, it is worth it. The Katadyn Combi filters water to .2 microns, which is as safe as you can get. Be sure to use a glass bottle, glass-lined thermos, or stainless steel bottle to carry your drinking water with you. Waterwise Systems also sells water distillers that are very good. In addition, the Rettin Company makes a good filter/ionizer that also gets our "thumbs up." (Remember to get a filter for your shower too, because the chlorine in tap water when heated is especially toxic.)

Pitch the plastic. Replace plastic wrap, plastic bags, and plastic storage containers with good old-fashioned wax paper and foil. Wax-paper sandwich bags are available in natural foods stores. Or just buy a roll of wax paper or foil. Wrap sandwiches with it and use it to cover glass bowls in the fridge. Then re-use it.

Go with glass. Look for Pyrex storage containers with rubber lids. These come in a variety of sizes and make a good choice for carrying a healthy lunch to work. Plastic containers and plastic wrap should never be heated in a microwave. In fact, avoid using microwaves if at all possible because microwaving alters the energy vibration of food. Repurpose (or "up-cycle") all your old plastic containers and yogurt tubs. Every workshop, mechanic, and gardener can use these for screws, nails, seeds, and small tools. Kids can play with them in the bathtub and sandbox. If they are overwhelming your kitchen, bid them "adieu" and toss into the recycle bin. Avoid buying more in the future.

Check your city's approved plastics for recycling. If you must purchase plastic products, check your city's recycling program and learn which plastics they recycle. Not every city recycles the same plastics. For example, your city might only recycle plastics with codes 2, 4 and 5.

Nix the non-stick. Replace non-stick cookware with stainless steel baking sheets, glass pans and casserole dishes, enamel cookware, or cast iron skillets. Teflon and other non-stick coatings decompose at high heat and pass into your body. A study done by the Environmental Working Group showed that Teflon pans preheated on "high" on an ordinary stovetop can reach temperatures of 700+ degrees F in three minutes. At the same time, studies by DuPont (the manufacturer) show that Teflon off-gasses toxic particulates at 446 degrees F! At 680 degrees F, no fewer than six toxic gasses are released—including carcinogens, pollutants, and other dangerous compounds. These fumes cause "polymer fume fever," which can disorient your brain. Long-term studies on these health hazards have not been conducted yet, but why wait?

Unplastic your utensils. Pitch plastic serving and cooking utensils (now that you've ditched your non-stick pans, there's no need for them anyway). Your cast iron skillet will be fine with the same wooden spoons and metal spatulas your grandma used. For the picnic set, replace plastic cups and plates with lightweight reusable bamboo ones. Avoid plastic as much as possible. But when you can't avoid it, do keep it away from the dishwasher and other heat sources.

Can the cans. Buy frozen veggies and soups in waxed cardboard boxes (better yet, make your own soup). *Consumer Reports* in December 2009 published results showing that virtually every one of 19 name-brand canned foods tested contained some BPA, which leaches from the material that lines cans. The tests included juice, green beans, and tuna. In fact, they even found BPA in foods packed in cans labeled "BPA-free." [290]

Clean green. Advertisers want you to believe you need a different product for every cleaning task—but, of course, you do not. There are a host of toxic chemicals in most cleaning products, and manufacturing them generates huge amounts of environmental waste. Wean yourself off standard household cleaners with a trip to the natural foods store, where you will find cleaning products made with naturally derived ingredients, ones without phosphates and other environmental pollutants. Or, you can go completely natural. Ask your grandma or cruise the Internet for easy, inexpensive, clean and green cleaners made from ingredients like baking soda, lemon juice, and white vinegar. They will leave your home clean and fresh with no toxic residue. Congratulate yourself for taking this step by buying a few glass spray bottles to hold your new green cleaners!

Avoid toxic chemicals in body care products. Using chemical-laden make-up, soaps, lotions, and other body care products daily can amount to an astonishing five pounds of toxic chemicals absorbed by your body each year. Among the worst offenders are parabens (*para-hydroxybenzoic acids*), the most widely-used preservatives in cosmetics. They are in everything from shampoo and soap to make-up, deodorant, and baby lotions. Parabens have even been detected in breast cancer tumors. [291]

When you bring chemicals into contact with your skin, they are taken up directly by your bloodstream. One study looked at 10,000 body care products and found that the average adult uses nine products daily—for a total of 126 unique chemical ingredients. Start reading the fine print on the back of shampoos, body lotions and cosmetics. You will be stunned by how many of them contain known toxic chemicals. Manufacturers say consumers are exposed to such small amounts that they are not dangerous, but researchers know better. Some European countries and Japan have banned many of these same chemicals to protect their consumers.

Chemical-free products for your body are predictably more expensive than others. But just like buying organic produce, wild salmon, and grass-fed beef, the return is worth the extra outlay to protect your health from these ubiquitous toxins.

Head back to your natural food store for skin products that are free of sodium laureth sulfate, parabens and petroleum products. Or just take a trip to your kitchen—coconut oil and olive oil make great skin moisturizers. One of Dr. Heilbron's patients slathers organic coconut oil on her skin every night. (No parabens in coconuts!) These safe, low-cost options will offset the little extra you pay for chemical-free cosmetics.

You will also discover that a lot of the products you thought you needed are actually unnecessary. Sticking to a few basic, natural products while eliminating the others will free up your budget as well as your toxic load. Finally, before you buy any body care product, go online to Campaign for Safe Cosmetics (www.safecosmetics.org) or Skin Deep Cosmetics Database of the Environmental Working Group (www.ewg.org/skindeep) to discover what is really in the products you use regularly or are considering for purchase.

Forget the fragrances. [292] Remove all air fresheners and scented dryer sheets, lotions, and candles from your house today—including anything with a fake "scent." The Natural Resources Defense Council released a study in 2007 that found most air fresheners and other scented products contain chemicals called *phthalates*. These are known hormone disruptors that affect reproductive development and are especially harmful to young children and babies. These toxic chemicals affect testosterone levels and produce abnormal genitals and decreased sperm production. The state of California says no fewer than five kinds of phthalates are "known to cause birth defects or reproductive harm," and advises pregnant women to stay away from them.

A study in the *American Journal of Respiratory and Critical Care Medicine* found that people using air fresheners and household cleaning sprays regularly have a stunning 30% to 50% higher incidence of asthma than people who did not use them. At the University of Washington, professor Anne Steinemann, PhD, did an analysis of some widely used scented products and discovered a whopping 100 unique volatile organic compounds, some of which are linked to cancer and problems with neurological, reproductive, and respiratory systems. [293]

Your local health food store and several online sources sell pure essential oils distilled from plants. You can put a drop of one of these oils on tissue and it will scent your home or car without harmful chemicals. Again, do your research to make sure the product you are purchasing is pure plant oil and has not been processed with alcohol or other chemicals. You can even use plant essence oils to scent your body instead of perfume or cologne. Because the oil is so concentrated, you must dilute it with a carrier oil before you put it on your skin. There is an entire branch of study called Unani Medicine that uses the pure essences of various plants to assist in bringing the body into balance. Whether you are interested in the metaphysical property of plants or you simply like the scent of real lilacs, pure plant essence oils are a non-toxic and inexpensive way to add pleasant scents to your environment.

PART TWO

THE 30-DAY BLOOD PRESSURE CURE PLAN

PHASE ONE:

DAYS 1 TO 10

Ground rules: Learn which foods you need to include in your diet—as well as those to leave out going forward. Write personal entries in your Success Planner every day.

DAY 1: MONITOR YOUR BLOOD PRESSURE

"If you don't know your blood pressure,
it's like not knowing the value of your company."

~Mehmet Oz, MD

Today is all about taking control of your own blood pressure readings. You'll learn why monitoring your own blood pressure is the first step toward curing hypertension, how to buy a home blood-pressure monitor, plus learn how and when to use it.

TAKING YOUR OWN BLOOD PRESSURE

As you learned in Chapter 4 in Part One, 25% of Americans with an official diagnosis of hypertension actually *do not* have it at all. How can this be? A new study confirms a quirky phenomenon called "white coat hypertension," in which the very presence of a doctor can send your blood pressure up.

This means that as many as 20 million hypertension patients may be taking drugs and modifying their diet and lifestyle for a condition they don't have. Could you be one of them? There's only one way to know for sure: by taking your own blood pressure in the comfort of your own home. Studies reveal that patients who track their blood pressure with home monitors receive the most accurate readings, thus eliminating the "white coat" effect.

HOME MONITORING HELPS LOWER BLOOD PRESSURE

Standard medical care is no match for a home blood pressure monitoring program for keeping hypertension in check, according to a randomized trial published online in *Circulation: Cardiovascular Quality and Outcomes.**

■ Nearly twice as many patients monitoring themselves at home reached their blood pressure goals after six months.

■ At six months, the average blood pressure of patients in the home monitoring group was significantly lower than in the usual care group. Those being home-monitored experienced a 12.4 mmHg larger drop in systolic blood pressure and a 5.7 mmHg larger drop in diastolic blood pressure than those in the usual care group.

■ The benefits of the home monitoring program were even better for patients with diabetes and/or chronic kidney disease (52% reached their target goal compared with 22% in usual medical care).

*Magid DJ, et al "A Pharmacist-led, American Heart Association Heart360 web-enabled home blood pressure monitoring program" http://www.medpagetoday.com/Cardiology/Hypertension/37694

HELPING TO REDUCE OR ELIMINATE YOUR MEDS

Home monitoring is also shown to be very effective in having the patient's medications adjusted to lower doses—or completely withdrawn. This can mean freedom from nasty side effects.

Home monitoring is valuable in another way: Keeping track of your blood pressure on a regular basis provides positive reinforcement for the good things you do, such as exercise, a better diet, and taking specific nutritional supplements that can lower blood pressure and keep you off drugs. When you see the positive effect these good habits are having on your readings, you are much more likely to stay with your healthy habits—and even add other positive behaviors. This, too, can result in having a drug dose reduced or completely eliminated.

PURCHASE A QUALITY MONITOR TODAY

Now is the time to buy your home blood-pressure monitor. You can order one online or pick it up at your nearest pharmacy. The brands and models for blood-pressure monitoring are endless. You can easily locate a decent monitor for around $50.

To be sure your monitor is reliable, take it with you to your next doctor's appointment and check its reading against the numbers the nurse gets on her sphygmomanometer. If both readings jibe, you can feel confident in taking your own at home.

Apple's new iHealth Blood Pressure Dock is made up of a blood pressure cuff with an attached cord that plugs into a plastic base where you then dock your iPhone, iPad, or iPod Touch. This allows you to look at the screen of your Apple device while taking your blood pressure and watching graphics that illustrate the testing process. Apple also makes the iHealth Wireless Blood Pressure Wrist Monitor. Simply put the small cuff around your wrist and start sending information wirelessly via Bluetooth to the iHealth app.

Whatever device or model you choose, make sure it's something you feel comfortable operating, as you'll be using it several times a day.

TAKING YOUR FIRST READING

Sit quietly for a couple of minutes and then start. Follow the manufacturer's directions for operating the monitor. The number at the top of the display is your systolic reading and the number beneath that is your diastolic reading.

- Your systolic reading is a measure of the pressure when your heart is beating.

- Your diastolic number is a measure of the pressure in your veins between heartbeats, when your heart is resting.

Take three or four readings, a minute or two apart, and on alternating arms. Then, average the readings for the most reliable number. Check your blood pressure three times a day: Morning, midday, and evening. Take the readings at about the same time every day.

MONITOR BOTH ARMS

We encourage you to take a reading on both arms, because the difference between each can be important. A new study [294] has discovered that a difference in blood pressure readings between the right and left arm in people with hypertension may indicate an increased risk of cardiovascular disease and death.

Even though hypertension guidelines recommending that blood pressure be checked in both arms date back to the 1930s, few doctors do it because of the extra time required. Now, this new study finds that when there is a difference of more than 10 mmHg in the systolic (top) reading between arms, it can signal a significantly higher risk of a fatal heart attack or stroke.

Note: If there is a significant difference in readings between your left and right side, bring this information to the attention of your physician immediately. A consistently noticeable difference in blood pressure numbers between the left and right sides of your body could be an indicator of some serious arterial blockage, and requires immediate medical attention.

KEEP A BLOOD PRESSURE LOG

Most blood pressure wrist monitors can store up to 99 readings, but it's still important to write these numbers down in your Success Planner so that you can see any trends easily. Recording these numbers in your Success Planner also makes it much easier to share these readings with your physician. In addition to the blood pressure numbers, also make note of the date, time and which wrist you are recording for each reading. Your emotional state is also of note, as is any caffeine use, recent exercise, and medication use.

Your blood pressure naturally fluctuates throughout the day and can vary depending on diet, physical exertion, climate, stress, sleep patterns, and other factors. Regular monitoring of your blood pressure can alert you to the effects, both positive and negative, that specific actions and foods have on your hypertension.

Enter the average of each reading in your health log so you have a record. This way you can tell at a glance how a particular food, beverage, or nutritional supplement affects your blood pressure.

This is a good habit to get into if you have hypertension; and it allows you to discuss your highs and lows with your doctor at checkup time.

WATCH YOUR NUMBERS IMPROVE

Self-monitoring is a terrific way to help you feel on top of your numbers and to take greater responsibility for your health. You will be able to tell your doctor what your blood pressure levels are when you take them in your own environment, where you are at ease. Monitoring your blood pressure also can help you and your healthcare provider determine the effectiveness of any treatment. As you try out new diet changes, exercises, and supplements, you can see for yourself how effective they are. Regular and consistent monitoring will allow you to detect any changes early, and react accordingly. Finally, reading your own blood pressure means fewer trips to the doctor's office to have him or her do it for you—and that keeps more money in your pocket. [295]

As you follow this plan, these readings will serve as motivation to keep you going. When you begin to see the effect of the positive changes you are making, you'll feel even more encouraged about taking charge of your health.

TODAY'S ACTION STEPS

- Order a blood-pressure monitor online or pick one up at your local pharmacy. Look for a monitor that attaches to your wrist, which is easier to use than one that attaches to your arm.

- Record your blood pressure three times a day: morning (upon waking), noon, and evening (before bedtime). Take three or four readings each time, alternating on your right and left side—then average them together.

- Record your numbers in your Success Planner, making note of your emotional state and caffeine use. Notice if your blood pressure changes with variables like the time of day, what you ate or drank, and your perceived stress level.

- Keep track of any significant changes in your diet and behavior and share them the next time you visit your doctor.

DAY 2: CAFFEINE SWAP

Coffee, anyone? "No thanks, I've had enough. One more cup and I'll jump to warp."

~Captain Janeway, Star Trek: Voyager

Your goal today is to reduce your caffeine intake; then monitor the effect this has on your blood pressure. Notice whether your reduced caffeine intake has a calming effect on your mind and body—and whether it helps you get a good night's sleep.

Today you also will learn how consuming caffeinated beverages can cause you stress, increase your heart rate and blood pressure, and even rob you of precious sleep. We will give you suggestions for coffee substitutes and motivation to incorporate them into your day.

TOO MUCH CAFFEINE?

It is well known that drinking caffeinated beverages constricts blood vessels, which raises blood pressure temporarily (for about an hour after consumption). But, if you "chain-drink" coffee or tea continuously throughout the day, your blood vessels never get a chance to relax, and that is not healthy.

Today, we are asking you to commit to swapping your caffeinated drinks with less stress-inducing alternatives. This step may seem extreme, but it is necessary for relieving your hypertension.

ELIMINATE AND MONITOR

Starting today, eliminate caffeine for five days and monitor your blood pressure diligently. Since we all react to caffeine differently, use this as an opportunity to observe the effect caffeine has on your body and blood pressure. After five days of caffeine abstinence and consistent blood pressure monitoring, you may gradually reintroduce caffeine. Start slowly, with just one cup of coffee or tea—or perhaps begin with decaf (which does contain a small amount of caffeine)—accompanied by monitoring your blood pressure 30 minutes to one hour after ingestion. If your blood pressure elevates, discontinue caffeine permanently. If not, increase your caffeine dosage and continue monitoring your blood pressure. In no case should your ingestion of coffee or tea go beyond four cups per day.

CAFFEINE STRESS

A study by researchers at Duke University Medical Center [296] found that caffeine exaggerates stress in people who consume it daily.

To determine the effects of caffeine on people as they go about their normal activities, the researchers enrolled a group of healthy, habitual coffee drinkers in a double blind, placebo-controlled study. That is, neither the participants nor the researchers knew when the participants were receiving caffeine or the placebo.

When the researchers compared the caffeine days with the placebo days, they discovered that caffeine consumption significantly raised systolic and diastolic blood pressure consistently throughout the day and night, and adrenaline levels rose by 32%. The researchers found that the elevated levels persisted as the evening progressed to bedtime.

"The caffeine we drink enhances the effects of the stresses we experience, so if we have a stressful job, drinking coffee makes our body respond more to the ordinary stresses we experience," said James D. Lane, PhD, associate research professor in the department of psychiatry and behavioral sciences at Duke.

If you already have high blood pressure, you should refrain from hyping yourself up further on caffeine. Much better for your health are calming drinks that will hydrate you without the stimulating effects of caffeine.

COFFEE SWAPS

Many coffee substitutes are made from roasted grains and are an acceptable alternative as you reduce your caffeine intake. Although they do not taste like coffee, these warm drinks are acceptable stand-ins for the comforting and familiar ritual of coffee drinking. Drinking these substitutes might make it a little bit easier to give up coffee for a few days—or permanently—if you notice that this lowers your blood pressure. (*Note:* Avoid products containing wheat if you are gluten-sensitive or are giving up wheat.)

LIST OF COFFEE SUBSTITUTES

Roasted grain beverages:

- **Dandy Blend.** There are many dandelion-based (or chicory-based) powdered coffee substitutes known as "dandelion coffee."

181

- **Pero.** Made from roasted barley, malted barley, chicory, and rye. It can be found in many health food stores and supermarkets.

- **Cafix.** Made from barley, malted barley, chicory, figs, and beet roots.

- **Teecino.** A blend of herbs brewed to produce strong coffee-like taste.

HIBISCUS TEA

Hibiscus tea (*Hibiscus sabdariffa*) tastes delicious and has been shown to reduce blood pressure. It is a well-respected traditional remedy for high blood pressure in many countries around the world. (See page145 for details.)

This tea can be brewed in the sun and can be enjoyed cold or hot. The tea is brewed from the flower blossoms (and sometimes the fruit) of the plant. Several brands make these available in single-serving tea bags.

While hibiscus tea produces reductions in blood pressure rather quickly, this effect is generally temporary, so it is wise to drink the tea on a regular basis. We are particularly fond of Hibiscus Superflower Tea produced by The Republic of Tea Company. "Red Zinger" by Celestial Seasonings is another popular brand of hibiscus tea. Note: Never discontinue any medication without speaking to your doctor first.

OTHER HERBAL TEAS

The shelves of your supermarket and natural food store are filled with a vast variety of non-caffeine herbal teas and beverages. Experiment until you find several that you are fond of.

TODAY'S ACTION STEPS

- Swap your favorite caffeinated drinks such as coffee, chai, energy drinks, "sports" drinks, and black tea for the non-caffeinated beverages suggested here for at least five days.

- Monitor your blood pressure 30 minutes to one hour after ingestion. If your blood pressure elevates, you should consider discontinuing caffeine permanently for the benefit of your blood pressure and cardiovascular health. If you notice no increase in your blood pressure, reintroduce your favorite caffeinated beverages and continue to monitor the effect they have on your blood pressure.

DAY 3: SODA AND ALCOHOL SWAP

"Life itself, when understood and utilized for what it is, is sweet."

~Benjamin Hoff, author of *The Tao of Pooh*

Today you are going to learn about why it is important to reduce your intake of sugar and sweeteners. Today you are going to learn why these sweeteners can harm your blood pressure—plus how abstaining from them can produce a positive effect on your blood pressure and overall health.

As you learned in Chapter Nine, refined carbohydrates in general are a secret cause of hypertension. The worst offenders, sugar and other sweeteners, such as high fructose corn syrup (HFCS), dominate the content of soft drinks and other sweet drinks. By eliminating these super-sweet beverages from your diet and switching to more "blood pressure friendly" drinks, you will be taking a giant step toward lowering your blood pressure and keeping it under control. In addition, since soda pop account, for 27% of the calories in the average American diet, you will be eliminating a majors source of weight gain.

LIQUID SUGAR SOURCES

Soda pop, alcohol, sweetened tea, and fruit juice are all examples of sugar-loaded beverages. Starting today, remove them from your diet entirely. You should also nix beverages labeled "diet" and "lite," because of the artificial sweeteners and harmful chemicals they contain. Diet sodas have been linked to depression, weight gain, and other health risks. [297,298,299] Even beverages labeled "100% fruit juice" can raise your blood pressure because of the high amounts of natural fruit sugar they contain. Likewise, you should abstain from wine, beer, and alcoholic beverages for the first 10 days of this plan (Phase One). If you are unwilling or unable to do this, you may have a dependency on alcohol, and you may benefit from professional treatment or a support group such as Alcoholics Anonymous. (Later in the plan you will be able to reintroduce moderate alcohol consumption as you monitor its effect on your blood pressure.)

While forgoing your daily soda may not seem like a big step, it may prove a difficult resolution to stick to. This is because, as you read in Chapter 9, sugar and sweets are addictive, just like alcohol and recreational drugs. Our brains have evolved to want sugar as an adaptation that leads to greater survival rates and reproductive success. [300] Not only is sugar the object of predisposed human desire, but sugar has been demonstrated to be physically addictive just like cocaine. Both satisfy the same reward center in the brain.

SUGAR INTAKE QUANTIFIED

Let's review the numbers presented in Chapter 9. On average, each person in the United States consumes 22 teaspoons of sugar daily, or 50 to175 pounds of sugar each year! Additionally, the intake of high fructose corn syrup (HFCS) represents another 50 pounds per person per year. This represents a 500% increase in sugar intake over the last 100 years. The consumption of soda pop and other sweetened beverages is a major source of this sugar intake, with each person in the United States averaging two sodas every day, or 56 gallons per year. However, drinking just one soda a day can add 15 pounds of fat to your body in one year, and increase your risk of diabetes by 85%! A single soda per day increases your risk of having a heart attack by 20%. And, if you drink two sodas per day, your risk of heart attack increases by a whopping 42%.

FRUIT JUICE AS LIQUID SUGAR SOURCE

Fruit juice raises blood pressure because it has been separated from the fibrous pulp of the fruit itself. This fiber slows the breakdown of fructose into glucose. Without the fiber, your body responds as quickly and in the same way to the fruit sugar as it does to any other sugar or sweetener: It elevates the blood sugar level, which increases damage to arteries and induces a corresponding surge in insulin levels, which exacerbates your hypertension. Instead of drinking juice, eat your fruit whole for a wealth of vitamins, minerals, antioxidants and other super-nutritious compounds.

HEALTHY SODA SWAPS

Water. The best thirst quencher you can give your body is clean water. Water is absolutely essential in all of your body's functions, yet most of us don't give ourselves adequate water. We recommend that you drink plenty of pure water daily (roughly half your body weight in ounces), which will hydrate your tissues and cells, aid in the healthy flow of electrolytes, and reduce blood sugar problems. This, in turn, will relieve your hypertension.

Avoid simply reaching for those nicely packaged bottles of water in the vending machines. The plastic that bottle is made from leaches into the water, contributing to hormone irregularities. If you store water in BPA-free plastic containers, this is probably acceptable. Making use of a glass jar or stainless steel bottle is the safest option.

Plain and simple—pure water is the best beverage you can drink, and can be transported just as neatly as a bottle of soda or juice. Staying adequately hydrated has numerous health benefits. While soda, alcohol, juice and other sweetened drinks pollute your body with sugar, sweeteners, and other chemicals—water simply rejuvenates. Planning now to have water accessible throughout your day is well worth the effort.

Beginning with water as a base, you can add a multitude of interesting flavors. Beginning on Day 11, you can also add a little fruit juice to your water for extra flavor. For these first 10 days, though, please avoid all fruit juices. Instead, try adding slices of fruit or veggies to give the water a little extra flavor. Cucumber slices transform the water into a cool, refreshing treat. Lemons add flavor as well as a boost of vitamin C. Add orange slices, watermelon, limes, or a few mint leaves from your garden. Be creative!

Add sparkle and extra fizz. If you've been a heavy soda drinker, you may enjoy the sensation of carbonation. You can still have your bubbles by drinking sparkling water, seltzer, club soda, or mineral water. Remember to read labels carefully and make sure you are buying only carbonated water and not getting any hidden chemical sweeteners! Also, beware the sodium content of mineral water. To ensure you are drinking quality carbonated water, you can easily make your own using a carbonation machine. If you decide to purchase such a machine—remember to throw away, as soon as possible, all the sweet syrups that come with it to avoid temptation.

Herbal teas. Lemon grass, mint, and ginger teas are wonderfully refreshing. Hibiscus tea is especially beneficial for those with hypertension. A Hawaiian native, the hibiscus flowers and fruit can be made into a tea that effectively lowers blood pressure. This effect is fast, but not long-lasting, so a daily habit may be beneficial. As you learned in Chapter Eleven, hibiscus tea may even be able to replace medication for hypertension, although you should always consult your doctor before discontinuing the use of any medications. If you enjoy the taste of hibiscus tea, we recommend two cups daily.

Fruit smoothies. Yogurt stabilizes your blood sugar and strengthens your immune system. Blend unsweetened yogurt with protein powder, a few frozen berries, and a splash of unsweetened almond milk or hemp milk. If you need it sweeter, add stevia to taste.

Black, green and white teas. Tea is one of nature's best medicines for hypertension. Black, green, and white teas contain flavonoids, which slow carbohydrate digestion, increase glucose uptake in muscle and fat cells, and protect insulin-producing beta cells in the pancreas from day-to-day damage. Tea also curbs your appetite, increases your metabolism, and boosts your endurance. Decaffeinated teas have the same health benefits.

To get the most from your tea, brew it from the leaf or twigs of the plant. Steep your tea for three to 10 minutes in piping hot—but not boiling—water. Drink it within one hour of brewing.

Coffee. This essential morning drink for many contains magnesium, polyphenols, and substances called quinides, all of which help to regulate blood sugar and insulin production. Brewed black coffee—hot or iced—is a great choice for diabetics. Avoid high-calorie cream and non-dairy creamers; instead, add a small amount of almond milk, hemp milk, or whole milk. Keep in mind, however, that you should only drink coffee after Day 5 if your daily readings indicate it has no adverse effect on your blood pressure.

Milk. The studies in Chapter 11 demonstrate that a proper balance of calcium in your diet reduces hypertension. Calcium is commonly obtained by drinking cow's milk. For those who are lactose intolerant, soy milk that has been fortified with calcium is an alternative. Remember to read those labels and avoid buying products that have been sweetened.

TODAY'S ACTION STEPS

- Get rid of any soda, diet drinks, fruit juice, and alcohol you have at home. This will eliminate the temptation to satisfy the cravings you will have for sugar.

- Plan for your new drinking habits by purchasing a water filter (see Chapter Twelve) and a glass or stainless steel water bottle to help you make this transition with ease.

DR. HEILBRON'S CASE STUDY: REVEREND GEOFFREY

"No more hypertension, no more medications, no more fatigue.
I can mow my lawn and don't fall asleep during sermons."

Geoffrey, an ordained minister, suffered high blood pressure, repeated blockages in his coronary arteries requiring seven stents, atrial fibrillation (a dangerous arrhythmia), elevated lead levels, and very low levels of the hormone cortisol.

After his seventh stent, Rev. Geoffrey came to Dr. Heilbron's clinic in a state of desperation. "Doc, you gotta help me," he pleaded. "I don't want to die."

His peak blood pressure (after exercise) was a dangerously high 220/92. Daily beta-blocker medication "controlled" his blood pressure to an average 152/77 (still too high). Though never formally diagnosed with Type 2 diabetes, Rev. Geoffrey's blood glucose level was 159 (normal is 100 or less) and his HbA1c level was 7.2% (normal is under 6.0%). He was clearly diabetic, which explains many of his cardiovascular problems.

I immediately placed him on *The 30-Day Blood Pressure Cure Plan* and monitored his progress regularly.

By the end of the 30 days, Rev. Geoffrey's blood pressure had dropped to 117/73, and averaged a healthy 123/73. This was without medication, because the health of his arteries had improved to the point where he was able to discontinue his beta-blocker. A stress test showed that his cardiovascular function was normal. As a bonus, his atrial fibrillation ceased and his heart beat was in a normal rhythm.

Rev. Geoffrey still needs to address his blood sugar issues. While his HbA1c dropped to 6.4% and his daily blood glucose readings averaged around 130, Type 2 diabetes continues to be a problem. I recommended that he begin *The 30-Day Diabetes Cure* plan right away.

Lab Results	Before the 30-Day Plan	After the 30-Day Plan
Total cholesterol	210	158
HDL cholesterol	35	48
LDL cholesterol	155	110
Triglycerides	78	64
Weight	188 lbs	180 lbs
Body Mass Index	22.4	21.5

DAY 4: ADD VEGETABLE JUICE TO YOUR DAILY DIET

"Let food be thy medicine and medicine be thy food."

~Hippocrates

Many vegetables possess substances that lower blood pressure naturally. Some of the most potent include: beetroot and beet tops, celery, spinach and other greens and carrots. These are all allies in the fight against high blood pressure. While eating these vegetables is beneficial to your health and blood pressure, juicing them can help bring your numbers down even faster.

DRINK YOUR VEGGIES

Today, we are going to teach you why it is important to add vegetable juice to your daily diet. Numerous studies show that vegetable juice can lower blood pressure as well as some medications—so, starting today, you're going to make the most of this healing liquid. We want you to experiment with juicing antioxidant-rich vegetables in yummy combinations. You should shoot for consuming six to eight ounces of fresh vegetable juice on *The 30-Day Blood Pressure Cure Plan* every day.

The goal is not to go on a "diet" for 30 days and then regress back to old ways of eating and living. Instead, this plan is about kick-starting a lifestyle change that will pay dividends for years to come. First, let us examine the benefits of drinking vegetable juice.

THE HEALTH BENEFITS OF VEGETABLE JUICE

Drinking fresh vegetable juice on a regular basis is one of the easiest, yet most powerful, ways to lower your blood pressure and boost your general health. Here are some of the health benefits that "drinking your veggies" can impart:

- Fills your stomach, leaving less room for hypertension-hurting foods and helps you lose weight in the process.

- Provides helpful vitamins and minerals, as nutrients from food are superior to supplements.

- Concentrated nutrition. One cup of vegetable juice equals approximately five cups of chopped vegetables. As a result, one cup of vegetable juice contains more health-giving phytonutrients than eating a salad or consuming a cup of leafy greens.

- Supports better blood sugar metabolism.

- Enhances disease-immunity.

- Reduces inflammation throughout the body.

- Supports healthy thyroid function.

- Supports a strong, steady, and regular heartbeat.

The best blood pressure healing vegetable drinks include some combination of carrots, celery, tomatoes, dandelion leaves, spinach, Swiss chard, parsley leaves and especially beets. What is it about these veggies that are so helpful in your quest for healthy blood pressure? Here are a few vital benefits:

Beets. The roots and green tops of beets are converted into nitric oxide, a gas that opens arteries wider, so blood flows with less pressure. Researchers have found that beet juice lowers blood pressure quickly, and that the effects last for 24 hours. [301] A study [302] showed that drinking a cup of nitrate-rich beetroot juice significantly lowered blood pressure in hypertensive individuals.

Cabbage contains a compound called *sulforaphane* that significantly improves not only blood pressure, but kidney function as well, [303] according to a new laboratory study published in the *American Journal of Hypertension.*

Carrots are full of healthful vitamins and minerals. Your body uses beta-carotene to make vitamin A, a powerful antioxidant.

Celery has long been used in Chinese medicine to lower blood pressure. Research also suggests it may help prevent arterial plaque buildup, and acts as an anti-inflammatory. Nearly every degenerative disease humans develop, including high blood pressure, has a link to inflammation. In many cases, high blood pressure is the result of arterial inflammation.

Dandelion leaves are a natural diuretic and are rich in potassium, which is necessary in balancing sodium intake and maintaining healthy blood pressure.

Ginger root has important active components that are thought to be volatile oils and pungent phenol compounds such as gingerols and shogaols. It can be juiced along with your favorite vegetables. Ginger may lower blood pressure too much [304] raising the risk of low blood pressure or irregular heartbeat in patients taking blood pressure medications—so consult your doctor.

Parsley leaves are packed with vitamins and recent studies [305] suggest that parsley helps relax blood vessels and thus improves circulation and lowers blood pressure.

Spinach contains folate and arterial-health-supporting peptides.

Swiss chard is high in antioxidants, which destroy free radicals and help guard against cardiovascular disease.

Tomatoes are an excellent source of lycopene (particularly when cooked), which has been shown to lower the risk of stroke.

HOW TO JUICE THESE VEGETABLES

Juicing your vegetables is an excellent way to get more produce into your diet, because veggie juice is nutrient dense and easy to drink. Just be sure to purchase "organic" vegetables since you'll be consuming the skins, which is where most pesticide residue dwells. You can easily consume several servings of vegetables in a very short time.

First, you're going to need a juicer—and the type you purchase will depend on the kind of juice you prefer. If you want to include all of the fiber in the vegetables you juice, you'll want an "all-in" juicer like the Vitamix blender (www.vitamix.com). This powerful machine pulverizes your veggies until they become a fiber-rich slurry. And since studies have shown that fiber protects against stroke, this is an easy way to up your fiber intake. However, not everyone likes the thick, mushy taste of fiber-rich juice. (Personally, we prefer to eat our fiber, rather than drank it.)

When it comes to juicers that filter out the fiber, you have a wider breadth to choose from. Between us, we have tried every major model on the market—and have been unhappy with the lot. The majority are underpowered, resulting in motor burnout or just slow going. Because their motors are so dinky, their feed spouts are small and limit the amount of produce you can insert. This means it can take up to 30 minutes to produce an 8-ounce glass of juice. And that doesn't even include the cleanup.

Then we discovered the Breville line of juicers (www.brevilleusa.com)—and it was like trading an old VW for a new Maserati. The Breville has a two-speed motor that is powerful (up to 2 hp!). Because the motor is so strong, the Breville engineers were able to add a feed spout that is almost three inches in diameter. This means you can grab a fistful of carrots or cram four or five stalks of kale into the wide spout without the motor bogging down. It just rips through the veggies with unbelievable speed and power. You can even pop in whole apples. Once upon a time, we had to pre-cut the vegetables before juicing, which added a lot of time. Not so with the Breville. In fact, the Breville makes juicing so much fun that you can produce a month's worth of juice (about five gallons) in about 90 minutes—and that includes cleanup. Since juicing every day can be a time-consuming and messy process, we prefer taking the bulk route and freezing a month's worth of fresh vegetable juice in ice tea bottles with screw tops. This way we are guaranteed a daily dose as soon as the bottle thaws. No muss, no fuss. You can purchase Breville's Juice Fountain Elite for about $300 online and from quality appliance stores such as Williams-Sonoma. Take it from us: This machine is worth every penny.

FORMULATING YOUR FAVORITE JUICE RECIPE

Generally speaking, leafy greens tend to be bitter, while carrots and beets are naturally sweet. Fresh ginger root can be quite spicy, so we suggest you start slow with it, and increase the amount as you get used to it.

Shoot for at least half of your amount to come from greens such as parsley, kale, celery, and spinach. Sweeten with an equal amount of carrot and beet juice. If you need a little extra sweetness, add some apple. We encourage you to experiment until you discover a mixture that is pleasurable and satisfying to you. Too get started, try making Jim's Blood Pressure-Lowering Veggie Juice (recipe on page 142 in Part One). If all this intimidates you a bit, you can ease into the daily juice habit by substituting a cold can of V8 juice until you decide to become more adventurous. According to a study published in the *Journal of the American Medical Association* in 2001, V8 juice lowers blood pressure significantly [306]—though probably not nearly as much as your own fresh-squeezed organic vegetable juice.

...OR ADD A "GREEN SMOOTHIE"

If you've ever had a "green smoothie" you know they are delicious and so good for you. All you need is a blender and some leafy greens. Mix water, ice, and a handful of leafy greens for a few seconds, pour into a glass and enjoy. Adding nuts, flax seeds, and other nutrients can make an even more powerfully healing drink. Right now you are abstaining from fruit and berries until you get your sugar craving under control. But, starting on Day 11 you can add them back into your diet—and your blender. Green drinks become naturally sweet treats by adding fruit, especially bananas and strawberries, although just about any fruit will sweeten the green concoction and make it a pleasure to drink. After Day 11, you can experiment with substituting coconut milk or juice for water.

When it comes to blenders, Vitamix is one of the best blenders on the market—and many green smoothie aficionados swear that it is "king of the hill." Its powerful motor allows you to blend all your ingredients—plus ice cubes—quickly, delivering a smoothie with an even, creamy texture. Any blender should be able to do the job, although it just may take a couple of minutes longer.

Green drinks are also made from dried-and-powdered grasses, including wheat grass and barley grass. Among other attributes, these grasses are high in omega-3, which is why grass-fed beef and dairy products are so good for you. A tall glass of green drink is better than a health insurance policy. Green drinks, powders, mixes, and supplements often contain one or more of the green superfoods—spirulina, chlorella, and barley grass. You can try them separately or find a mix that has all three.

Spirulina: A tiny single-celled algae that grows in warm water, spirulina contains 65% protein—the highest of any food—and contributes to the proper functioning of your pancreas, liver, and entire immune system.

Chlorella: This freshwater algae is loaded with protein—380% more than soybeans. It is extremely rich in vitamins and minerals, and contains nine essential amino acids. It is bursting with magnesium, which is essential for balanced blood sugar, optimal blood pressure, and healthy nerve and muscle action.

Barley grass: By weight, barley grass packs 500% more iron than spinach—and has 1,000% more calcium than milk. It is also an anti-inflammatory. Plus, evidence is building that barley grass can protect against heart disease and stroke by keeping the blood naturally thin.

TIPS FOR DRINKING YOUR GREENS

- Pill or powder? Pills you swallow, which is easy. Powders you mix with water, vegetable juice, milk, or soymilk.

- Just a couple of spoonfuls of your favorite green powder in your water bottle, sipped throughout the day can make a difference; or add green powder to a smoothie (my favorite choice). You may notice physical improvements within days or weeks.

- Browse the internet or your local health food store for these highly recommended brands and purchase a month's supply: Boku Super Food, Hawaiian Spirulina by Nutrex-Hawaii, New Chapter's Berry Green, Marine Phytoplankton by Ocean's Alive, Greens+, Emerald Energy Original and NanoGreens by Biopharmacy.

TODAY'S ACTION STEPS

- Make a shopping list of the high blood pressure-healing organic vegetables and buy them next time you go to the market.

- Experiment with juicing, blending, and mixing veggie juice, green smoothies, and green drinks. Commit to making green drinks a part of your diet.

- Monitor your blood pressure and record any changes to your blood pressure.

DAY 5: ADD TWO SERVINGS OF VEGETABLES TO EACH MEAL

"I grow my own vegetables and herbs. I like being able to tell people that the lunch I'm serving started out as a seed in my yard."

~Curtis Stone, chef, author and television host of *Top Chef Masters*

As you read in yesterday's entry, vegetables produce a powerfully beneficial effect on hypertension. That's why, starting today, we want you to eat two servings of vegetables at each meal. (See meal recipes on page 196.)

THE BLOOD PRESSURE BENEFITS OF VEGETABLES

While vegetable *juice* can exert a healing effect on your blood pressure, you also need to eat your veggies—and the more you eat, the better for you. In addition to the many nutrients they contain, eating whole vegetables adds valuable fiber to your diet. Vegetables are the healthful slow carbs that your body needs to regulate your blood sugar, repair any damage and regenerate new cells.

Vegetables, in their natural state, are a time-release source of energy, containing many of the essential nutrients your body requires to operate at peak efficiency. By remembering to eat two servings of veggies at each meal, you will know that your cells are receiving proper nutrition.

Of course, you will want to make sure you're eating the best quality vegetables available. We recommend you choose organic produce because of its superior nutritional content, as well as the absence of toxic pesticide residues. It may have a higher price tag, but if you consider the health benefits you are receiving from organic produce, it is a bargain compared with the health-destroying effects of chemically grown crops (also referred to as "conventionally raised").

While fresh vegetables are ideal, frozen organic vegetables are an acceptable substitute. We recommend that you stay away from canned veggies because a good percentage of nutrients are destroyed in the canning process. Also, many food cans are lined with bisphenol A (BPA) plastic, a known toxin.

If your food budget is feeling the pinch and it is impractical for you to go 100% organic, then at the very least buy organic versions of celery, collard greens, kale, lettuce, spinach, and bell peppers. These are the vegetables that are most heavily sprayed with pesticides. Generally speaking, a crop that grows above the ground is likely to be sprayed with pesticides several times per season—unless it is organically grown. (See "The New Dirty Dozen" list below.)

Of course, one of the best ways to ensure that your produce is fresh and clean and organically grown is to grow your own. Even if you live in a small apartment in the city, you can grow salad greens and herbs in pots on the balcony. And everyone with a tiny bit of kitchen space can grow countertop sprouts and herbs.

THE NEW DIRTY DOZEN PLUS™

Here is a list from the Environmental Working Group (*www.ewg.org/foodnews*) of 14 fruits and veggies you should always buy organic. Due to their potentially high pesticide residue or possible use of genetically modified seeds, it can be hazardous to your health to consume the conventionally grown versions:

1. Apples
2. Celery
3. Strawberries
4. Peaches
5. Spinach
6. Nectarines (imported)
7. Grapes
8. Sweet bell peppers
9. Potatoes
10. Hot Peppers
11. Lettuce
12. Kale/collard greens
13. Summer squash
14. Cherry tomatoes

ALWAYS Buy Organic

THE CLEAN 15™

Fruits and veggies that have an outer covering to protect them from external contaminants, such as corn, watermelon and other melons, are less likely to be harmful to you even if they have been sprayed with pesticides. This outer husk provides some protection. Below is a list, also from the Environmental Working Group (www.ewg.org) of fruits and veggies that are generally safe to consume, after washing, even when they are conventionally grown:

1. Onions
2. Sweet corn

3.   Pineapple

4.   Avocado

5.   Asparagus

6.   Sweet peas (frozen)

7.   Mangoes

8.   Eggplant

9.   Cantaloupe

10.   Kiwi

11.   Cabbage

12.   Watermelon

13.   Sweet potatoes

14.   Grapefruit

15.   Mushrooms

After you've stocked your refrigerator and freezer full of tasty, colorful organic veggies, keep your eyes and ears pealed for exciting and unusual ways to prepare and serve them.

EAT VEGGIES RAW

One of the fastest and easiest ways to get more fresh vegetables into your diet to help lower your blood pressure is to eat them raw. Many fresh veggies are delightful when eaten raw—either in salads or as yummy between-meal snacks. Delicious raw vegetables include:

- Carrots
- Cucumbers
- Celery
- Tomatoes
- Bean sprouts
- Bell peppers
- Onions

EAT RAW

Each of these vegetables is bursting with its own unique flavor, which you will begin to recognize and enjoy more as you become accustomed to eating them raw. Try putting them straight onto your lunch or dinner plate. Alternatively, you can whip up (or buy) a healthy dip, such as hummus or babaganush (eggplant dip). We also recommend dipping your vegetables in our Fatigue-Free Spinach Pesto recipe, listed below.

MAKING THE MOST OF YOUR VEGGIES

To preserve their nutrients, we suggest you keep vegetables in the fridge whole and prepare them just before they are to be incorporated into recipes for meals.

Dice, slice, and grate them to add to salads and soups. Add them to the grill when you're grilling meat. Stir them into your morning eggs for a delicious frittata. Roast them, steam them, or mash them up and make your own vegetable burgers.

Use vegetables to add flavor, texture, nutrients, fiber (which can lower blood pressure dramatically on its own), and color to your meals. Besides the recipes in this book, Jim's web site My-HealingKitchen.com has a wealth of good recipes to get you started.

ENJOY THESE RECIPES

Fatigue-Free Spinach Pesto Recipe

Ingredients

- 3 clove garlic, chopped

- ½ cup extra virgin olive oil

- 4 cups spinach, fresh

- ¼ cup shallots, chopped

- ½ cup pine nuts

Instructions

Combine all ingredients in a food processor and blend. Season with sea salt and pepper to taste.

Farmers Market Salad with Balsamic Vinaigrette Recipe

Ingredients

- 1 pound greens (arugula, cress, radicchio, frisee)

- 1 bunch radishes, peeled and sliced

- 1 sweet pepper, sliced

- 1 carrot, sliced

- ½ small red onion, sliced

- ⅛ cup balsamic vinegar

- ½ tablespoon Dijon mustard

- 1 clove garlic, minced

- 1 sprig of fresh minced basil or tarragon (optional)

- ¼ cup extra virgin olive oil

Instructions

1. Combine last five ingredients for the dressing except for the olive oil. Whisk in oil slowly and set aside.

2. Arrange the greens and veggies in a large salad bowl and either toss with the vinaigrette and serve immediately or serve with the vinaigrette on the side.

Vitality-Building Roasted Broccoli with Dried Cherries and Walnuts

Ingredients

- 2 small bunches of broccoli

- 1 tablespoon coconut or grape seed oil

- dash of sea salt and pepper to taste

- ¼ cup dried unsweetened cherries

- ½ cup walnuts, crushed

Instructions

1. Preheat the oven to 450 degrees.

2. Peel the broccoli stems with a vegetable peeler and cut the broccoli stalks in halves or quarters (slicing lengthwise).

3. Sprinkle the broccoli with oil.

4. Bake for 10–15 minutes.

5. Add the cherries and nuts and bake for 5–7 minutes more.

For more recipes, visit www.myhealingkitchen.com.

TODAY'S ACTION STEPS

- Search online for vegetable-based recipes that appeal to you. Create a menu for the week that features a few of these meals and dishes.

- Make a shopping list of these vegetables and ingredients so you will be ready to prepare them. The idea here is to start small with a couple of vegetables you're confident you can prepare and slowly, build a repertoire of favorite vegetable side dishes along the way. Visit www.localharvest.org to find a farmer's market near you.

- If you are trying to save money and need to buy conventionally grown vegetables, buy only those listed in the "Clean 15," because they are either grown with minimal use of pesticides, or have an outer covering that can be removed.

- All the veggies listed in the "Dirty Dozen" should be purchased organically to reduce your pesticide consumption. Don't be afraid of frozen vegetables—quite often, their nutritional value rivals that of fresh because they have been processed immediately. It is not uncommon for fresh produce to sit out on display in the supermarket for up to a week or longer. For the freshest produce (much of it picked the same day), we recommend a trip to the local farmer's market.

DAY 6: TAKE A BREAK FROM SUGAR AND SWEETS

"We don't need sugar to live, and we don't need it as a society."

~Dr. Mehmet Oz

Today you will begin to cut down and eliminate the sugar, sweets, and sweeteners in your diet. Eliminating your consumption of sugar and sweets will reset your metabolism, balance your hormones, and give you a strong foundation for your new dietary habits.

TOO MUCH SUGAR

The overconsumption of refined carbohydrates and sugar is a major cause of high blood pressure. In fact, refined carbs may be responsible for 90% of the hypertension doctors maintain is "idiopathic," or of unknown cause. Consuming sweets and other refined carbohydrates raises your insulin levels—and insulin makes your body retain sodium and fluid, which raises blood pressure. On the other hand, refraining from sweets—and refined carbohydrates in general—causes the body to release sodium and fluid through the urine via action of the kidneys (the process called natriuresis). Natriuresis lowers the concentration of sodium in the blood and also tends to lower blood volume because water follows sodium out of the body. Many diuretic drugs take advantage of this mechanism to treat hypertension. Current medical advice tells us to reduce our consumption of sodium in an attempt to lower blood pressure, but the real culprits responsible are sugar, sweets, and a high carbohydrate diet.

On Day 3, you took the first step toward reducing the sugar in your diet by giving up sodas and other sweetened beverages. Today you will finish the job by eliminating sugar and sweets.

Incredibly, the average American consumes over 22 teaspoons of added sugar each day. When you consider that the vast majority of the processed foods we buy and eat contain added sugars, that amount makes sense. This includes everything from fruit juice and frozen meals to bread, baked goods, and condiments. There is simply no way the human metabolism can process this much glucose, sucrose, and fructose. As a result, the hormonal system is thrown completely out of whack. Insulin levels remain high throughout the entire day and night, causing the body to retain fluid and elevate blood pressure.

WHY WE CRAVE SUGAR

Ninety-nine percent of human evolution took place in a hunter-gatherer setting; only in the last 10,000 years have cultivated foods been available for human consumption. So, humans have mainly consumed fats and proteins, with a smattering of fruits, nuts, and roots when gathered.

Because high-energy, high-sugar foods were scarce in a hunter-gatherer setting, humans are wired to crave them—cravings that persist today. Yet, we now live with an abundance of these foods, which we eat to excess.

Additionally, sugar is as physically addictive as cocaine, stimulating the reward center of the human brain when consumed. Food manufacturers realize this and design products loaded with sugar and sweeteners to "hook" us.

BEWARE OF HIGH-FRUCTOSE CORN SYRUP

One of the most widespread sweeteners is high fructose corn syrup (HFCS). It is in every type of processed food and beverage. In fact, it is used so frequently that HFCS has been deemed the leading source of calories in the American diet. [302] HFCS is highly processed, a potent package of glucose and fructose unimpeded by any fiber or protein and that HFCS is converted directly into blood glucose by our bodies, immediately upon consumption. That means it is turned into fat at a faster rate than normal sugar. What's more, studies have shown that HFCS doesn't stop hunger—so these calories won't make you feel full. Essentially, our bodies don't recognize the calories in HFCS, so we naturally eat more.

SUGARS TO AVOID

When you are reading food labels, keep in mind that sugar goes by many names. Here is a list of a few common forms of sugar, all of which are best to avoid:

- agave syrup
- barley malt syrup
- brown sugar
- dextrose
- fruit juice
- glucose
- high fructose corn syrup
- maltodextrin
- maltose

- raw sugar
- sugar beet syrup
- turbinado sugar

HEALTHIER SUGAR SWAPS

Beginning today, your goal is to eliminate sugar, sweeteners, and all foods and beverages that contain them, in order to break your continual need for "something sweet." If you find this very difficult at first, don't be dissuaded. If you must initially have a little sweetener for your coffee or tea, there are two sweeteners you can use that do not trigger your body's insulin response. They are stevia and xylitol.

Stevia. Known in South America as the "sweet herb," stevia (steviol glycoside rebaudioside) has been used for over 400 years without ill effects. It has been used widely in Japan for more than 20 years and is rivaling Equal and Sweet'N Low in popularity, as more people in the US are using it as a natural sugar substitute. It is naturally 200 to 300 times sweeter than sugar, so just a small amount will do. It contains zero calories and will not spike your blood glucose.

Xylitol was discovered in the late 19th century and has been used extensively in Europe since World War II. It is fairly new in the US market, but is rapidly gaining popularity as more people become aware of its unique health benefits. The body does not require insulin to metabolize xylitol, which means it produces a lower glycemic response than sucrose or glucose. It is 100% natural and can be found in fruit, vegetables, and mushrooms. It also occurs naturally in our bodies, with up to 15 grams of xylitol manufactured daily during normal metabolism in an average size adult. It can be found in gums, mints, candies, toothpaste, and as a pure sweetener from selected outlets or online.

These alternative sweeteners are healthful and will not affect your blood pressure negatively. Artificial sweeteners such as aspartame, however, have been linked to health problems ranging from brain tumors to fatty liver disease.

RESETTING YOUR METABOLISM

Eliminating sugar cold turkey for a period of two weeks will reset your body's metabolism so that your insulin levels drop to normal and your sensitivity to sugar will return. This means that your taste buds will become more sensitive to the natural sugars that occur in all fruits and vegetables.

SUGAR-CRAVING "RESCUES"

When the body craves the sugar and sweeteners that have been eliminated, there are a few quick "rescues" that will curb your craving while maintaining your new diet. Making use of these "rescues" will ease the transition into eliminating sugar:

Ice cubes. Sometimes all it takes to curb a sugar craving is something in your mouth, so grab some ice cubes and pop one in your mouth. The frozen ice may be all you need to put those pesky cravings aside.

Dark chocolate. Instead of grabbing a milk chocolate candy bar, reach for a slice or two of dark chocolate that contains 80% pure cocoa, which means it has a high level of antioxidants and a low amount of sugar. Plus, dark chocolate also contains magnesium, an important mineral for blood sugar balance because it helps cells respond to insulin.

Frozen grapes. Grapes are naturally sweet and just one or two will curb a sugar craving. Simply put a bag of grapes in the freezer overnight and they are ready to eat the next day. Grapes are high in vitamins C and K and contain fiber and potassium, making them a much healthier choice than candy or other sweets.

TODAY'S ACTION STEPS

- Starting today, eliminate all sugar, sweets, and sweeteners from your diet. Carefully read the labels of packaged and processed foods in your fridge and cupboards, and eliminate those products you find that contain sugar and other sweeteners.

- For the sake of your blood pressure, your weight, and your general health, avoid buying packaged, processed foods and beverages that contain sweeteners. Choose whole, unprocessed foods instead.

- Realize that the first three to seven days of going cold turkey will be the most challenging. After this period, your sugar cravings and "sweet tooth" will diminish. To make it through this initial period, you can defeat a particularly strong sugar craving by reaching for ice cubes, a couple frozen grapes, or a tiny piece of dark chocolate.

DR. HEILBRON'S CASE STUDY: BILL

*"I can't believe how good I feel. I thought I'd be on those medications for life.
Now I'm back on the golf course. It's like a miracle!"*

The nurses called Bill "Mr. Pitt" because of his remarkable resemblance to the actor Brad Pitt. But Bill's health problems were no fantasy. As a retired bank president, he was used to stress. He came to me with an uncontrolled blood pressure of 141/104 despite being on four blood pressure medications: a calcium channel blocker (*verapamil*, 240 mg twice a day)…an ACE inhibitor (*Enalapril*, 20 mg twice a day)…a direct rennin inhibitor (*Tekturna*, 300 mg twice a day)…and a diuretic (*HCTZ, hydrochlorothiazide* 25 mg twice a day)

That wasn't the worst of it. Bill also had metastatic prostate cancer and was told he only had 2 to 6 weeks to live. (This was January 2012—a year before he started our program.) He also suffered from polycythemia vera, (a blood disease) for which he had to have a pint of blood drawn every few weeks accompanied by a chemotherapeutic drug. He also had a history of parotid (salivary gland) cancer and had three central blood clots in his lungs. Because of his lung condition, Bill experienced severe oxygen-deficiency, requiring him to use supplemental oxygen constantly. When he arrived at our clinic, he was unable to walk 10 feet without stopping because of shortness of breath. Tests also revealed that he had an extremely high lead level and very low cortisol. Many of his blood values were abnormal.

After completing our program, Bill was able to run on the treadmill without oxygen, his blood pressure became normal (110/75) off medications, his polycythemia vera completely went away, and he no longer had to take anything for it. Additionally, his prostate cancer went into remission, his blood clots cleared, and he plays golf again. He is thrilled.

Lab Results	Before the 30-Day Plan	After the 30-Day Plan
Lead	70	2
Mercury	11	1
Cadmium	49	1
Arsenic	49	1
Cortisol	11 (low)	24
Progesterone	0	3.41
Estrogen (normal 30-40)	242	16
Hematocrit	0	31
HDL cholesterol	48.5 (very high)	43 (normal)

DAY 7: PROTEIN SWAP

"Calories from protein affect your brain, your appetite control center, so you are more satiated."

~Mark Hyman, MD

Today, you are going to improve your blood pressure and your overall health by choosing clean, high-quality animal and vegetable protein. Our bodies need protein to build nerves, tissues, bones, and to create new cells. Protein also helps our bodies generate hormones and amino acids. But the kind of protein we choose to eat can either harm or heal our blood pressure.

ALL MEAT IS NOT CREATED EQUAL

Some meat is terrible quality—filled with hormones, antibiotics, preservatives, and other harmful chemicals. Think processed meat products, cold cuts, bacon, and greasy sausage, plus junky hotdogs. Scratch these off your grocery list permanently.

Equally bad for your health are animal products that come from large factory farms where animals are penned up in crowded conditions that are a breeding ground for disease. They are fed an unnatural diet designed to speed up production of meat, eggs, and milk. These animals are routinely injected with antibiotics to control the diseases and parasites that breed in these disgusting, unhygienic conditions. Hormone injections are given to unnaturally speed the animal's growth so that its body can turn a profit more quickly. Scientists are now even experimenting with altering the genes of factory-farmed animals. This type of protein is not good for your health and contributes to inflammation, which is the source of high blood pressure.

You can avoid these bad-for-you products by reading labels carefully. Look for "grass-fed," "hormone-free," "organic" and "free-range" on labels. This will usually protect you from purchasing inhumanely raised animal products. Ask questions of your butcher and fishmonger. Learn where your food comes from. Get to know small, health conscious, compassionate ranchers who will sell their products directly to you from the farm.

In addition to being a clean source of protein, naturally raised grass-fed and free-range animal products are high in omega-3, the essential fatty acids that lower inflammation and are beneficial for cardiovascular health. Shop for fish that is "wild" or "wild-caught," and avoid anything that is "farmed." Ask your fishmonger for fish and seafood that has not been factory farmed or altered in any way.

Stay away from protein sources that are preserved or processed. This includes deli meats, hot dogs, bacon, sausage, jerky, canned meat and meat products, plus sandwich meats. Besides containing poor-quality animal sources, these products usually contain chemicals and preservatives such as nitrates and nitrites, which have been linked to cancer (nitrates and nitrites are known carcinogens). Canned meats and the meats used in products such as canned chili and soup should also generally be avoided due to the same reasons. Note, however, that not all canned meats suffer from such issues and are safe to consume. Such products are typically found in health-food aisles or stores. When in doubt, read the label. And if you are not certain, buy fresh.

SHOP FOR HIGH-QUALITY EGGS AND DAIRY

Just as all meat is not created equal, the same is true for eggs, milk, cheese, and yogurt. As part of your hypertension-healing plan, you're going to move away from poor-quality eggs and dairy products and toward the products that are better for your health, heart, and blood pressure.

Eggs are an excellent, inexpensive source of protein—especially when they come from free-range chickens that are fed an organic diet and allowed to peck at omega-3-rich grasses, weeds, and wild herbs.

In fact, a new study shows that a protein contained in eggs reduces blood pressure as much as the popular antihypertensive drug *captopril* in laboratory animals. These egg proteins have been shown to produce effects similar to ACE inhibitor drugs. [307]

This new finding about eggs and high blood pressure add to the positive nutritional image of eggs. Once regarded as a food to avoid, numerous research studies have concluded that eggs can be eaten without raising blood cholesterol levels.

Milk and dairy products from pasture-fed cows are also good sources of omega-3 fats. When shopping, look for organic, hormone-free milk, yogurt, cheese, cottage cheese, sour cream, butter, and other dairy products. Not only do they have more flavor, but they are much better for your health.

WHY ANIMAL PROTEIN?

Animal protein sources are complete proteins, meaning that they contain the full range of amino acids, which are the building blocks and repair agents of your body's muscle tissue. These sources include meat, fish, seafood and poultry, as well as eggs and milk and some products made from milk.

Plant proteins are incomplete, lacking in some of the essential amino acids. Incomplete plant proteins can be combined with other complementary plant proteins to create a complete protein. For example, the combination of beans and rice is the best-known example of pairing two incomplete plant proteins to create a meal that provides all the essential amino acids.

WHAT TO DO IF YOU ARE VEGETARIAN

If you choose to live a vegetarian lifestyle, it is important to teach yourself how to combine two or more incomplete complementary proteins to create a complete protein and assure your body gets all the nutrition it requires. Here are the most popular pairings of plant proteins that create all the essential amino acids:

Protein	Pair With...
Beans	Brown rice
Beans	Corn
Soybeans	Rice
Hummus	Pita bread
Chickpeas	Rice
Tofu	Sesame seeds
Barley	Lentils
Peanut butter	on multigrain toast
Oatmeal	Soy milk
Toasted cheese	Whole wheat bread
Cornbread	Beans
Farro	Crumbled feta

PROTEIN POWDERS

If you are concerned about getting enough quality protein in your diet, you might be interested in protein powder. Made from spirulina (blue-green algae) or whey (a milk by-product), protein powders are a quick and easy way to increase your daily consumption of protein. Add a scoop of powder to yogurt or almond milk for a quick, protein-rich drink. Starting on Day 15, you can make a delicious, high-protein fruit smoothie (or even vegetable juice blend) that makes a great breakfast or afternoon pick-me-up.

Protein powders vary greatly in quality and ingredients. Read labels to ensure you are getting a quality product with no added chemicals or sugars.

TODAY'S ACTION STEPS

- Remove all junky protein from your home and diet.

- Buy only organic, free-range eggs, milk, cheese, and yogurt. Speak with the butcher and ask for grass-fed, hormone-free chicken and turkey, bison and beef. If you must buy canned from time to time, consider products by Pleasant Hill Grain (www.PleasantHillGrain.com), which has an excellent reputation.

- Purchase wild Alaskan salmon (either fresh or canned) and other wild-caught seafood products. Your body and your blood pressure will thank you. Our favorite source is http://www.vitalchoice.com.

DAY 8: SMART CARBOHYDRATES SWAP

*"If we are creating ourselves all the time, then it is
never too late to begin creating the bodies we want, instead
of the ones we mistakenly assume we are stuck with."*

~Deepak Chopra, MD

Now it is time to replace the refined carbohydrates in your diet with natural and unprocessed "slow" carbs which will stabilize your body's glucose and insulin levels. This will allow your hypertension to reverse and can reduce the damage your body sustains when subjected to a diet high in refined carbohydrates.

CARBOHYDRATES AND METABOLISM

So far, we have talked a lot about the unhealthful role that refined carbohydrates—especially sugar and other sweeteners—play in exacerbating hypertension. While doctors and government officials continue to advise the public to adopt a low-sodium, low-fat diet and dutifully take drugs to reduce high blood pressure, these recommendations are scientifically unfounded. As you read in Chapter Nine, refined carbohydrates are the true culprits in the majority of hypertension cases.

Today, we are going to focus on eliminating the many sources of refined carbohydrates in your diet, such as bread and baked goods, crackers, pancakes, pasta, and refined white rice. White potatoes, although unrefined in their natural state, also digest like refined carbohydrates and can spike blood sugar and insulin.

If these foods make up the bulk of your current diet, it may be daunting to consider eliminating all refined carbohydrates. But take heart. Not only does your body not need refined carbohydrates as an energy source, these foods are very likely at the root of your hypertension problem. Reducing refined carbohydrate intake is absolutely essential in reversing hypertension.

Refined carbohydrates are foods that originally existed in a whole state, such as grains like corn, wheat, and rice. However, during processing they have been stripped of their fiber, nutrients, and oils. Lacking fiber, the starch that is left is quickly converted into glucose in the bloodstream during digestion. This sudden spike in blood glucose elevates insulin levels—and, as we've seen, insulin encourages the kidneys to retain sodium and fluid, which elevates blood pressure.

DOES YOUR BODY "NEED" CARBOHYDRATES?

Our bodies need energy to function. But this energy does not need to be obtained from refined carbohydrates. In fact, while protein and fats are absolutely essential for human health, the same can't be said for carbohydrates. There is no such thing as an "essential carbohydrate." Actually, the diet that humans evolved on was quite low in carbohydrates. As you learned in Chapter Nine, humans evolved on a diet that consisted of mostly fat and protein with only a small fraction coming from carbohydrates in the form of roots, grasses, and wild fruits and berries.

In truth, the human body can get along just fine without carbs. In the absence of carbohydrates, the liver breaks down fatty acids to produce molecules called ketones, which provide adequate glucose and fuel for brain function. The liver can also synthesize glucose from protein. And glycerol, a derivative of stored body fat and triglycerides, can be utilized as energy by the body.

Studies have shown that both the heart and the brain operate more efficiently when the body obtains its energy from fat and protein, and ketones are the source of energy. However, because it requires fewer calories to break down carbohydrates into glucose (compared with fat and protein), our metabolism uses glucose for fuel first. Unfortunately, when there is a steady stream of these carbohydrates available to our body (as is the case with our modern diet), the glucose from these carbs becomes our main source of energy and our body fat remains intact, or actually increases.

FAST VS. SLOW CARBS

Not all carbohydrates are bad for us. It is specifically the refined carbohydrates, in addition to the general overabundance of carbohydrates in the Western diet, that contribute to hypertension (as well as obesity, Type 2 diabetes, kidney disease, cardiovascular diseases, and various other metabolic problems).

Fast carbs. These are carbohydrate crops that have been processed to remove the fiber, nutrients, and oil originally present. This "fast" carb now consists of a few, simple carbohydrate molecules that are converted quickly into glucose in your bloodstream. "Fast" carbs are also referred to as "simple" and "refined" carbohydrates. They are the main component of the following foods, which you should eliminate from your diet starting today. Doing so will lower your blood pressure naturally and may even allow your doctor to reduce or completely eliminate your antihypertensive medication. Considering the adverse side effects of these drugs, that's not a bad trade-off.

Slow carbs. These are carbohydrate foods in their natural state that have not been processed, or may have been processed very lightly. As such, they retain all of their natural fiber, nutrients, and oils, which slow down their conversion into glucose during the digestion process. Glucose is therefore released more slowly and evenly, eliminating the roller coaster highs and lows in energy and mental acuity that characterize refined carbohydrates. The fiber and oil also keep your hunger satisfied longer, so you're less likely to be hungry after eating, as is the case with refined carbs.

NEW STUDY: FIBER-RICH DIET PREVENTS STROKE

Getting more fiber into your diet could very well protect you from having a stroke by lowering your blood pressure. That's the finding from a recent meta-analysis of eight large cohort studies involving 200,000 people that was conducted by the University of Leeds in the UK.

"We found that with each additional 7 grams of fiber per day consumed, risk of stroke was reduced by about 7%," said Victoria J. Burley, PhD. Previous studies have shown that dietary fiber may help reduce stroke risk factors, including high blood pressure and elevated LDL-cholesterol levels. [308] This 7% reduction may not sound significant until you realize the average adult only eats 15 grams of dietary fiber per day, compared with the 25 grams recommended by USDA Dietary Guidelines for Americans. And some say (us included) that this recommendation is still too low.

If Americans tripled their daily fiber intake to 45 grams, this would result in a 20% reduction in stroke risk—which is quite significant, indeed. And the more fiber we add, the lower our stroke risk and blood pressure would be.

Top sources of fiber are beans (all kinds), peas, artichokes, whole grains such as barley, bulgur and oat bran, raspberries, blackberries, and prunes.

Avoiding refined grains—such as white flour, white pasta, and white rice—and replacing them with whole grains is a great way to boost the amount of fiber in your diet.

A WORD ABOUT GLUTEN

Most baked goods, even those that are labeled "whole wheat" or "whole grain" contain gluten protein. Gluten can cause a range of health problems—including depression, inflammatory bowel disease, hives, chronic bloating, joint pain, and fatigue. It is estimated that up to one-third of the population is sensitive to the gluten in wheat, but most don't know it. The gluten in GMO crops is especially harmful. Even if you are not allergic to this modified wheat, it can still cause inflammation throughout your body. Inflammation and tissue damage can contribute to a variety of chronic diseases—such as arthritis, diabetes, and heart disease. (You will learn more about gluten-free whole grains on Day 19.)

EASY "SLOW CARB" SWAPS

On Day 5, you began eating fresh vegetables every day. These healthful veggies are the healing foods that should replace "The Top 10 Worst Fast Carb Foods" (see the box on page 92) that may still be in your diet. Eat less of them—and more of these:

- Broccoli

- Spinach

- Cauliflower

- Horseradish

- Collard greens

- Brussel sprouts

- Cabbage

- Bok choy

On Day 17, you'll add in legumes…and on Day 19, you'll add in whole grains.

THE GLYCEMIC INDEX AND GLYCEMIC LOAD

Another tool to aid you in avoiding fast carbs is the Glycemic Index (GI). The higher a food's GI, the faster it breaks down into blood glucose in the bloodstream. The lower its GI, the more slowly it is converted into blood sugar.

The Glycemic Load (GL) of a food includes both a food's GI rating, as well as the total amount of carbohydrates in the food.

Refer to the Glycemic Index in Appendix B (beginning on page 312) to determine whether a carbohydrate food is fast or slow.

TODAY'S ACTION STEPS

- Comb through your cupboards and fridge, removing all products that contain refined carbohydrates. This includes bread, muffins, chips, crackers, pasta, pancake mix, pre-packaged frozen meals, fruit juice, ketchup, and salad dressing. Now that you understand just how harmful these refined carbohydrates can be to your blood pressure and overall health, you can feel extremely proud of yourself for eliminating them from your diet.

- For the next two weeks, avoid all wheat products and foods containing gluten.

- Monitor how you feel in order to determine whether you may have gluten sensitivity.

DAY 9: EAT BREAKFAST EVERY DAY

"Healthy citizens are the greatest assets any country can have."

~Winston Churchill

Add breakfast today—and every day hereafter. If you are already a breakfast eater, we want you to upgrade to a healthier low-carb, high-protein breakfast. Add eggs and familiarize yourself with some alternative high-quality protein sources. Quick breakfast tips and recipes will keep you going on mornings when you are short on time or low on inspiration. You're going to learn how easy it is to add protein-rich smoothies to your breakfast repertoire (see Healing Breakfast Suggestions in Appendix F, beginning on page 327).

THE MOST IMPORTANT MEAL OF THE DAY

When asked, "What is the most important meal of the day?" most people know the answer: "Breakfast!" And yet, when asked, "What meal do you most often skip?" most give the very same answer: "Breakfast."

The right high-protein breakfast can help stabilize your blood sugar, reduce your insulin load, lower your blood pressure, control your weight, satisfy your hunger until lunch and provide your brain and body with the fuel you need to take on a new day. Breakfast also helps jumpstart metabolism. It is interesting to note that most fit, healthy people are enthusiastic breakfast-eaters, while many overweight people tend to skip this vital meal.

COMPONENTS OF A HEALTHY BREAKFAST

High-quality protein is the most important component of a healthy breakfast. Unless you're a vegetarian, you'll want to add good quality meat and dairy products from free-range or cage-free animals that have been grass-fed and organically raised. High-quality breakfast proteins include:

- Turkey bacon
- Turkey sausage
- Wild Alaskan salmon
- Omega-3 eggs
- Almond butter
- Greek yogurt
- Chia seeds
- Cottage cheese

These proteins can be mixed and matched with fruits and veggies in any combination you find appealing. Just remember to exclude fruits and grains until Day 15. Here are some hypertension-healing combinations you can make today:

- Veggie omelet with turkey sausage
- Frittata with veggies and ricotta cheese
- Crustless quiche with veggies and turkey bacon
- Boiled eggs with turkey bacon
- Scrambled eggs with veggies and salmon bacon
- Plain yogurt sprinkled with chia seeds

What about those mornings when you just don't have time for breakfast? Try blending this fast, high-protein Tangerine Green Tea Smoothie:

Ingredients

- 1 cup green tea
- 1 cup plain yogurt
- ½ teaspoon vanilla extract
- 2 tangerines, juice of
- 1 grapefruit, juice of

Instructions

Combine all ingredients in a blender and mix until smooth.

Chill for 10–15 minutes.

Eating protein in the morning will improve your health, your well-being and your life. For many, the morning routine is just too rushed. However, with just a little planning, you can enjoy a delicious and nutritious breakfast every morning, even when you're pressed for time.

BETTER BREAKFAST TIPS

Plan ahead. Prep tomorrow's breakfast while you make tonight's dinner. Since you're already in the kitchen, take a few extra minutes to plan and prepare the ingredients for the next morning. If you're making a veggie–protein smoothie, wash and prepare all the vegetables and place them together in a covered bowl, ready to toss into the blender in the morning. Prepare similarly if you're planning to cook a frittata. The veggies will be ready and waiting to toss into your morning eggs.

Prepare tomorrow's breakfast tonight. While tonight's dinner cooks, you can also be preparing tomorrow's breakfast. This will help you save cooking and cleaning time.

Set the stage for success. Before you go to bed, set your dining table with your favorite mug and dishes. Placemats, tablecloths, candles, flowers, or an inspiring book all make welcoming additions to the breakfast table. Make your table an inviting place, ready and waiting for your morning meal. Lay out your tea or coffee substitute-making supplies. Set your alarm 15 to 20 minutes earlier and make space to nourish your body and soul in the morning.

Make mornings peaceful. Turn off the electronics and stretch and breathe your way into a new day. Enjoy the process of making delicious food. While you wait for your eggs to cook or your smoothie to blend, stretch. Take a few deep breaths. This will help both brain and body wake up in a peaceful and relaxing way. Once you sit down, try to focus on your food and let it nourish you.

Change the scenery. As much as a peaceful routine and smart planning make mornings easier, it is also important not to get stuck in our habits. Shake up your morning routine by changing your morning view. Have breakfast near a window, so you can watch the changing sky. When possible, dine outside on a porch or patio. Switch up placemats and dishes. Make breakfast fun for yourself and others.

TODAY'S ACTION STEPS

- Make breakfast an important part of each morning, striving for a high-protein breakfast made up of animal products that are high-quality, organic, free-range, and pasture-raised. Eggs are a healthy breakfast staple that can be combined with good-quality dairy products and fresh vegetables.

- Plan tomorrow's breakfast as you make dinner tonight, and prep as much of it as you can before you go to bed.

- Set your alarm clock early enough so you have time to awaken in a leisurely way—stretch, breathe deeply, meditate, and then sit down to a healthy, high-protein, restorative breakfast.

DR. HEILBRON'S CASE STUDY: HELENE

"I feel so much better—and my whole family is doing better."

When Helene came to our clinic, her blood pressure was 151/100—even though she was on a high dose beta-blocker (*labetolol*). "This stress is going to kill me," she told me. And from the looks of her blood pressure, she was right. She works for the government and was under a lot of stress. She suffered terrible lung problems as well as allergies. She felt terrible. "I can't live like this."

Tests showed that she had severely low cortisol and high levels of lead.

Lab Results	Before the 30-Day Plan	After the 30-Day Plan
Lead	12	.2
Mercury	9.4	0
Arsenic	85	11
TSH	5.92	1.33
Cortisol	2.9 (very low)	17
Progesterone	0	3.41
Blood sugar	202 (very high)	92 (normal)

After completing *The 30-Day Blood Pressure Cure Plan*, she was able to discontinue her beta-blocker. Without the medication, her blood pressure was a very healthy 118/76.

After undergoing a series of intravenous chelation treatments, Helene's lead and cortisol levels normalized—as did her life. She feels so much better. Her allergies and lung problems have resolved. She remains medication-free to this day.

"Doc, you saved my life," she says with a beaming smile.

DAY 10: ELIMINATE TOXIC FOOD INGREDIENTS

"Education, whatever else it should or should not be, must be an inoculation against the poisons of life and an adequate equipment in knowledge and skill for meeting the chances of life."

~Havelock Ellis, MD, pioneering British physician, 1859-1939

Food companies add lots of unhealthful ingredients to their products. These chemicals are used to extend the shelf life of their products, add color and texture, improve flavor, boost their profits, and/or create food cravings in you. What these questionable ingredients are *not* designed to do is to nourish your body. In many cases, these artificial ingredients can be quite harmful. Learning to read labels carefully will help you avoid ingredients that raise blood pressure and diminish your health.

PROTECT YOURSELF

The easiest way to protect yourself and your family from toxic ingredients is to avoid as much processed food as you possibly can. Foods that come directly from nature don't have an ingredients list. An egg is an egg. An almond is an almond. Water is water. Because of this, some nutritionists say that the most healthful foods are "single ingredient" foods.

Still, there are times when you might want to use certain processed foods. While we don't recommend that you make a habit of this, there are some processed foods on the market that contain organic and healthful ingredients. When consumers demand healthy ingredients in our foods, food companies will get the message and provide us with better products.

Here is an at-a-glance list of the 11 "worst of the worst" food product ingredients, in our opinion (not necessarily ranked in order of the harm they do). Read labels carefully. Do *not* purchase or consume any products that contain these substances:

TOP 11 WORST TOXIC FOOD INGREDIENTS

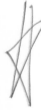

1.   Agave nectar
2.   Artificial food coloring
3.   Aspartame and other artificial sweeteners
4.   BHA and BHT (preservatives)
5.   High fructose corn syrup (HFCS)
6.   Monosodium glutamate (MSG)

7.   Potassium bromate

8.   Recombinant bovine growth hormone (rBGH) in milk and other dairy products

9.   Refined vegetable oils (including those made from corn, safflower, soybeans, and canola)

10.   Sodium benzoate

11.   Sodium nitrite and sodium nitrate

The eleven toxic food ingredients listed above are commonly found in processed foods. Descriptions of each toxic ingredient follows, along with explanations as to why it is thought to be harmful, other names it may masquerade as ("AKA"), and in which foods the ingredient(s) may be found. Again, read labels carefully. Do not purchase or consume any food products that contain these substances.

Note that trans fats—liquid vegetable oils chemically altered into more solid fats, which are used by the food industry instead of more expensive animal fats—should be considered toxic as well. We discuss them in detail on pages 65–67.

AGAVE NECTAR

What it is: This highly processed sweetener is derived from the agave cactus plant. Most agave sold in the US comes from Mexico.

Why it is harmful: Many consumers believe agave nectar is a healthful sweetener, but it is anything but. Agave nectar contains the highest amount of fructose (55% to 97%) of all the commercial sweeteners, including HFCS (which averages 55% fructose).

Contrary to what many health experts and the majority of consumers believe, fructose is not inherently evil. In fact, fructose is the natural sugar found in fruits and vegetables. The health problems associated with fructose arise when it is extracted from fruits and vegetables and isolated from the fiber that slows its digestion. This allows a person to over-consume fructose easily, particularly with fruit juice. For example, the amount of fructose in a can of soda or glass of juice is equal to the amount in approximately 10 to 12 apples or oranges. Over-consumption of fructose has been shown to increase insulin resistance, the precursor to Type 2 diabetes. The liver converts fructose to fat. Fructose, consumed in quantities greater than 25 grams a day (the equivalent of five teaspoons), has been shown to elevate uric acid levels, which causes chronic, low-level inflammation throughout the body, and may cause gout. It is also a main cause of fatty liver disease. Fructose overconsumption also leads to weight gain, elevated blood sugar and triglycerides, and high blood pressure.

A.K.A.: Agave syrup

Found in: Ice cream, energy bars and cereals, ketchup and other sauces and condiments. Agave is also sold by itself as a "healthy" sweetener.

ARTIFICIAL FOOD COLORING

What it is: Food product manufacturers add dyes to make bland-colored products look more appealing.

Why it is harmful: Artificial food dyes were originally synthesized from coal tar—and now they are derived from petroleum. They have long been controversial and are one of the most widely used additives in food products today. Many food dyes have been banned because of their adverse effects on laboratory animals. Studies have confirmed that nine dyes currently approved for use in the US raise health concerns.

According to the Center for Science in the Public Interest's (CSPI) study on food dyes, "The three most widely used dyes, Red 40, Yellow 5, and Yellow 6, are contaminated with known carcinogens. Another dye, Red 3, has been acknowledged for years by the Food and Drug Administration to be a carcinogen, yet it is still in the food supply." CPSI further reports that these nine food dyes are linked to many health issues including hyperactivity, ADHD, allergic reactions, and cancer.

A large-scale study conducted by the British government found that a variety of common food dyes, as well as the preservative sodium benzoate, increased hyperactivity and behavioral problems in children, while also decreasing their attention spans. The study was published in 2007 in the British medical journal *Lancet*.

While the European Union has mandatory labeling regulations in place to inform consumers of the health risks, the US has no such labeling requirements at this time.

A.K.A.: Caramel color, FD&C Blue #1, Brilliant Blue FCF, Bright blue, Blue #2, Ingtotine, Royal Blue, Red #3, Erythrosine, FD&C Red #40, Allura Red AC, Yellow #5 and #6, FD&C Green #3, Fast Green, Sea Green, as well as other names.

Found in: Beverages, candy, baked goods, cereals, energy bars, puddings, jams, bread, macaroni and cheese, deli meat, frostings, condiments, fast food, ice cream, sherbet, sorbet. These dyes are also added to raw meat and fish to make them appear "fresher."

ASPARTAME

What it is: One of the most commonly used artificial sweeteners.

Why it is harmful: Aspartame is an excitotoxin, which is a neurotoxic chemical additive shown to harm nerve cells by overexciting them, sometimes to the point of cell death. Regularly consuming excitotoxins destroys significant numbers of brain cells and can lead to serious health problems, including neurological disorders. (The two other common excitotoxins used in food are *monosodium glutamate (MSG)* and *l-cysteine*, which is used as a dough conditioner.) In addition, regular consumption of aspartame has been shown to stimulate the appetite and contribute to weight gain and obesity.

Aspartame and *aspartic acid* are also believed to be carcinogenic. They produce neurotoxic effects such as headaches, dizziness, blurry vision, and gastrointestinal disturbances.

Aspartame contains *10% methanol*, which is broken down by the body into the toxic by-products formic acid and formaldehyde. [309] Formaldehyde is considered to be a potent nerve toxin and carcinogen, which may explain why aspartame accounts for more reports to the FDA of adverse reactions than all other foods and food additives combined.

A.K.A.: NutraSweet, Equal, Canderel, Spoonful, NatraTaste, AminoSweet, and others.

Found in: Over 6,000 products contain asparatame, including diet and sugar-free sodas and drinks, sugar-free chewing gum, yogurt, breath mints, instant breakfasts, frozen desserts, juice beverages, and gelatins. Common in products labeled "lite," "diet" and "low-fat."

Avoid its cousins: Splenda (sucralose), Sweet'N Low (saccharine).

BHA AND BHT

What it is: Butylated hydroxyanisole (BHA) and butylated hydrozyttoluene (BHT) are preservative chemicals used to prevent oxidation and extend the shelf life of many grocery items.

Why it is harmful: BHA and BHT are *oxidants,* which form potentially cancer-causing reactive compounds in the body. The International Agency for Research on Cancer considers BHA to be possibly carcinogenic to humans. The State of California has listed it as a known carcinogen.

Found in: Packaging materials, cereals, sausage, hot dogs, meat patties, chewing gum, potato chips, beer, butter, vegetable oils, cosmetics, and animal feed.

HIGH FRUCTOSE CORN SYRUP (HFCS)

What it is: This is a highly processed sweetener made from cornstarch. The starch is separated from the corn kernel, and then converted into corn syrup through a process called acid *hydrolysis.*

Why it is harmful: Nearly all HFCS is made from genetically *bona fide* corn, which creates health concerns of its own. HFCS is absorbed by your blood stream much more rapidly than sugar. This results in massive spikes in insulin—our body's major fat storage hormone. In turn, this leads to a host of problems, both immediate and long term: increase in appetite, weight gain, Type 2 diabetes, heart disease, and cancer, among other chronic conditions. [310] Its use is so widespread that it is the number one source of calories in the US diet.

HFCS is a major contributor to cardiovascular disease, arthritis, insulin resistance, and elevated triglycerides and LDL cholesterol. In 2009, mercury was found in nearly half of all samples taken of HFCS. [311] The HFCS came from three different manufacturers, including popular brands such as Quaker, Hunt's, Kraft, Yoplait, Nutri-Grain, and Smucker's. Mercury is a heavy metal and is considered a potent brain toxin. The presence of mercury-contaminated caustic soda in the production of HFCS is common. [312] Americans consume an average of 12 teaspoons of HFCS per day per person.

A.K.A.: Corn sugar, glucose/fructose syrup, high-fructose maize syrup, iso-glucose, and fruit fructose.

Found in: HFCS is inexpensive, and as such is often the preferred sweetener used by the processed food industry. It's found in soda pop, sports drinks, sweet teas, sweetened juices, salad dressings, breads, cereals, yogurts, soups, lunch meats, pizza sauce, and condiments such as ketchup.

MONOSODIUM GLUTAMATE (MSG)

What it is: MSG is one of the most common food additives. It is an amino acid used as a flavor-enhancer in processed foods. It is also used in some restaurants.

Why it is harmful: Like aspartame, MSG is an excitotoxin, shown to harm nerve cells. Regularly consuming excitotoxins such as MSG can lead to serious health problems, including neurological disorders. (L-cystene and aspartame are two other excitotoxins to avoid.) Regular consumption of MSG also stimulates the appetite contributing to weight gain and obesity. Common side effects of eating foods with MSG include headaches, numbness, and heart palpitations.

A.K.A.: MSG has many aliases, including hydrolyzed vegetable protein, hydrolyzed plant protein, vegetable protein extract, yeast extract, glutamate, glutamic acid, sodium caseinate, textured protein, soy protein isolates, barley malt, calcium caseinate, and malt extract.

Found in: Processed foods such as salad dressings, low-fat yogurt, canned meats, frozen entrees, potato chips, canned soups, instant soup powder, canned stews, and flavored crackers.

POTASSIUM BROMATE

What it is: Potassium bromate is a form of bromide, a chemical compound. It is used as an additive to increase the volume in some breads, baked goods and flours.

Why it is harmful: Potassium bromate is banned in the EU, Canada, and several other countries. It has been shown to cause cancer in animals. Bromide is also known to disrupt the thyroid gland's endocrine functioning system. The state of California requires that all baked goods made with bromate carry a cancer warning label. However, it is not regulated throughout the rest of the US. Since 1991, the FDA has asked bakers to voluntarily cease its use.

A.K.A.: Bromic acid, potassium salt, bromated flour, "enriched flour."

Found in: Some commercial baked goods in the US. It's also common in flour mixes and baking mixes. It is also an ingredient in some mouthwashes and toothpastes.

RECOMBINANT BOVINE GROWTH HORMONE (rBGH)

What it is: Created by the Monsanto Corporation, rBGH is a genetically engineered version of the natural growth hormone produced by cows. rBGH is used to hasten lactation and boost milk production in dairy cows.

Why it is harmful: In the US, milk containing rBGH is not required to be labeled. Milk from cows who have received rBGH contains high levels of insulin-like growth factor (IGF-1), excess levels of which have been implicated as a major cause of breast, colon, and prostate cancers.

Dairy cows given rBGH have an increased risk of mastitis (inflammation of the udder). When a cow has mastitis, pus and blood are secreted into the milk. Cows are given antibiotics to try to prevent or treat mastitis. This leads to antibiotic resistance, which is tied to the spread of virulent and potentially deadly staph infections such as MRSA. These germs and the antibiotics used to treat them can also get into the milk. Hormones in food have also been linked to the onset of early puberty for girls.

Consumer protest encouraged such companies as Dannon and General Mills, Walmart, Starbucks, and Publix to phase out dairy products containing the hormones rBST and rBGH.

A.K.A.: Recombinant bovine somatotropin (rBST).

Found in: Dairy products that aren't specifically labeled "No rBGH or rBST."

REFINED VEGETABLE OILS

What it is: There are many different kinds of commercially refined vegetable oils, including soybean oil, corn oil, safflower oil, canola oil, and peanut oil.

Why it is harmful: Intensive mechanical and chemical processes are used to extract the oil from the seeds of plants. The refining process also uses chemical solvents and high temperatures. The oils are then typically deodorized and bleached. This refining process removes the natural vitamins and minerals from the seeds and creates a product that has been shown to easily oxidize and become rancid, leading to the formation of free radicals, which are linked to cancer, rapid aging, and other health concerns.

Refined vegetable oils are also high in omega-6 fatty acid, which neutralizes the benefits of omega-3s in your diet, and causes inflammation in the body. The oxidation effect has also been shown to contribute to DNA damage, elevated blood triglycerides and impaired insulin response. Additionally, many refined vegetable oils are hydrogenated. This process creates trans fatty acids, which are known to contribute to heart disease and some cancers.

A.K.A.: Partially hydrogenated vegetable oil, cooking oil, shortening, margarine.

Found in: Many, if not most, processed foods and baked goods such as crackers and granola bars use these vegetable oils. They also are sold as cooking oils and margarines.

SODIUM BENZOATE

What it is: Sodium benzoate is a chemical created from the interaction of benzoic acid (found in low levels in some fruits) and sodium hydroxide.

Why it is harmful: Sodium benzoate prevents your body from receiving nutrients by depriving mitochondria cells of oxygen, sometimes completely shutting them down in the process. Without these cells functioning properly, your immune system cannot fight off infections, which can eventually lead to cancer. It has been linked to a number of disturbing health issues, including personality disorders, brain damage, autism, and gastrointestinal problems.

Found in: Carbonated beverages such as soda pop, salad dressings, condiments, jams, and fruit juices.

SODIUM NITRITE AND SODIUM NITRATE

What they are: These two closely related chemicals are used to preserve meat. They are present in most canned meats and in many dried meats, cold cuts, and bacons.

Why they are harmful: When added to meat, the nitrates are readily converted to nitrosamines, which are associated with an increased risk of certain types of cancers. This chemical reaction occurs most readily at high temperatures. In a 2007 analysis, The World Cancer Research Fund revealed that consuming 1.8 ounces of processed meat every day increases your cancer risk by 20%.

A.K.A.: Soda niter, chile saltpeter

Found in: Cured meats, bacon, ham, salami, corned beef and hot dogs, paté, pickled pig's feet, canned meat (such as Vienna sausages and deviled ham), smoked salmon, dried fish jerky.

TODAY'S ACTION STEPS

- Become a careful label reader. Keep an eye peeled for any and all of these toxic ingredients while shopping.

- Remove any processed food products from your cupboards that contain any of the 10 harmful ingredients listed for this day. Then, the next time you go shopping, seek out real food, including fresh and frozen organically grown vegetables, lean and clean proteins that are cage-free, pasture-raised and free range, and dairy products that are labeled "organic" and hormone-free. Refuse to purchase products that contain toxic materials.

- "Vote" with your dollars by refusing to buy any food products that contain unwholesome and toxic ingredients. Food manufacturers and marketers keep a very careful record of sales, so your personal boycott will show up on their radar very quickly. When enough of us say no, they will change their ways and give us the products we want. Your every purchase decision is important and can make a difference. Shop wisely and you can change the world.

THE 30-DAY BLOOD PRESSURE CURE PLAN

CONGRATULATIONS!

WELCOME TO PHASE TWO:

DAYS 11 TO 20

Ground rules: No restaurant dining. Continue to abstain from bread, baked goods, wheat and other gluten-containing products. Reintroduce healthful alcohol swaps. Continue to make personal entries in your Success Planner every day.

DAY 11: HEALTHY FAT SWAP AND OIL CHANGE

"Your diet is a bank account. Good food choices are good investments."

~Bethenny Frankel, author, talk-show host

Your task for today is to clear your kitchen of artery-clogging vegetable oils and trans-fats, plus all foods containing them. Swap the harmful fats for healthful oils such as coconut, cold-pressed extra virgin olive oil and—yes!—butter. We also will explore why you shouldn't be afraid of saturated fats and discover the best sources of omega-3 fatty acids from both animal and plant sources.

MEET THE GOOD FATS

Way back in the 1930s, a Harvard graduate and dentist named Dr. Weston A. Price took a trip around the world. His mission was to study indigenous cultures and observe the effects that their natural diets had on their health. He discovered that, although native populations in various parts of the world ate very different foods, there were some interesting similarities in their diets and their general health. Dr. Price discovered that all healthy populations had at least one source of saturated animal fat and protein in their diets. Many of these diets contained at least 10 times the animal fat recommended by more "civilized" cultures, yet these populations did not suffer from the heart disease, digestive problems, cancer, or obesity rates plaguing their "modern" cousins. In fact, these conditions did not exist in these primitive cultures.

Contrary to what you may have been told, here are some surprising facts about the health benefits of saturated fats:

- Saturated fats help our bones absorb calcium.
- Saturated fats support our immune systems.
- Saturated fats provide essential strength to cell membranes.
- Saturated fats help balance our hormones.
- Saturated fats contribute to a healthy nervous system.
- Saturated fats lower lipoprotein (a), or Lp (a), a significant factor in the development of heart disease.
- Saturated fats protect the liver from toxins, including alcohol.
- Saturated fats help the body utilize essential fatty acids—especially omega-3s.

Numerous studies show that saturated fats are vital for good health. Try adding the following foods and ingredients into your meals and recipes because they are concentrated sources of healthful fats and/or beneficial cholesterol:

1. Avocado (including its oil)

2. Raw nuts and seeds, including their oils

3. Cold-water wild-caught fish

4. Organic cage-free eggs

5. Organic free-range chicken

6. Grass-fed beef

7. Virgin coconut oil

8. Organic red palm oil

9. Cold-pressed olive oil

10. Whole butter

Be sure to consume saturated fats from whole foods that have been minimally processed. These beneficial cholesterols and fats contribute to healthy blood pressure and cardiovascular wellness. The danger comes when we consume fats that have been damaged in the refining process by heat, oxygen, and man-made chemicals.

THE BAD FATS

In addition to the consumption of saturated fats, Dr. Price noticed that native populations had an absence of sugar and polyunsaturated fats. Diets high in sugar and easily oxidized oils—such as polyunsaturated vegetable oils—are extremely inflammatory and contribute to heart disease. Here's how: Polyunsaturated fats spoil (oxidize) easily and must be treated with care. These oils should never be heated or used in cooking because they become unstable and are prone to oxidation. Polyunsaturated fatty acids have two or more pairs of double bonds and consequently lack four or more hydrogen atoms. The unpaired electrons make these fats highly reactive and easily oxidized, which lead to free radical damage and blood pressure-hurting inflammation. We advise that you reduce your consumption of polyunsaturated fats found in margarine, salad dressing, and vegetable oils including corn, canola, cottonseed, flaxseed, grape seed, safflower, soybean, and sunflower.

Trans-fats, which are made by passing hydrogen into cheap vegetable oils so they are solid at room temperature, are by far the worst fat for your heart and blood vessels—yet they are hidden in a large percentage of US food products under coded names such as "partially hydrogenated vegetable oil" and "vegetable shortening."

Trans-fats are commonly found in many processed foods, including commercially baked goods, icing, margarine, and "snack" foods such as potato chips, cookies, crackers, and microwavable popcorn. They are even commonly used in some vegan products. Trans-fats are also widely used in fast foods and fried foods, such as French fries and fried chicken. We recommend you avoid them entirely.

HEAT STABILITY OR "SMOKE POINT"

When oil begins to smoke at high temperatures, it is a sign that it has a low smoke point and is therefore not stable or recommended for high heat. The oxidation that occurs at these temperatures will create free radical molecules in the body, which are highly inflammatory. This is how they contribute to high blood pressure.

Coconut oil and palm oil is good for high-heat cooking because it remains stable when heated. Olive oil, on the other hand, becomes unstable and therefore unhealthful when heated to a high temperature. For this reason, olive oil is one of those healthy fats that are best consumed raw, and should not be used for frying (although light sautéing is fine).

TODAY'S ACTION STEPS

- Remove any harmful cooking oils from your home. This includes vegetable oils like corn, canola, cottonseed, flaxseed, grape seed, safflower, soybean, and sunflower.

- Buy healthful cooking oils such as coconut oil and palm oil that have a high "smoke point." Say goodbye to margarine and shortening.

- Read labels on food products like mayonnaise and salad dressing and avoid anything that lists harmful fats.

- Look through your pantry for commercially baked goods, icing, margarine, and "snack" foods like potato chips, cookies, crackers, and microwavable popcorn. Throw away any food in your fridge or pantry that contains health-damaging oils.

- If you don't have them already, purchase a jar of coconut oil and a bottle of extra virgin olive oil.

DAY 12: SNACK TWICE DAILY

"Enough is as good as a feast."

~Joshua Sylvester, English poet (1563–1618)

Between-meal snacking keeps your energy balanced, which means your blood sugar will remain stable. When you skip healthful snacks between meals, you are likely to reach for sugary snacks and fast carbs which will trigger insulin spikes. Eating two healthful snacks each day will curb carbohydrate cravings and stabilize a high blood pressure healing diet.

THE PERFECT SNACK

The perfect snacks combine a protein food, a healthful fat source, and a low-glycemic carbohydrate (such as vegetables or whole grains). Any snack should at least combine either fat or protein with a low-glycemic carbohydrate. Aim for 100 to 150 calories per snack.

Snacking is absolutely vital because it helps you stay one step ahead of your hunger. Snack twice a day—even if you aren't hungry. Once your stomach starts growling and your brain screams for food, you'll gobble whatever is handy. So your best strategy is to pack your snacks at home and keep them close at hand at work and when you're traveling. Here are some examples:

Nuts and seeds. These snacks are rich in fiber, essential nutrients, and healthy monounsaturated fats—and they won't spike your blood sugar. Nuts and seeds are high in fiber, vitamins, minerals, and antioxidants. Seven grams of fiber reduces the risk of stroke by 7%. Their portability and versatility make nuts a great snack food. Nuts are also a versatile, high protein food. Ounce for ounce, nuts contain nearly twice as much protein as lean meat and, unlike many protein sources, nuts don't require refrigeration.

In a Harvard University study, nuts were shown to reduce the risk of developing cardiovascular disease and Type 2 diabetes by helping to control glucose levels and improving the body's insulin response. The study involving 83,000 women showed that those who frequently ate walnuts, almonds, peanuts, pecans, cashews, pistachios, Brazil nuts, hazelnuts, pine nuts, or macadamia nuts were 27% less likely to develop diabetes than women who rarely ate nuts. As an added benefit, the women who ate nuts also tended to lose body fat.

You can eat nuts out of hand, add them to stir-frys, roast them, sprinkle them on your salad, and mix them with yogurt and berries. To enjoy nuts and seeds in another form, purée them in your food processor and make your own nut butter to use as a dip for your veggie or fruit slices. Even try adding a few nuts to your veggie drink.

Almonds. These nuts are especially good at keeping blood sugar levels under control. According to a study published in the *Journal of Nutrition*, their high antioxidant content helps neutralize free radicals caused by chronically high glucose levels. And a study published in the medical journal *Metabolism* reported that almonds not only have a low GI, but actually help lower the GI of the entire meal eaten. They're also rich in the antioxidant vitamin E.

Try almonds lightly toasted and sprinkled on yogurt, or buy natural almond butter and spread it on celery sticks. Whole grain bread or sliced apples (after Day 12) are delectable snacks when spread with a little almond butter. Have a few almonds between breakfast and lunch to keep your energy and blood sugar stable.

More health benefits: The monounsaturated fats in almonds also help lower LDL cholesterol and reduce the risk for cardiovascular disease. According to a study published in the *British Journal of Nutrition*, eating almonds instead of other fats reduced LDL by 8% to 12%.

Walnuts. These nuts are exceptionally high in omega-3 essential fatty acids—and have the lowest ratio of omega-6 to omega-3 of any nut (4.2 to 1). Numerous studies show that a diet rich in omega-3s helps prevent the blood clotting and plaque build-up that can lead to atherosclerosis. And omega-3s also improve the ratio of HDL cholesterol to LDL cholesterol, while reducing inflammation. Walnuts and apples are a classic combo eaten by hand or mixed into yogurt with a generous sprinkle of cinnamon—and it's a fantastically healthful snack.

- A Spanish study involving high-cholesterol adults found those who ate walnuts drove down their total cholesterol by 4.4% to 7.4% and their LDL by 6.4% to 10%. A quarter cup of walnuts provides an astonishing 90.8% of your daily omega-3 needs.

- Eating antioxidant-rich nuts also lowers your risk for coronary heart disease. According to a study published in the *British Journal of Nutrition*, walnuts, pecans and chestnuts are also exceptionally high in antioxidants.

- Another study published in the research journal *Phytochemistry* identified 16 different antioxidant polyphenols in walnuts they describe as "remarkable."

- Four large studies—the Adventist Health Study, Iowa Women's Study, the Nurses' Health Study, and the Physician's Study—found that those who ate nuts at least four times a week lowered their risk for coronary heart disease by an amazing 37%. [313]

Peanuts. Although technically a legume, peanuts contain *oleic acid*, the same healthy fat found in olive oil. Peanuts are high in vitamin E and a great source of antioxidants. A study published in the journal *Food Chemistry* found that peanuts contain high concentrations of the antioxidant polyphenol *p-coumaric acid*. Slow roasting (170 degrees for 20 minutes) can increase the levels by 22%.

Peanuts are also high in *resveratrol*, an antioxidant found in red grapes and red wine and linked to the "French Paradox," which maintains that eating a diet high in certain fats, the way the French do, can actually benefit your heart. According to a study published in the *Journal of*

Agricultural and Food Chemistry, resveratrol improves blood flow to the brain by as much as 30%, significantly reducing the risk of stroke. [314]

Dress up fruits and vegetables. Adding cheese to fresh produce equals great snacking. Try sliced apples with a pinky-sized piece of sharp cheddar, celery sticks with cottage cheese or peanut butter, pears and bleu cheese, or raw broccoli with goat cheese. These fiber-plus-protein combos are endless and so are the nutritional benefits. Fruits and veggies are the ultimate slow carb foods because their fiber slows down carbohydrate break-down into blood sugar. The result is that you receive a steady-sustained supply of energy. The protein and good fats digest even more slowly, so you feel full sooner and hunger is abated for longer. In addition, a protein snack will perk up your brain and mental functions.

Dipping permitted. Making your own hummus is as easy as opening a can, and this yummy dip brings together several healing foods: Chickpeas, olive oil, and the sesame-seed "butter" called *tahini,* along with lemon juice and garlic. Yogurt also makes a perfect base for a dip—add herbs, a dash of hot sauce and some curry powder (all of which are beneficial for healthy blood sugar). Another satisfying dip can be made by seeding and dicing cucumbers, stirring them into yogurt with fresh chopped mint or dill and cracked pepper. And try warmed refried beans as a dip for raw veggies. These dips are perfect with raw carrot sticks, bell peppers, celery and/or radishes (called *crudités* in gourmet circles).

Sweet surprise. A small square of high-quality dark chocolate (containing at least 75% to 85% cocoa solids) is quite healthful in small amounts of about 150 calories due to the cacao bean's antioxidants, called *polyphenols*. In Italian research reported in the September 2008 *Journal of Nutrition,* a group of healthy people were given a daily dose of either white or dark chocolate and measured their blood sugar. The dark chocolate group showed 10% greater insulin sensitivity and 45% less insulin resistance than the white chocolate group, thanks to the higher concentration of polyphenols. [315]

Popcorn snack. Popcorn is a *bona fide* whole grain that's loaded with fiber. Reject microwave popcorn. It's bathed in toxic chemicals, artificial flavors, and excess salt. Movie theatre popcorn is also off-limits due to its high omega-6 oils and salt content. Buy your own popcorn (organic is best) and pop it in an inexpensive air popper. Try adding chili powder, garlic powder, dry mustard, cinnamon, or herbs like basil or oregano. Pack some in a sealed container and take to work for a snack.

Other snack suggestions. Other savory snacks to keep your blood sugar stable while providing a bounty of healing nutrients include: A few canned sardines in olive oil (or a forkful or two of canned salmon) with a smear of soft cheese (after Day 12, you can eat these on whole grain crackers). A mid-day hard-boiled egg. Cottage cheese with cinnamon. Toasted garbanzo beans sprinkled with spices. Let your imagination run wild!

Assume that virtually every snack food—in a bag or packaging or stocked in a vending machine, convenience store, or snack-food aisle at the grocery store—has HFCS or other added sweeteners, plus trans-fats, polyunsaturated vegetable oils like soybean or canola, refined white flour, excessive salt, and myriad chemicals used as preservatives, stabilizers, dough conditioners, artificial colors, and artificial flavors.

JUNKY SNACKS CAN MASQUERADE AS "HEALTH FOOD"

Most so-called energy bars (including granola bars) are high in processed soy products (much harder for the body to metabolize than traditional soy foods such as miso and tempeh), as well as sweeteners and refined carbohydrates such as rice "crisps" and highly concentrated fruit syrups.

"Yogurt-covered" raisins and dried banana chips are sweeter than candy. Rice cakes may be low in calories, but they're really just another refined and processed fast carb. Cheese-flavored or spice-flavored "puffs" are nothing more than damaging fats filled with air, fake colors and added flavors. "Natural" potato chips are potatoes minus their healing fiber that have been fried in polyunsaturated oils and salted for maximum fulfillment. Even innocent-sounding "whole grain" pretzels and crackers turn into a rush of sugar in your blood.

Always avoid HFCS: The most popular sugar substitute is high fructose corn syrup, the sweetener of choice in soft drinks and snack foods.

Dr. Robert Lustig, Professor of Pediatrics in the Division of Endocrinology at the University of California, San Francisco, has discovered a number of subtle differences from regular cane sugar in the way our bodies respond to HFCS. Chief among them is that HFCS calories are stored immediately as fat in a much higher ratio than plain old sugar. Nearly one-third of HFCS calories don't even line up to be converted into energy—they move directly into fat storage. It also creates a range of waste products for your liver to process that ordinary sugar does not. The resulting toxin build-up includes uric acid, which pushes up blood pressure and causes gout, a painful inflammatory condition.

BE PREPARED

Having your refrigerator stocked with sliced vegetables, vegetable juice, boiled eggs and home-made nut butter will make grabbing a healthful snack easy. Never leave home without carrying a supply of healthful food—one of the biggest traps that people fall into. If you're unprepared when hunger strikes, you will reach for anything. Always travel with your own supply of food and water (or other healthful beverage). A small baggie of mixed nuts travels well. So does a hard-boiled egg, chunks of cheese, and raw veggie slices. If you keep good snacks on hand, you won't be tempted to ruin your health with fast food and "fast" carb snacks.

TODAY'S ACTION STEPS

- Prepare tomorrow's mid-morning and midday snacks tonight. Slice up some vegetables, boil some eggs, and put some nuts into bags to grab on your way out the door.

- Remember: The ideal snack contains 100 to150 calories and includes fat and protein with a fiber-rich complex carbohydrate.
- Refer to Appendix G (beginning on page 339) for more snack ideas—and then write a shopping list for items that will comprise these healthful snacks.

DR. HEILBRON'S CASE STUDY: EDUARDO

"I have had high blood pressure since high school.
I want to get off these prescription blood pressure pills."

Eduardo is an ultra-high-stress stock broker. When he first came to our clinic, his blood pressure was 140/100, despite being on an angiotensin-converting enzyme blocker (Diovan).

He told me that he has had hypertension since he was in high school. Because he had such a long history of high blood pressure, his heart muscle had become thickened (left ventricular hypertrophy), placing him in danger of congestive heart failure. Scans also revealed that he had a buildup of calcium in his heart valves.

Like many of the patients who come to our clinic, test, showed that he had high levels of lead and low levels of cortisol.

Lab Results	Before the 30-Day Plan	After the 30-Day Plan
Lead	4.3	.3
Mercury	6.7	0
Cortisol	14	21
Body Age	61 (actual)	49 (measured)
Cholesterol	285	199
Blood Sugar	135	88
HDL	72	60
LDL	165	98
Triglycerides	305	125
Testosterone	110	755

After completing *The 30-Day Blood Pressure Cure* plan, Eduardo's blood pressure normalized at 110/70 and we removed his blood pressure medication.

After receiving intravenous chelation therapy, he displayed a low level of lead and normal cortisol activity. Scans showed that the calcium buildup in his heart valves was gone—and his heart function normalized. His energy has improved and he has never been happier.

DAY 13: ADD HEALING LUNCHES

"I believe in stopping work and eating lunch."

~L'Wren Scott, fashion designer

Like breakfast and snacks, the ideal lunch includes a combination of protein, healthy fat, and fiber-rich complex carbohydrates. Providing your system with enough protein is particularly important in order to stabilize your blood sugar throughout the day. Build your healthful lunch around protein, always including at least two servings of vegetables and a healthy fat.

The typical lunch, such as fast food, hotdogs, sandwiches with cold cuts, and pizza are all damaging to blood pressure. These foods are packed with unhealthful proteins, fats, and refined carbs that raise blood pressure and endanger cardiovascular health.

PUTTING IT ALL TOGETHER

The key to assembling a hypertension-healing lunch is to include *lean* protein, *healthful* fat and vegetables. These groups can be combined in countless ways in order to become fantastic, blood pressure-healing lunches. Having a variety of lunches that travel easily will encourage you to stick to *The 30-Day Blood Pressure Cure Plan* because you will be sure to enjoy the meal. More benefits of brown bagging your lunch are increased economy, assurance of food safety, no waiting in lines, and more free time in which to take a walk. Preparedness will serve you well!

PROTEIN AND HEALTHY FATS

Just as you were encouraged in Day Nine to build your breakfast around protein, we recommend that you build your lunch on protein and healthy fat as well. This may include meat such as beef, chicken, or fish. Nuts and hard-boiled eggs are also healthful sources of protein and fat that are easily transportable. Use extra-virgin olive oil as a dressing.

Beef, bison, and chicken. Choose free-range beef, bison, and chicken for the most healthful effects. Health studies that have focused exclusively on grass-fed, naturally raised cattle, bison and free-range chickens all find them excellent sources of high-quality protein and beneficial omega-3 fats. In fact, pasture-raised cattle contain up to four times more omega-3s than grain-fed beef. [316] Grass-fed beef is also lower in calories—one of its many health advantages over its grain-fed, factory feedlot counterpart.

Fish. Varieties of fish such as wild salmon, sardines, and anchovies contain healthful omega-3 fats. Remember that omega-3 fats lower inflammation and are beneficial for cardiovascular health, proper blood sugar metabolism, and reducing cancer risk. Your brain also benefits from these EFAs. Studies show that people with a diet high in omega-3s are less likely to fall victim to depression, schizophrenia, attention deficit disorder, and Alzheimer's disease.

VEGETABLES

Vegetables are a healthy source of complex carbohydrates. Whether you eat them as salad, steamed, sautéed, baked, or stir-fried, vegetables help to provide the steady release of glucose energy to your brain and body. These fiber and nutrients slow down the conversion of the carbohydrates in the vegetables to blood glucose, preventing glucose and insulin spikes. Providing your body with a complete lunch will ensure the steady release of nutrients into the bloodstream throughout the afternoon, eliminating cravings for fast-carb, high-sugar snacking before dinner. A healthful lunch will also help maintain your blood pressure at a healthy level.

Refer to Appendix H (beginning on page 343) for more lunch ideas.

TODAY'S ACTION STEPS

Think about lunch possibilities that combine protein and fiber and create a list of them. Add to this list in the days ahead to get in the habit of identifying ideal blood pressure-healing lunches.

- Before you go to bed tonight, assemble and pack a nutritious lunch for yourself for tomorrow. Another option is to prepare enough for your hypertension-healing dinner that you will have leftovers for lunch.

- Remember to store your food in a safe material, such as glass. (While it is acceptable to carry food in plastic containers, never use them for microwaving. The plastic releases toxic substances as they are heated.)

DAY 14: CLIMB OFF THE COUCH

"Walking is the best possible exercise."

~Thomas Jefferson

If you aren't already active, today is the day when you will incorporate some physical activity into your hypertension-healing plan. Begin with a very simple activity that you are sure you can do, such as walking or yoga, which will provide your body with the blood pressure-lowering benefits of moderate exercise. Make a commitment to yourself to be consistent so you can build this workout into a regular daily habit. Record your blood pressure reading immediately after your exercise so you'll see how much benefit you gain. Seeing your success will encourage you to keep at it.

THE HEALING POWER OF EXERCISE

Now that you have begun to incorporate the important dietary changes that are helping to reverse your hypertension, it is time to kick it up another notch with some physical activity.

After diet, regular physical activity is the most important tool in controlling your high blood pressure. In fact, studies show that moderate activity may be more beneficial in alleviating hypertension than intense aerobic activity. In one clinical trial, jogging only two miles a day allowed hypertension patients to come off their anti-hypertension medication *completely*. [317] Even slow-paced activities such as yoga, tai chi, and walking can have the same benefit. These gentle activities stimulate the production of nitric oxide in your bloodstream when you work up a sweat. Nitric oxide is a natural bio-gas that relaxes blood vessels so they can open wider (dilate), allowing easier blood flow and lower blood pressure. This is how nitric oxide protects the heart and cardiovascular system from injury during exercise. [318] To achieve these impressive benefits, all you need is a minimum of 30 minutes of physical activity every day. Study after study shows that this is some of the best "medicine" for conquering hypertension.

THE "KAIZEN" SECRET OF SUCCESS

Of course, it is neither necessary nor advisable to start out with 30 minutes of activity. The most important first step of any exercise program is to create a new habit—and the best way to do this is by utilizing what the Japanese call "kaizen." The term literally means "continuous improvement."

Kaizen is about building good habits so they become incorporated in your daily life. Recognizing that habits must be nurtured, kaizen is based on the principle of starting small. In fact, it recommends that you start with the *smallest* action that you are absolutely sure you can perform and commit to.

For example, if you want to start a running program, yet you haven't run in a long time—or ever—kaizen suggests that you start by walking. This is a very practical approach because if you have been inactive for a long period of time, running for 30 minutes is going to be painful and difficult. In fact, it will be so painful and difficult that most people quit on the spot and never attempt it again.

Kaizen takes a much smarter—and more successful—approach. It realizes that repetition is the basis of building a habit and that "slow and steady wins every time." So, in the beginning, kaizen asks you to commit to a habit that you are 100% sure you can perform—no matter how "stupidly small" it appears. For example, if you have doubts that you can commit to 30 minutes of walking per day, ask yourself what you are absolutely sure you can commit to. For some people, this will be walking for a mere five to 10 minutes. For others, it might be walking to the mailbox and turning around. People who feel they have no willpower at all might only be willing to commit to putting on their walking/running shoes and lacing them up. That's it. And believe it or not, that is enough.

You see, the whole idea is to get a good habit started. Putting your walking/running shoes on at the same time of the day for a week or so will give you the encouragement to take the next step—which might simply be walking out to the mailbox and turning around. Doing this for a while can encourage you to walk around the block. Once you do this, it's just a matter of slowly increasing your time and distance until you are walking for 30 minutes or maybe an hour.

The kaizen approach is wise and practical. It realizes that the most important factor in achieving success is building success-oriented habits. Neuroscientists tell us that every time we perform a repetition, we actually create and reinforce a "groove" in our brain—and this groove makes it easier to continue with the good habit. That's the power of kaizen. Remember: Mighty oaks grow from tiny acorns.

KAIZEN IN THE REAL WORLD

Motivational speaker and publisher of *Success* magazine, Darren Hardy likes to tell this story to illustrate the power of kaizen:

One of the women that worked for me—her name was Beverly—just returned to work after having her second child. She was having a hard time losing her "baby weight" and was chatting with a friend who just signed up to run a half-marathon. I overheard Beverly saying how much she wished that she could run a half-marathon.

"Beverly, you could run a half-marathon," I said.

"Oh, there's no way," she replied. "I get winded just going up a small flight of stairs."

So I said: "Beverly, if I could show you how to run a half-marathon and never experience pain in the process, would you take me up on it?"

"That's impossible," she replied. "The very *idea* of a half-marathon gives me pain."

"Okay," I told her, "I will create a plan that will have you running a half marathon in nine months—and you will never experience any pain."

"You're on," she said. And here's the plan I created for her:

I asked Beverly to get in a car and map out a one-mile loop around her house. Then I asked her to walk this loop just three times over a period of two weeks. And she did that easily.

Then I told her to walk it three times per week for an additional two weeks. And she had no trouble doing that.

Then I told her to start a slow jog until you become breathless. "As soon as you become breathless, just walk the rest of the way," I said.

Using this technique, Beverly was able to jog a quarter of a mile. In a short time, she was able to jog a half-mile. It took her three weeks to get up to three-quarters of a mile; and almost two months before she could run a full mile.

Now, a half-marathon is more than 13 miles. And if it took Beverly two months to run a mile, you're probably thinking that she isn't ever going to make 13 miles. But you'd be wrong.

I asked Beverly to just increase her distance by ⅛ of a mile each time she went out for a jog. That's only 300 steps. Well, at the end of six months, she was running nine miles. And at the end of nine months, she was running 13 ½ miles. Result? She ran her half-marathon.

Since then, Beverly has run four *full* marathons—and she lost 50 pounds in the process. Running is her new passion and she can't wait to lace up her Nikes. It has changed everything in her life. She looks fantastic…has energy to spare for her kids…she's sexy and attractive to her husband…and she is loaded with self-confidence!

TAP INTO THE "COMPOUND EFFECT"

It's a fact of life: The longer you do something, the longer you are more likely to do it. We humans, after all, are creatures of habit.

If you reach for a cigarette every time you feel stressed or need to relax, that is what you will always do. If your first act when you get home from work is to pop a cold beer, you will look forward to that all day and will keep doing it. If you watch TV on the couch every evening accompanied by a bowl of ice cream, missing even one night will make you irritable, sad, and uncomfortable.

Habits are like automatic behaviors. They don't require us to be very conscious. There are no decisions to be made. And no willpower is needed. We just keep doing the same thing over and over, until one day we encounter the accumulated consequences of our actions. We may discover that we have added 50 pounds to our weight. We may receive a cancer diagnosis. We may have a heart attack.

The good news is that healthy habits, such as regular physical activity, can become just as automatic. All it takes is getting started and sticking with it for a minimum of seven days. After that, the power of habit begins to take over—and it gets easier with each passing day. The habit has a power of its own.

It doesn't take much time or effort for an exercise program to have a positive effect on your hypertension and overall health. Overcoming your genetic impulse to conserve energy by climbing off that couch will reward you quickly.

Remember to drink plenty of water before, during, and after your workout. This will keep your body hydrated and assist the removal of toxins from your body.

Start off slowly with your exercise routine. Warm up your body for five to ten minutes before you really get going. Monitor your blood pressure before and after your walk or workout. This will help you find the best level of activity for your body now. Your blood pressure should remain below 220/120 immediately after your workout.

While exercising, remember that you want to aim for activity that puts your heart rate at 65% to 85% of your maximum heart rate. To calculate your maximum target rate, subtract your age from 220. If you are 50 years old, your maximum heart rate is 170, so you should aim for 110 to 145 beats per minute.

WALKING 101

As presented in the *Journal of Hypertension*, walking for 10 minutes four times a day reduces your systolic blood pressure by the same 5 mmHg as walking for a continuous 40 minutes does—and the benefits of breaking up your activity actually last longer.

Consider your walk to be personal "me time" for de-stressing and relaxing. Many people enjoy listening to music as they walk and digital MP3 players such as the iPod are perfect for this. You can download your favorite music at iTunes online. Or you may prefer listening to a good book. Choose from thousands of bestsellers and classics available through Audible (www.audible.com). Listening to books is a great way to increase your intelligence and boost your vocabulary. Many audiobooks, especially novels and works of fiction, are read by very talented actors who can transport you into their own private world of imaginable drama. This is a great way to nourish your body and your mind. By listening during the one-hour walk, you could easily "read" 30 or more books in a year.

FIND THE RIGHT EXERCISE

After a few weeks of regular walking, you will find yourself feeling stronger and fit enough to be up to the challenge. Dr. Wanpen Vongpatanasin, MD, of the Texas Southwestern Medical Center in Dallas, suggests that a simple blood pressure check every few weeks will provide you with adequate information to assess whether the intensity of your exercise routine is appropriate.

Consult your doctor if you have questions about your blood pressure readings, and he or she can help you find the most appropriate type of exercise for you.

STAYING MOTIVATED

Developing a new habit can be challenging, but there are many things you can do to remind and encourage yourself to get your body activated. Be consistent. Try to go through your exercise at the same time every day. If you are a morning person, take your walk after your morning cup of hibiscus tea. If you have a busy work schedule, utilize your lunch break every day, or hit the gym every day on your way home.

Prepare yourself. Set out your walking shoes and clothes each night before bed. Have your gym bag packed and ready to go before you go to bed each night.

Find a buddy. Having an exercise friend for support and company will make this exercise routine even more meaningful. Building up your community around a healthy lifestyle is a good idea. Just remember to rely on yourself and our own motivation; if your friend bows out of your activity every now and then, don't let it stop you.

Accessorize. Dress in layers that can be removed as exercising raises your body temperature. Wear gloves and cover your ears if it is chilly outside. Sunglasses will protect your eyes from harmful sunrays, dust, and pollen. A fanny pack to hold your ID, cell phone, and water will free your hands for unrestricted movement. Comfortable and supportive shoes will also benefit your body in your new exercise habit. As you begin your walking program, one accessory *not* to have with you is weights. For now, the focus should be on developing a routine that's easy for you to maintain and one that's not strenuous.

Log your time and readings. Keeping track of your progress will keep you motivated. You can use a pedometer to track the number of steps you take during your walk. Or, you can record your distances. Also, be sure to monitor your blood pressure and log those readings in your Success Planner.

Keep getting better. As you build up your strength and stamina, try for a landmark that extends your walk. Increase your pace or practice a session of yoga. Change the location or difficulty of your workout if you need to add a little interest.

TODAY'S ACTION STEPS

- Commit to climbing off the couch today. Decide on the minimal action you are 100% sure you will do (no matter how easy) and do it. It may be as simple as lacing up your walking shoes. Just make sure you do it for at least a week.

- When you can trust your commitment to this action, take it to the next level. Remember, willpower is like a muscle. The more you work it, the stronger it gets. Use it or lose it.

- Be sure to keep a log of your daily progress. You may wish to call a friend or family member and invite him or her to start this new exercise habit with you.

DAY 15: REINTRODUCE FRUITS AND BERRIES

*"Taste every fruit of every tree in the garden at least once.
It is an insult to creation not to experience it fully."*

~Stephen Fry, British comedian

It is finally time to reintroduce fruit into your diet. On Day 6, we asked you to take a break from sugar and sweeteners in order to reset your metabolism and begin to drop your blood pressure. Today, we will show you how to incorporate naturally sweet fruits and berries into your diet. By now, your taste buds will be sensitized to delicate sugars, so a little will go a long way. Learn to appreciate fruit as a satisfying dessert and an excellent addition to your breakfast and protein smoothies.

THE HEALTH BENEFITS OF FRUITS AND BERRIES

Add the sweet flavors of fruits into your diet. Continue to abstain from processed fruit juice because, stripped of its fiber, the natural sugar in fruit juice (fructose) is speedily converted into blood glucose. As a refined carbohydrate, the sugar in fruit juice contributes to glucose and insulin spikes in your blood stream, increasing your blood pressure.

Fruits and berries contain beneficial antioxidants. Antioxidants neutralize free radicals present in the body. Free radicals cause inflammation in the body whenever present, and inflammation leads to high blood pressure. So, choosing fruits and berries (such as blueberries, red grapes, oranges, pineapples, and peaches) high in antioxidants will help heal your blood pressure.

When you eat a piece of fruit in its whole form, you also consume the fiber, nutrients, and oils that slow down the conversion of fruit sugar (fructose) into blood glucose. This is why it is usually better to consume fruit whole—and never just its juice. Another way to mitigate the insulin-spiking effect of fruit is to combine the fruit with a protein source. Protein sources such as nuts or nut butters, yogurt, and cottage cheese mesh well with the flavors of fruits and berries. These combinations make great breakfast and snack options.

BUY ONLY FRESH OR FROZEN

Canned fruits often contain extra sugar, either because it has been added by the processing company or from the concentration of the fruit, itself. If the fruit is packed in unsweetened juice, that is still very high in sugar, and the natural acids in the fruits can accelerate the leaching of BPA or metals from the can into your food.

Dried fruits should be avoided as well, because they are concentrated sources of fruit sugar and are often processed with chemicals. Drying your own, however, is a great way to utilize your fruit. If you buy fruit when it is in season and dry the excess, you will save on your budget and enjoy a greater variety of fruit options throughout the winter months. Remember that the sugars in the fruit you dry, raisins for example, will be concentrated. So, keep that in mind as you continue to consciously balance your sugar intake.

THE 10 BEST HYPERTENSION-HEALING FRUITS

Look for these top 10 highly beneficial fruits and berries on your next shopping trip. Most are probably old favorites, but now you will learn just how they can help reduce your blood pressure and benefit your overall health.

1. **Blueberries.** This little gem is packed with antioxidant vitamins. Specifically, blueberries contain anthyocyanins, which are a type of flavonoid. Flavonoids are antioxidants. While other foods contain antioxidants, such as dark chocolate, red wine, and tea, researchers at the University of East Anglia in England found that the anthocyanins in blueberries lower blood pressure more effectively than those in other foods. [319] Anthocyanins can also be found in black currants, blood oranges, and eggplant. Keep these fruits in mind while shopping, as well.

2. **Apples.** They contain beneficial natural compounds that have been shown to lower blood pressure, in addition to lowering the risk of prostate cancer. In red apples, these compounds include ellagic acid, hesperidin, and quercetin. Green apples contain chlorophyll, antioxidant vitamin C, and lutein.

3. **Cherries.** These sweet and sour nuggets contain ellagic acid and quercetin, two nutrients that help eliminate toxins from the body. Cherries also contain anti-inflammatory properties and have been linked to improved joint function for those suffering from arthritis.

4. **Green grapes.** These contain chlorophyll, fiber, zeaxanthin, folate, and vitamin C—nutrients that help to reduce blood pressure. Grapes also support the digestive and immune systems.

5. **Red grapes.** These small, sweet orbs contain compounds that have been shown to lower the risk of high blood pressure and heart disease. They are rich in fiber, antioxidants, and resveratrol. Red grapes and red wine both contain this restorative compound.

6. **Grapefruit.** This popular citrus fruit helps prevent arterial plaque buildup by flushing LDL cholesterol from arteries.

7. **Oranges, lemons, and tangerines.** All three are loaded with vitamin C. The antioxidants in oranges help support the liver. Oranges also contain potassium, flavonoids, lycopene and zeaxanthin. If consumed regularly, these nutrients help combat high blood pressure.

8. **Peaches.** These golden globes contain beta-carotene and a host of antioxidants that are good for lowering blood pressure. The natural beta-glucans and lignans found in this fruit encourage healthy blood pressure and fortify the immune system. In addition, eating peaches helps balance hormone levels.

9. **Pineapples.** This tropical fruit contains antioxidants and blood pressure-lowering potassium.

10. **Avocados and olives.** Even though they grow on trees, avocados and olives are often not thought of as fruits because they are not sweet. However, both are high in monounsaturated fat, a beneficial fat that helps lower blood pressure

COMBINING PROTEIN WITH FRUIT

Remember that your meals and snacks should have protein and healthy fat, as well as a healthy carbohydrate source. When enjoying fruits and berries, remember to combine them with foods containing protein and fats, such as cheese, nuts, yogurt, or protein powder. Add flavor by sprinkling spices such as ground cloves, cinnamon, allspice, or cardamom. Chopped fresh mint or dill are also refreshing.

Here are a few combination ideas:

- Apple and cheese slices

- Berries and yogurt

- Fruit and nuts

- Fruit slices dipped in unsweetened almond butter

- Chopped fruit and cottage cheese

"POWER SMOOTHIE"

Serves: 2

Prep. Time: 10 minutes

This smoothie is packed with protein, fiber, and nutrition. It's naturally sweet, whips up in minutes, and is easily transported for sipping during your commute or later in the morning.

Ingredients:

- 2 cups berries—strawberries, blueberries, blackberries, or raspberries in any combination, fresh or frozen

- 1 cup plain Greek yogurt

- 2 tablespoons whey protein powder or spirulina powder

- 1 to 2 tablespoons of ground flaxseed (1 might be easier on your digestive tract to start)

- A few ice cubes (omit if you use frozen berries)

- Water, as needed to thin consistency

Instructions:

- Place all ingredients in blender and blend until smooth. Drink immediately or transfer to a thermos bottle for easy transport. Get prepared by making a bigger batch and freeze the leftovers in ice cube trays. Transfer frozen "smoothie cubes" to zip-lock bags and store in the freezer. When needed, pop a few cubes into the blender, add a little water and you're good to go!

TODAY'S ACTION STEPS

- Fix yourself a delicious fruit snack as a reward for making it to Day 15. Incorporate protein into healthful combinations of fruit, allowing your body to benefit from the bountiful nutrition of fruit without over-consuming sugars.

- Stock your kitchen with a supply of fruits and berries, then try out some delicious combinations.

DR. HEILBRON'S CASE STUDY: KEVIN

*"I really wanted to be off those medications. I was willing to do anything
to cure my high blood pressure. I'm so happy I did this program."*

Kevin was a New York executive until his health began to fail. He realized he needed to
make some important lifestyle changes, so he left the business world and studied massage
therapy with the goal of becoming a "healer." He drank four cups of coffee a day.

When he came to our clinic, Kevin's blood pressure was a very high 168/113, despite being on
two antihypertensive medications. He also experienced chest pains upon exertion (angina).

Lab Results	Before the 30-Day Plan	After the 30-Day Plan
Lead	24	6.7
Mercury	13	2.5
Cholesterol	294	197
HDL	31	60
LDL	178	101
Triglycerides	345	136
Blood Sugar (fasting)	102	81

Kevin undertook *The 30-Day Blood Pressure Cure Plan* with zeal—and it paid off for him.
His blood pressure dropped to 110/70—and he was able to completely eliminate his medications. In addition, his angina vanished.

Today, Kevin's blood pressure continues to be normal and he is medication-free. Needless
to say he is very, very happy. He no longer needs coffee or other sources of caffeine. His
biological age improved from 70 to 67.

DAY 16: PRACTICE CONSCIOUS DINING

"One cannot think well, love well, sleep well, if one has not dined well."

~ Virginia Woolf, English author (1882–1941)

Today you are going to learn how to practice conscious dining to slow down your meal and minimize overeating. You will see how to make mealtime more of a sensual, pleasurable experience by applying all five senses while you eat. One way to do this is to chew slowly, placing your fork down after each bite. You will learn how to minimize distractions and focus just on eating. The goal today is to replace mere "eating" with relaxed, conscious dining.

SLOWING DOWN

Americans have become accustomed to eating while on the run. Too many of us are used to gobbling down our food as fast as possible while in a car, at a desk, or while walking from one place to another. Although on-the-go eating is sometimes unavoidable, more often than not it is simply a habit. When this habit is replaced with slow, conscious dining, we reap the benefits of more enjoyment from our food—and we eat less of it.

DINE—DON'T JUST EAT

In a world of fast food, paper plates and microwave meals, dining seems to have taken a back seat to just eating. Too often, mealtime is rushed through, rather than savored.

There is a big difference between eating and dining. All animals eat to sustain their bodies. But eating with awareness and conscious enjoyment turns this basic act of survival into an opportunity to add social grace and refined pleasure to our mealtimes.

It is no coincidence that people who describe their eating habits as "dining" also tend to be less likely to be obese than those who eat on the run. When we make our meals small celebrations, we are more likely to chew, taste, and savor our food. Eating slowly and with more awareness allows our bodies the opportunity to extract more nutrients from our food. It also allows intake-regulating hormones to signal when we are full.

PREPARE YOUR OWN MEALS

Cooking for yourself also adds to the pleasure. Take time to plan, shop for, and prepare your own meals. This way, you will have complete control over your menu, the ingredients and the safety and flavor of your meals. This is a period of transition where you will move toward more healthful foods and learn to prepare them in ways you find more personally satisfying. Although the ultimate responsibility for your new food choices lies with you, it is helpful to bring those close to you along on your new journey. When preparing your own meals:

- Take time to plan each meal ahead of time.

- Give yourself enough time to prepare your meal.

- Cook with your spouse, children, roommate, or a friend.

Adding creative preparation, sufficient time and planning, plus including your partner or friends will encourage success in your new, healthier lifestyle.

KEEP THE CONVERSATION PLEASANT

Dining with others can sometimes encourage heated discussions that can turn divisive or even confrontational. Whether you are dining with friends or family, keep the conversation pleasant and light so as not to lose your focus on slow, mindful eating. Mealtime should be relaxed and fun, whether with friends, or at home with a spouse or children. Limit criticisms, business details, nagging, and lectures so that you and your fellow diners can concentrate on mindful eating. This can be difficult if you have children who refuse to eat what is served to them, or who are causing trouble at the table. Still, it is best to focus as best you can on enjoying your meal, and let other things go. Redirecting conversation can be artfully done, always remembering to keep it light, fun, and pleasant.

RECOGNIZE WHEN YOU ARE FULL

Check in with your stomach often. Eat only when your body is hungry. There is a difference between physical hunger and emotional eating, stress eating, addictive eating, eating from boredom, or appetite. Practice recognizing true hunger from mere appetite—the craving for a specific food or flavor—by following these steps, which are useful when battling food cravings between meals:

- Close your eyes.

- Breathe deeply.

- Place a hand on your stomach.

- Focus your attention on your digestive system, and assess whether you are hungry or not.

Never deprive yourself of the food and nourishment your body and brain need. Skipping meals, low caloric intake, imbalanced meals, and nutrient deficiencies can damage your metabolism and may lead to binge eating, blood sugar spikes, hormonal imbalances, and other problems.

Eat enough to nourish your body and to train yourself to stop eating when you have had enough, but are not "full." Eat at a measured pace to give your brain the time it needs to process that your stomach is full.

FOCUS ON YOUR MEAL

Treat your senses. Creating a meal comprised of foods that represent a variety of colors, shapes, textures, and flavors enhances your dining experience. Really notice your food. Feast your eyes on your meal before you take your first bite. Take a deep breath to savor the aroma of the blending favors. Engage as many of your senses in the process as possible. Eat slowly and mindfully.

Give thanks. There is no religious affiliation needed to appreciate the earth, the farmers, plus all the other people who helped make your meal possible. When someone is gracious enough to cook for you, always thank the chef, even when that chef is you. Remember that there are millions of people around the world who cannot eat because they do not have food. Feel your gratitude with every bite.

Digestion begins in the mouth. Slow down and really enjoy the flavors and textures on your tongue. Enzymes in your saliva begin the digestion process. Thoroughly chew every bite in order to facilitate full extraction of taste and nutrients.

PRACTICE CONSCIOUS DINING

You can practice conscious dining with small morsels of food. Really taste and experience a single sunflower seed or bean sprout. Get in the habit of letting both food and beverages spend a little time in your mouth. *Enjoy your food.* We spend so much time avoiding certain foods or viewing food as the enemy that we forget it can be pleasurable and healing at the same time.

TODAY'S ACTION STEPS

- Plan, create, and enjoy a wonderful dining experience. Pay attention to detail. Set the table. Create a relaxing atmosphere and start dining instead of just eating.

- Relax before you begin your meal. Practice conscious dining by focusing on your meal and enjoying your food. Slow down and try to make your meal last for 20 or even 30 minutes.

- Recognize when you have had enough.

- Write a little about your dining experience in your Success Planner.

DAY 17: ADD MORE BEANS AND OTHER LEGUMES

"Whole foods feed your cells as needed, and as a result, you have loads of stable energy that powers you through the day.

~Kathy Freston, healthy-living author

Beans and other legumes are among the best foods you can eat to help lower your blood pressure. Beans increase insulin sensitivity, lower blood glucose levels, add precious fiber, and fill you up on fewer calories. Eat beans as often as you can—at least one serving daily—for maximum blood pressure and weight loss benefits. Beans can be eaten at breakfast, lunch, and dinner—and even as a snack.

THE MANY BENEFITS OF BEANS

Beans are your best food friend, whether you are reversing your hypertension, lowering your blood sugar, whittling your waistline or trimming your grocery expenses. They are low in fat, full of nutrients, high in protein, loaded with fiber, and low in cost. They can be prepared in a myriad of styles and cuisines, so they always add variety to your meals.

You have already read about some of the benefits of beans in Chapter Thirteen and on Day 7 of this 30-day Plan—so you know how beneficial they can be. The next step is to eat more of them. Here are a few suggestions:

BEANS AT BREAKFAST

Beans are a breakfast staple in Mexico and in the southwestern part of the US. Perhaps you already eat beans with breakfast, but if not, today is a good time to start. Pinto and black beans are easy to incorporate into your breakfast because they pair so deliciously with most hot, savory breakfast items such as eggs, vegetables, avocados, and cheese. They also taste good with whole grain tortillas. Add a huge scoop of salsa, which will give the dish even more flavor and double as a serving of vegetables.

If you are not already a bean eater, it's time to start. Try a small serving of black beans or refried beans as a side dish, and then build up to making beans your main dish.

The cheapest and easiest way to add beans to your breakfast is to make a batch ahead of time and store them in your fridge or freezer to be used as needed. Beans are easy to prepare from scratch—simply sort, soak, and boil. Season your beans to taste by adding a bit of salt, herbs, or spices.

Alternately, you can open a can of refried black beans, heat a half-cup portion and enjoy with scrambled eggs and some avocado slices for healthy fat. You may wish to sauté some tomatoes, onions, and spicy chilies in butter or olive oil, add them to a serving of beans, and melt a little grated cheese on top.

BEANS FOR LUNCH

Bean burritos (use only whole grain tortillas, such as Ezekiel brand), bean soup, and bean salad are all good lunch options. Bean burritos and bean soups are delicious served piping hot. If you are packing a lunch and cannot heat your beans, try bean salads tossed in olive oil and vinegar. A small container of beans, or a bean burrito, makes for a portable lunch. If you have not yet become comfortable with the idea of beans as a main dish, try eating a small scoop alongside your regular lunch.

BEANS FOR DINNER

Beans and other legumes shine at dinnertime because there are so many ways to prepare and enjoy them straight from the stovetop, crockpot, or the oven. Each food culture has its own distinctive recipes for beans, uniquely seasoned with spices typical of the region. These cultural flavors mean you can eat beans in many ways, without tiring of them. It also means that whatever your food preference, you can flavor your beans to reflect it. If you like Mexican food, add cilantro, onion, chile (green or red), and cheese. If you enjoy Indian food, flavor your kidney beans or lentils with curry powder and garam masala. For a Moroccan flair, choose lima beans flavored with cumin, cinnamon, and pepper. The goal is to find the beans and flavors you enjoy so this new habit will become a lifestyle change that will continue to keep your blood pressure low for years to come.

An easy way to add beans for people who don't like them is to purée and mix into soups or sauces. The beans will add thickness, but negligible flavor.

SNACK ON BEANS AND OTHER LEGUMES

Few people think of beans as between-meal snacks, but edamame, hummus, and various bean dips can help you snack your way to healthy blood pressure. Also try roasting chickpeas or other large bean, with a spray of oil and a shake of spices at 400°F for 30 minutes.

Edamame. These are green soybeans which are harvested while still young. They grow as pods with peas inside. They are eaten by squeezing the beans out with your fingers, making them great snack foods for days when you need a portable snack that is easily eaten straight from a container. Edamame is available at most grocery stores and can be purchased either frozen or fresh. Edamame requires little effort to prepare. Simply boil or steam and then sprinkle them with salt.

Hummus. This popular Middle Eastern favorite consists of mashed garbanzo beans (chickpeas) mixed with a spoonful of tahini (crushed sesame seed paste), lemon juice, olive oil and sea salt. This dip is a healthy snack on its own, but becomes even more nutritious when paired with sliced fresh vegetables (called crudités).

Bean dip. Dips can be made from any kind of bean you choose. All healthy bean dips are basically mashed beans with seasoning. A creamy consistency is easy to attain with a blender or food processor. Add a little bit of extra virgin olive oil and lemon and season to taste. For a creamier bean dip, try mixing in Greek yogurt. Eat with whole grain pita triangles or raw, sweet red bell peppers and other sliced raw vegetables.

TODAY'S ACTION STEPS

- Eat at least one extra serving of beans or other legumes every day. Breakfast, lunch, dinner, and snack time are all opportunities to eat beans.

- Add beans in the morning, pack them for lunch, and build your dinners around your favorite beans and spices. Try snacking on edamame, hummus, and bean dips.

- If you have no beans in the house, head to the store and pick up six cans of various beans (or bean soups). Just make sure the label says "BPA-free," which means that, if the can is lined, it is safe from the toxic chemical compound bisphenol A.

- Use some of the suggestions above to include them in your very next meal. Gradually build up to preparing your own beans from scratch in a crockpot, pressure cooker or on the stove.

DAY 18: SIT LESS, MOVE MORE

"Physical fitness is not only one of the most important keys to a healthy body, it is the basis of dynamic and creative intellectual activity."

~John F. Kennedy

Sitting is the new smoking. Several studies have shown how sitting for long periods of time adversely affect our health. Today, you are going to learn how to alter your daily habits in small ways that can turn a sedentary life into a more active and healthy lifestyle.

We modern humans live in a very different world than our ancestors. New technologies have made possible the tasks of securing food, shelter, and other resources with a minimum of physical activity. In fact, most Americans spend the majority of their time sitting. Consider the difference between our hunter-gatherer ancestors, who constructed their own shelters, hunted for their own food and engaged in a myriad of other activities necessary to maintain their physical existence, and the typical American, who commutes to work, sits at a desk all day, then drives home to watch television on the couch and go to bed. This has become extremely dangerous for our health. New studies show that sitting all day is as bad for our cardiovascular system as smoking. [320]

The physical inactivity of our society contributes significantly to our increasingly unhealthy bodies, particularly higher blood pressure. Today, go through your day consciously aware of how often (or how little) you walk around, stretch your body and physically exert yourself.

ACTIVATE YOUR HABITS

Practice some physical activity at least once per hour. Here are some ways to incorporate a little movement into routine activities:

Take the stairs. Instead of riding passively to your office in an elevator, activate your body by taking the stairs. If this is physically challenging for you, take it a flight at a time. If your office or destination is on the fourth floor, climb the first flight of stairs and take the elevator the rest of the way during the first week. During the second week, climb the first two flights of stairs and use the elevator for the second two. As you feel your body becoming more conditioned, add flights of stairs until you are climbing all the way to your office or destination. Choose climbing the stairs whenever possible. Remember that you are changing your daily habits, and that every time you choose to be more active, you reinforce your new habit.

Park and walk. Instead of seeking out the parking space nearest the door, park farther away. This will increase the distance you walk, and will increase your health at the same time.

Moderate exercise, especially in the form of walking, is particularly effective at reducing blood pressure.

Time your "activity break." If you work at a desk, set up timers on your computer to go off at five minutes before every hour. When the alarm goes off, get up, stretch, do a few heel raises and squats, walk, do something physical. Research has shown that taking frequent short activity breaks throughout the day helps to reverse much of the damage caused by sitting. As an added bonus, this habit can also increase productivity and creative thought.

Take a stand. Many desk-bound workers are choosing to stand, instead of sit. They elevate their keyboard and computer screen with a lectern or podium. (A sturdy box will do in a pinch.) Or, consider a standing desk (www.geekdesk.com) or a treadmill desk (www.trekdesk.com). If you are not ready to go this far yet, have brief meetings standing up. Unless there is a compelling reason to sit, keep standing and invite those around you to do the same. A meeting where everyone stands might also benefit your schedule—as there will be more incentive to move things along. Standing meetings are always more brief.

If you must sit, sit erect. Use those abdominal muscles. Suck in your tummy and drop your shoulders. Do not cross your legs. You want your blood to be able to circulate unimpeded. Arrange your computer monitor and keyboard so that they are at the optimal position when you are sitting erect. Use pop-up reminders on your computer screen or Post-it Notes on your monitor frame to remind yourself to drop your shoulders, pull in your tummy, and breathe deeply.

Have a ball. Active sitting is a term that describes sitting in a way that requires more use of the body's core muscles. The Evolution Chair (actually a large, sturdy air-filled ball) is one of our favorite ways to engage in "active sitting." It encourages good posture, balance, and builds core strength. You can learn more at www.evolutionchair.com.

Invite your co-workers to a "moving meeting." If you need to have a longer discussion or brainstorming session with a co-worker, consider taking a walk together. New scenery will stimulate new thoughts and the exercise will be good for both your minds and bodies.

Do more housework. Fire your maid! Dishwashing, vacuuming, window washing, bed making, mopping, and other cleaning activities can help strengthen your body and burn calories. Put on some music and add some fancy footwork to your chores. Dance your way to a cleaner home and a healthier body.

Do the horizontal bop. Sex has to be one of the most fun ways to add more activity to your day. The health benefits are myriad. One of the "reasons" couples give for a dwindling sex life is that they are "too tired." Yet these same people often skip sleep while they stare at flickering screens. If you want more intimacy in your relationship, it's up to you to turn up the heat. Turn off the TV, shut down the computer, and take your sweetheart to bed.

Get creative. Use your imagination and creativity to come up with new ways to add more physical activity to your day. Remember, becoming more active can have a contagious effect on your coworkers and friends. Seeing you moving just might inspire them to get off their duffs, too. The late Jack LaLanne, who was fit and healthy right up until his death at age 96, made a habit of flicking light switches on and off with his toes. Add more movement into your day, and over time these new actions will become helpful habits.

Walk and chat. Instead of lounging on the couch while talking on the phone to a friend, try walking around the house or yard. If you take lots of calls while at work, get up and pace instead of sitting in your chair.

TODAY'S ACTION STEPS

- Choose at least two routine activities and add in more movement. Try to get up and move at least once an hour.

- Take the stairs, park and walk, get out of your desk, sit up straight, practice active sitting, try meetings where everyone stands instead of sitting, walk and talk with people at the same time, do more housework, have more sex, move in a different way and take phone calls while pacing the room.

DR. HEILBRON'S CASE STUDY: MARIE

"I feel 90% better!"

When Marie came to our clinic, she had very high blood pressure and she felt very bad. Her migraine headaches weren't helping either. Our first reading showed 166/114. Still, she did not want to take prescription medications.

Normally, I would prescribe a medication temporarily to bring down her blood pressure. But Marie was adamant that she didn't want to use a drug. So I started her on *The 30-Day Blood Pressure Cure Plan* right away.

Test showed that she also had very high lead levels (Marie loves to paint). In fact, her levels were off the scale (lead: 24; mercury: 9.9; arsenic: 13). So I also started her on our protocol of oral and intravenous chelation therapy.

Marie's cortisol was also very low (4) and, as a result, she had little to no energy. Her cholesterol was also mildly elevated at 205, her triglycerides were 75, HDL was 62, and her LDL cholesterol was 128.

The 30-Day Blood Pressure Cure Plan worked like a charm for Marie. Her blood pressure normalized at a perfect 120/80—and it is still there today without any medication.

After completing combined oral and IV chelation treatments, her lead, mercury, and arsenic levels dropped into the normal range.

Marie's total cholesterol is now a healthy 193; her triglycerides are 77; her HDL is 54; and her LDL 124.

Her cortisol level is now a healthy 17—and she has lots of energy. Marie is thrilled to be painting again—without any more headaches.

DAY 19: REINTRODUCE WHOLE GRAINS

"Our deep respect for the land and its harvest
is the legacy of generations of farmers who put food on our tables,
preserved our landscape, and inspired us with a powerful work ethic."

~William Shakespeare

Today, you are going to add whole grains to your high blood pressure-healing diet. Whole grains are a good source of protein, fiber, and other nutrients. Eaten in their whole form, these grains will add flavor, depth, and versatility to your diet. Continue to eliminate from your diet all refined grain products such as breakfast cereals, bread and baked goods, chips and snacks, cookies and the like—plus any non-organic whole grains that contain gluten and genetically modified organisms (GMOs).

AVOIDING GLUTEN

Up until now, we have asked you to stay away from grains, especially wheat. This addressed the problem of overconsumption of carbohydrates, and helped you develop new eating habits. Avoiding wheat products may have also helped an undiagnosed allergic response to the gluten in modern, genetically modified grain. Continue to refrain from eating wheat products and also avoid these other gluten-containing crops: Barley, bulgur, farro, kamut, rye, semolina, spelt, and triticale. Be aware that gluten is an ingredient in many manufactured food products, such as sauces, candies, and condiments, so keep reading labels. (Of course, you shouldn't be buying those products anymore anyway.)

KEEP IT "WHOLE"

Eating whole foods can be good for your blood pressure. The fiber slows down the digestion of carbohydrate into blood glucose. By eating the whole grain, you also receive the benefit of the other nutrients it contains. Remember that the process of refining the grain strips it of fiber, oil, and nutrients. Choose healthy grains in their whole form instead.

GLUTEN-FREE WHOLE GRAINS

Although wheat may be one of the most mainstream and common grains available, there is a wide variety of other grains that are healing to your health and high blood pressure.

Here is a list of the top 10 gluten-free whole grains, as well as a few ideas for incorporating them into your diet:

Quinoa. Technically a seed, quinoa comes in several varieties, making it a colorful addition to your diet. Quinoa has one of the highest protein contents when compared with grains. It is also a complete protein, which means it contains all nine essential amino acids. Quinoa is high in fiber as well.

How to use: Preparation of quinoa is simple—just boil until all water is absorbed. Once cooked, quinoa can be flavored as either a sweet or savory dish. While quinoa can serve as a substitute for rice and pasta, it also makes a wonderful hot cereal. Season your quinoa cereal with cinnamon for an additional high blood pressure-healing effect. Quinoa also makes a satisfying main or side dish when combined with chopped vegetables.

Amaranth. This is another good whole grain source of protein, having an especially high level of the amino acid lycine. Use amaranth flour for pancakes and baking.

How to use: Combine with corn in order to get a complete range of essential amino acids.

Oats. Whole oats are naturally gluten-free, but are often wheat-contaminated during harvesting and for processing. Read labels to ensure you buy a gluten-free product.

How to use: Oats can be used in homemade granola and granola bars. Cooked thick-rolled oats are delicious as a cold or hot breakfast cereal, especially when sprinkled with cinnamon, allspice, cocoa, or cardamom. Labels such as "steel-cut" and "old-fashioned" suggest that the oats are whole, but read labels carefully to ensure you are choosing a whole grain.

Wild rice. This colorful and delicious variety is technically a grass. It is a good protein source, but needs to be paired with another food high in lysine content in order to provide a complete protein.

How to use: Rice forms the base for a wide variety of dishes. Simply substitute wild rice in your favorite recipes, or experiment with other recipes you find at www.myhealingkitchen.com. Combine with foods such as organic chicken, beef, beans, and dairy to create meals with a full complement of essential amino acids.

Buckwheat. This whole grain contains a high concentration of amino acids, especially lysine, threonine, and tryptophan.

How to use: Cook this grain as a hot breakfast cereal commonly known as porridge. Sauté onions and garlic and mix into cooked buckwheat for a savory dish. Or, use buckwheat flour for pasta, pancakes, and baking. Buckwheat gives an earthy flavor to the food. It has also become the base for some gluten-free beers.

Millet. This African staple was one of the first cultivated crops. It contains high levels of B vitamins, calcium, magnesium, iron, lysine, niacin, riboflavin, phosphorus, and manganese.

How to use: Millet serves as a rice substitute with a nutty flavor. Millet can become a side dish, a dessert ingredient, or a breakfast cereal.

Corn. A highly versatile grain and vegetable. Use only organic, non-GMO varieties. Blue corn is more likely to be available in an organic, non-GMO form.

How to use: Add beans and squash to corn, completing the trifecta Native Americans know as the "Three Sisters." This combination contains all the basic nutrients your body needs. Non-GMO cornstarch can be used to thicken sauces in place of wheat flour. Organic corn flour can be used in cooking and baking as well.

Montina. Also known as "Indian rice grass," this grain was a Native American staple prior to the introduction of maize (corn). It is also high in protein and fiber.

How to use: Montina flour is a wonderful gluten-free whole grain substitute for wheat flour. It has a woodsy flavor.

Sorghum. Widely grown in India and Africa, this grain is high in protein and fiber, though especially full of antioxidants.

How to use: Its mild flavor makes sorghum flour a great substitute for wheat flour in cooking. Sorghum beer is also gluten-free.

Teff. This small, nutrient-packed African grass seed is high in calcium, iron, potassium, phosphorus, zinc and all the B-vitamins (except B-12). Teff is high in protein and contains all the essential amino acids.

How to use: After being cooked, teff has a sticky texture and a nutty flavor. Try cooked teff with steamed greens or with stew.

WHOLE GRAINS AT MEALTIME

Here are a few ideas for incorporating whole grains into your meals and snacks:

- **Whole grain hot cereals.** Oatmeal, quinoa, brown rice, and buckwheat all make deliciously satisfying hot breakfast cereals. Add cinnamon, fresh berries, nuts, almond extract and/or unsweetened yogurt for extra flavor.

- **Whole grain bread.** Whole grains can be used individually or in combinations as flour for baking bread. Try spreading almond butter on a slice of whole grain toast in order to get a complete serving of protein, complex carbs, and healthy fats in one serving.

- **Whole grain pasta.** Many mainstream grocery stores now carry gluten-free whole grain pasta products. Or, you could experiment with making homemade whole grain pastas. Find healthy pasta recipes at www.myhealingkitchen.com.

- **Homemade granola.** Oats and millet can be used to make homemade granola. It only takes a little plain yogurt, nuts, and some fresh berries to transform plain whole grains into a delicious breakfast or snack. Adding a small amount of healthy fat from coconut oil or olive oil is another option.

BAKING FOR YOUR BLOOD PRESSURE

Options for cooking and baking without raising your blood pressure are plentiful. To avoid the high omega-6 content of vegetable oil, substitute applesauce. Use real butter or coconut oil instead of shortening. Choose from a wide range of whole grain flours, particularly Bob's Red Mill brand, to substitute for wheat flour, or grind your own flour using a coffee grinder.

TODAY'S ACTION STEPS

- Treat yourself to whole grains today. Prepare a blood pressure-healing meal that incorporates this grain, and enjoy the reintroduction of whole grains into your diet. Continue to experiment with whole, non-gluten, non-GMO grains by incorporating these grains into your hypertension-healing meals.

- Eat whole grain cereals, bread, pasta, and granola.

- Become familiar with ways to cook quinoa, amaranth, oats, wild rice, buckwheat, millet, corn, montina, sorghum, and teff. Enjoy baked goods made from gluten-free, whole grain flour.

- Substitute applesauce for vegetable oil and use butter and olive oil instead of shortening.

DAY 20: ADD FERMENTED FOODS

"If you walk into a gourmet food store and start thinking about the nature of the foods that we elevate on the gourmet pedestal, almost all of them are the products of fermentation."

~Sandor Katz, author and fermentation revivalist

Fermented foods, such as yogurt, kefir, sauerkraut, and kim-chee, boost your immunity from infection and illness, lower your blood sugar levels, and ease your blood pressure. Including fermented foods in your diet will strengthen the army of good bacteria in your GI track, which is where much of the nutrients are extracted from your food—and where much of your immune system carries out its function.

CONSUME FERMENTED FOODS EVERY DAY

Disturbances in gut flora appear to be a significant factor in the development of heart disease, as well as in many other chronic health problems. [321] Fermented foods are an important source of vitamin K2, which plays a crucial role in protecting your heart and brain. The best way to increase the strength and population of beneficial bacteria in your gut is by including some naturally fermented foods in your diet. Yogurt is a commonly used probiotic, but it is only one in a long list of foods that provide beneficial bacteria.

POPULAR FERMENTED DAIRY FOODS

Yogurt. The secret of yogurt's beneficial properties is the bacteria it contains, called probiotics. When milk is kept warm until the lactose (milk sugar) turns to lactic acid and ferments, an ideal environment is provided for these good bacteria to multiply. Eating yogurt is like sending in the cavalry to reinforce the good guy bacteria in your GI tract, where most infections are fought. These beneficial bugs also control and destroy the "bad-guy" bacteria, such as *e. coli, salmonella, listeria, Campylobacter,* and *clostridium perfringens* (which are responsible for food poisoning and other health problems), so they don't overwhelm your body and ruin your health.

If you are not making your own yogurt, purchase Greek yogurt that contains living cultures and sweeten to taste with nuts, fruits, and berries. To assure your yogurt is of the highest quality, we recommend that you make your own. Try Jim Healthy's Homemade Yogurt Recipe in Chapter Twelve.

Kefir. This is fermented milk made with live, active cultures that has a tart flavor and creamy texture. Try swapping it for milk as a beverage or use it in dressings and sauces. A glass of kefir makes an especially satisfying and protein-rich snack. Buy plain, unsweetened kefir and blend it with berries to make a healthy smoothie.

Raw cheese. Popular probiotic-rich cheeses include gouda, edam, cheddar, feta, provolone, and gruyere. You can find raw cheese at most health food stores. Look for the words "probiotic" on the label and take care that you are buying organic cheese made from raw, hormone-free milk.

FERMENTED VEGETABLES

Sauerkraut. Traditionally fermented in lactic acid bacteria, the bacteria naturally found within the cabbage leaves (green, red, Savoy or Napa), sauerkraut is a powerful probiotic. Its tangy flavor is a welcome garnish, side dish, or even a snack. When purchasing commercial sauerkraut, make sure it has not been pasteurized, which destroys the bacterial content. Making your own sauerkraut is surprisingly easy and a lot of fun. For foolproof sauerkraut, see *Real Food Fermentation,* a wonderful book by Alex Lewin (Quarry Books, 2012). Beware of so-called "new kraut," which looks and tastes like sauerkraut but doesn't have probiotics. Lastly, check labels when purchasing sauerkraut, as some brands add sugar.

Kim-chi (kimchee). This spicy condiment is made with cabbage, red pepper, and white radishes. It has been called Korean sauerkraut. It can be eaten fresh or fermented. The most popular version is pickled, and with good reason. It turns out that the fermented version has a more positive impact on health. Because it is fermented and seasoned with hot chili, garlic, and sometimes ginger, it helps to lower blood pressure. Alex Lewin's book, mentioned above, contains easy directions and wonderful recipes for kim-chi as well.

FERMENTED SOY FOODS

Two popular choices…

Tofu (soybean curd). Perhaps the most popular soy food, tofu contains large amounts of protein, iron, and calcium. It is a versatile protein source that can be marinated, sliced, cubed and used hot or cold, as the center of a meal or as an accent. If you're using tofu as a meat substitute, buy extra firm tofu—freezing it before cooking will give tofu more of a "meaty" texture.

Miso paste. You can quickly make a delicious miso soup by dissolving miso paste in hot—not boiling—water, adding a strip of kombu seaweed, sliced spring onions and cubed tofu.

Check out the many choices of fermented soy foods in your local natural food store, such as tempeh (fermented soybean mixture typically bound in the shape of a patty) and soybean pastes.

SOY TIPS

Shoppers' note: Always buy organic, non-GMO soy products that are minimally processed. It's best to enjoy soy as it is traditionally consumed in Asia: Either as soybeans themselves (Japanese edamame) or in the healing fermented foods known as tofu, tempeh, and miso. Avoid all gimmicky soy products such as soy hot dogs and burgers, soy "meat" products, and Tofurkey.

TODAY'S ACTION STEPS

- Try to go beyond relying on yogurt for probiotics and branch out. Add fermented vegetables and sauerkraut to your diet. If you are unfamiliar with fermented soy products, experiment with natto, tempeh, or miso paste. While it might be tempting to simply purchase probiotic supplements instead, be aware that they vary widely in quality and are not considered as effective as eating probiotic foods.

- The next time you are at the grocery store, pick up a couple of probiotic-rich foods that sound appealing. Once you have become used to eating them at meal or snack times, try choosing a fermented food that seems more exotic to you and see if you can incorporate it into your new lifestyle.

THE 30-DAY BLOOD PRESSURE CURE PLAN

ALMOST THERE!

PHASE THREE:

DAYS 21 TO 30

Ground rules: Increase your focus on your lifestyle while maintaining the changes you've made thus far to your diet. Build on the momentum of your increased movement and make being active a priority. Record your progress in your Success Planner.

DAY 21: SLEEP LONGER AND BETTER

"A well-spent day brings happy sleep."

~Leonardo da Vinci

Quality sleep reduces blood pressure, so if you have trouble sleeping this chapter is for you. Today you are going to learn how to practice proper "bedroom hygiene." You will be incorporating the best fall-asleep techniques and relaxation exercises we have found.

HEALTH BENEFITS OF SOUND SLEEP

When we sleep, our mind and body rest, repair, regenerate, and heal. During deep sleep, blood pressure drops up to 20 points, arterial walls relax, and the immune system gathers its strength. Brain function and mood are both greatly improved with quality sleep in adequate amounts. Sleep also helps to reduce the levels of stress and inflammation in your body. During sleep, respiration, heart rate, blood pressure, and the body's stress hormone levels are lowered.

BETTER SLEEP LOWERS BLOOD PRESSURE

A study at Harvard, published in the *Journal of Sleep*, found that when those who usually slept seven hours or less per night increased their sleep by an average of just 35 minutes nightly, their blood pressure dropped by between eight and 14 points. [322] That's on a par with or significantly better than most antihypertensive medications.

But getting proper enough sleep may be easier said than done for many people. Today, we're going to teach you some proven techniques that can improve the duration and quality of your sleep. Getting eight hours of quality sleep every night for a week is your immediate goal. (Of course, we want eight hours of quality sleep to be part of your life from now on.) Monitor your blood pressure throughout the week so you can observe any improvements in your blood pressure as a result of sleeping better.

FALLING ASLEEP FAST

Most people think going to bed earlier will solve their sleep problems. Unfortunately, for many people, once they are in bed they experience great difficulty in falling asleep. Chapter Fifteen contains many suggestions to help you sleep. Here are some additional ideas:

Wind down earlier. Begin winding down at least an hour before bedtime. Turn off the computer and put household chores on hold. Turn down the house lights. Turn off the television and put on some soft, calming music. Put on your most comfortable nightclothes, relax and read an uplifting book. Some people find that a hot bath accompanied by the aroma of lavender oil makes them quite drowsy.

Stay on schedule. Make sure you are in bed at a certain time each night. Consistency reinforces your body's sleep cycle and makes it easier both to fall asleep at night and to wake up refreshed the next morning.

Be careful what you eat and drink. Alcohol can compromise the quality of your sleep, especially when consumed later in the evening. Even though alcohol might help you relax initially, its long-term effect usually disrupts sleep in a few hours. Having an overfull belly can also cause you to toss and turn. So, eat early, avoid spicy foods and put down your fork before you feel full. If you drink caffeine, make your cutoff deadline earlier—at least six hours before your bedtime. People who are particularly sensitive to caffeine may find they have trouble falling asleep if coffee or tea is consumed any later.

Get natural help from magnesium. Foods rich in magnesium, which aids in the relaxation process, improve the quality of sleep. These foods include halibut, nuts, oatmeal and oat bran, pumpkin seeds, and artichokes. You also may choose to take a powdered magnesium supplement called Natural Calm (www.calmnatural.com) just before bedtime. Some people find it helps them sleep better.

Set the stage. Your bedroom should be reserved for sleep and sex only. Make sure your sleeping surroundings are cozy and comfortable, welcoming and supportive. Keep televisions, phones (as much as is possible), computers and other electronic devices out of the bedroom because their flickering screens make it difficult for the brain to relax. In addition, the electromagnetic energy and subtle noise they emit can upset your sleep, even if you don't think you are sensitive.

Keep your bedroom peaceful. If you have an issue with your partner, have your discussion in the living room, preferably in the daytime. Agree that you won't go to bed angry—and make an appointment to resolve your disagreement later.

Minimize your stress levels. As advised above, avoid television news and stressful conversations at bedtime. Uncontrolled stress, worry and anger will surely disrupt your sleep. Each can elevate your blood pressure and trigger unhealthy behaviors that contribute further to your high blood pressure. To neutralize the stress you may have accumulated during the day, add meditation, deep breathing exercises and making a "gratitude list" to your evening routine. Studies have shown that counting your blessings can make you happier and improves both your health and your sleep.[323] The so-called "moving meditations," including tai chi, qi gong, and yoga, can also be helpful for managing your stress levels.

TREAT SLEEP APNEA

When fatty tissue in the throat obstructs airways during sleep, your breathing may be interrupted for brief periods during the night. If you snore, are overweight, and/or your spouse says you stop breathing during the night, you might have sleep apnea. Work with your doctor to devise a treatment plan including losing weight, using a special type of mouth guard prepared by your dentist, sleeping on your side instead of your back or stomach, or using a continuous positive airway pressure (CPAP) machine during sleep.

A more permanent solution is a quick outpatient surgery called the Pillar Procedure, in which small polyester rods are surgically inserted in your soft palate to make it stiffer so that it stops fluttering.

A WORD ABOUT SLEEPING PILLS

Most medical research agrees that pharmaceutical sleep medications can be addictive and harmful to your health in the long run. That said, they do have their place. Sleep deprivation is far more dangerous and harmful. It raises your blood sugar levels, elevates blood pressure, and triggers unhealthful behaviors such as uncontrolled eating and excessive alcohol consumption. Millions of people in the US are walking—and driving—around every day deprived of sleep. Sleep deprivation is a major cause of accidents, injury, and loss of productivity. If you are plagued by chronic insomnia, have a discussion with your physician about a sleep aid for short-term relief.

TODAY'S ACTION STEPS

- Try to get eight hours of sleep tonight by going to bed earlier and practicing some of the techniques presented today that help you fall asleep quickly.

- What is your ideal bedtime each night? Try to begin relaxing one hour before you hit the hay.

- Review the section on sleep in Chapter Fifteen. Pay attention to what you eat and drink. Remove electronics from your bedroom. Keep your bedroom peaceful and cozy. Manage your stress levels. Devise and stick to a sleep routine that works for you.

- Record the number of hours you slept, including when you went to bed and woke up, in your Success Planner.

DR. HEILBRON'S CASE STUDY: MARY

"You saved my life."

Mary, an executive assistant with the state court, had very high blood pressure (168/88) when she first came to see me. She had just had a heart attack and was told she would suffer from heart disease for the rest of her life, as well as require prescription medications. Her previous doctors could not explain why she had experienced a heart attack at such a young age (59)—because she had normal cholesterol, ate correctly, and exercised regularly.

She had a long history of cardiovascular problems and had been seen by many doctors, including numerous visits to the emergency room and hospital stays. Needless to say, she also was on several prescription medications, including *atenolol, lisinopril,* Plavix, Lipitor, and *nitroglycerine.*

As with many of the patients I see, Mary's lead levels tested very high (12; best is zero, acceptable is less than 2). Experience told me that metal toxicity was the underlying cause of her cardiovascular problems.

I immediately placed Mary on *The 30-Day Blood Pressure Cure Plan* and scheduled a series of intravenous chelation treatments in combination with our oral chelation program. Her lead levels reduced from 12 to 4, mercury from 6 to 4, and arsenic from 8 to 6.

After completing our program, her blood pressure normalized at 129/76 and I was able to withdraw all of her medications. The chelation treatments brought her lead levels back into the normal range.

"I have my life back. I was so scared that because none of the other doctors could find the cause, I felt that at any moment I could have another heart attack. Thank you, Dr. Heilbron."

DAY 22: REDUCE DEPRESSION AND BOREDOM

"The two enemies of human happiness are pain and boredom."

~Arthur Schopenhauer, German philosopher, 1788–1860

The past three weeks of *The 30-Day Blood Pressure Cure* plan have provided you with ways for reducing your high blood pressure by developing habits for a healthful lifestyle. Today, we will expand the conversation to include your emotional health and wellness. Numerous studies show that chronic depression can elevate blood pressure, [324] so look for ways to perk up your moods. For starters, make sure you're getting enough omega-3 essential fatty acids, tryptophan, B vitamins, calcium, and magnesium. Look to pets, friends, support systems, and social networks to decrease isolation and reduce boredom. Regular exercise is a powerful antidepressant as well.

Depression is a common malady that can be brought on in many ways, such as brain chemistry imbalances and sensitivity to gloomy weather. Depression raises your blood pressure by increasing your stress and anxiety levels. While the standard conventional treatment is usually medication, most mild depression can be alleviated with a healthful diet and lifestyle, and perhaps nutritional supplements and/or herbs.

DIET AND DEPRESSION

Just as we have demonstrated that the overconsumption of refined carbohydrates is the most common culprit responsible for high blood pressure, poor diet can be a major factor in developing depression. When chronic, depression and stress elevate glucose levels in the blood stream. This is why depressed individuals are often insulin resistant. As discussed on Day 6, elevated levels of insulin can damage arteries and the kidneys, leading to serious medical conditions.

Some depression can be traced to an imbalance of serotonin in the brain and dopamine, two chemicals that affect mood, thoughts, and self-esteem. When your diet lacks the proper nutritional components to support the conversion of one chemical to another in the brain, you can end up with a chronic imbalance in your brain chemistry as well as the rest of your metabolism. Debilitating disease *and* serious depression can result.

Certain vitamins, minerals, amino acids, and essential fats play a major role in maintaining healthy brain chemistry. These vitamins, minerals, amino acids, and essential fats are found in naturally raised meat, egg, fish, and dairy products—plus whole grains, leafy green vegetables, soy foods, nuts, and seeds. Here is a list of these nutrients and how to increase their presence in your diet:

Omega-3 essential fatty acids. Omega-3s, plus the essential fatty acid omega-6 (when taken in the right proportion to omega-3), can help fight off depression. [325] Additionally, omega-3s are anti-inflammatory and help reduce blood pressure. Omega-3 deficiency is a heavily researched topic and research scientists have identified it as a major factor in dozens of medical conditions and serious ills. Combined with our overconsumption of omega-6 fatty acids in our modern diet, low intake of omega-3 is a recipe for a major health disaster. (This is because omega-6 and omega-3 compete for the same pathways in the body. When there is excessive omega-6 in the diet due to overconsumption of processed foods, it overwhelms the omega-3 and causes a dangerous deficiency.) Rich sources of beneficial omega-3 fats include wild Alaskan salmon, anchovies and sardines, flax and other seeds, avocados, plus walnuts and pecans. Products from grass-fed animals, such as eggs, beef, milk, and cheese, are also good sources of omega-3s.

Tryptophan. This essential amino acid is especially good for elevating serotonin levels in the brain. A 1992 study reported in the *International Journal of Neuroscience* confirms that tryptophan can stimulate the proper function of serotonin in the brain, thus alleviating mild depression. [326] Tryptophan actually increases serotonin levels, and has the advantage of doing it without the adverse side effects associated with antidepressant drugs.

Tryptophan can be added into your diet through the supplement 5-hydroxy tryptophan (5-HTP). Serotonin is made from the amino acid 5-HTP, which, itself, is made from tryptophan. More than 25 clinical studies comparing 5-HTP and SSRI antidepressants showed that this supplement is just as effective—and sometimes even better. [327] Other studies show that 5-HTP helps induce sleep and limit appetite, as well as improves mood by increasing serotonin. Look for a quality product and follow directions on the label. Turkey is also an excellent food source of the amino acid tryptophan.

B vitamins, calcium, and magnesium. These vitamins and minerals are important in maintaining balanced brain chemistry. They are found in products from grass-fed animals, such as eggs, beef, milk and cheese, as well as nuts and seeds (such as sesame). Non-dairy sources of calcium include dark green vegetables such as kale and broccoli, nuts and seeds.

EXERCISE DEPRESSION OUT OF YOUR SYSTEM

Depression is a vicious cycle. Depression causes inaction, and inactivity worsens depression. We have encouraged you throughout *The 30-Day Blood Pressure Cure* to become more active in order to heal your high blood pressure, but exercise will also benefit your mental and emotional health. Here are some depression-healing ways to work more physical activity into your daily life:

Get outdoors. Simply climbing off the couch and getting outside is a great way to become more active. The cloistered habitats we have created are increasingly removed from the beauty and healing power of the natural world. Next time you're feeling down in the dumps, perk yourself up by going for a walk around the neighborhood or a hike in the woods or participating in some other physical activity outdoors.

Take a sun bath. Lack of sunlight can be a factor in the development of depression. Melatonin, a neurotransmitter that helps control sleep, may overproduce in people who spend too much time indoors or in the dark. This imbalance can cause fatigue, lethargy, and depression. Poor indoor air quality may also affect mood.

Develop a social network. People suffering from depression tend to isolate themselves, but this can further increase depression. Reach out to a friend whose company you have been missing, or invite a family member to visit. Even picking up the phone and having a meaningful conversation with a friend or family member can reduce feelings of isolation. (Sorry, Facebook doesn't count.) Participating in a community event, volunteering for an organization you support, or taking a class at your local community college are more ways to reduce your isolation and perk yourself up.

Develop positive self-talk. People suffering from depression often maintain a negative inner discourse about their worth, capabilities, and value. It is important to understand that you can change these negative thoughts with a little practice and perseverance. Thinking about yourself in a positive way will actually make you feel better about yourself and can reduce depression. Start by becoming more aware. Sit quietly and listen to your inner self-talk. Note how you feel about yourself and your abilities. Pay special attention to your attitudes. If you notice a lot of negative thoughts, devise a plan to transform them. Don't be afraid to ask for professional help if you feel you need it.

Practice deep breathing. There is a strong link between depression and a lack of oxygen to the brain. When we slump, it is difficult to fill our diaphragm with air. Our breathing becomes shallow and our brain may actually be deprived of the optimal amount of oxygen needed. Shallow breathing also signals the brain that we may be in danger, thus causing even more anxiety. Deep breathing breaks this cycle.

Here is a simple breathing exercise you can try right now: Sit or stand tall with good posture. Hold your head high. Lower your shoulders and look straight ahead. Inhale deeply through your nose, first expanding your lower abdomen, and then filling your lungs all the way to the top. Hold that breath for a second or two. Exhale slowly through your mouth until both your diaphragm and lungs are empty. Repeat for five minutes.

Volunteer yourself. Your actions have a direct and powerful effect on your physical health, emotional well-being, and the lives of those around you. Every positive action, however small, increases your ability to create more happiness for yourself and others.

Begin to lift the cloud of depression by smiling and waving to your neighbor—or to strangers—the next time you cross paths. Offer to tend a child for an hour or two for a harried parent you know, or volunteer in a classroom at your local elementary school or help run an activity for your house of worship. Choose an organization you support and begin to volunteer regularly. Find community events or organizations to volunteer for, such as your local library.

Continue your adult education. Another way to get out of the house, interact with more people and engage your mind is to sign up for an educational class. This could be anything from a yoga class at your community center to a literature class at your community college. Follow an old passion or discover a new one, while making new friends at the same time.

Spend time with animals. Interacting with animals reduces stress and depression. Perhaps you want to commit to a pet of your own, or maybe a better fit would be volunteering at your local animal shelter. Consider volunteering at a horse rescue center or pet-sitting for a friend. Erecting a bird feeder will provide the simple pleasure of viewing your local birds.

Get better sleep. In Chapter 14 and on Day 21 you learned that poor sleep is linked to depression and high blood pressure. Researchers, led by Dr. Rosa Maria Bruno, of the National Research Council Institute of Clinical Physiology, University of Pisa (Italy), found a link between poor sleep quality and resistant hypertension. "In women, poor sleep quality was strongly related to anxiety and depression and resistant hypertension." Make sure your room is dark and quiet, and that you have relaxed your body sufficiently prior to lying down. This will aid in better sleep.

All of these suggestions for optimizing your mood will help in your journey to heal high blood pressure. By increasing your activity level and social interactions, and by consuming foods rich in mood-enhancing nutrients, you are also lowering your blood pressure and increasing health.

TODAY'S ACTION STEPS

- Give your emotional health a boost today. Add depression-reversing foods to your diet. Consume more omega-3s, tryptophan, B vitamins, calcium, and magnesium.

- Turn the television off and get outside for some sun and exercise.

- Interact with more people by signing up for a class or volunteer activity. Spend time with family and friends.

- Develop positive inner narratives and perform breathing exercises.

- There is plenty you can do to cheer yourself up. Give these easy tips a try today!

DAY 23: STEP UP YOUR ACTIVITY LEVEL

"When you work out or you're doing anything active, it's more fun as a group. You may lose track of the time, and the next thing you know, you're working out for two hours because you're having fun."

~Lebron James, basketball star

Now it is time to add more time, distance, and challenging physical activity to your exercise routine. Over the last three weeks you have been strengthening your health by adding more physical activity to your daily routine. You began daily activity on Day 14. Then, on Day 18 you adopted the habit of getting up and moving for a few minutes at least once every hour. Now you are ready to pick up a new activity or sport. The more you exert your body, the stronger and more capable it will become.

TALK TO YOUR DOCTOR FIRST

Before you increase your activity level, discuss this with your doctor. Bring your Success Planner to the meeting so you can talk about your blood pressure readings, plus your new diet and lifestyle improvements. Involve your doctor in your decision to increase the intensity of your workouts to be certain there is no danger. Once you have been cleared to step up your level of activity, decide how you will implement the intensity increase.

GETTING STRONGER

Notice how easy your daily walk has become. This means your muscles and lungs have adjusted to a greater amount of exertion. So now you are ready for a longer distance or faster pace. You may also notice the increased flexibility and endurance of your body during yoga class or whichever activity you have adopted. This means you might be ready for an additional weekly class or a class of higher difficulty.

No matter how you do it, it is time to extend your current exercise routine. If you feel like your exercise routine is great as it is, but that your body is ready for a higher intensity, consider making your daily routine more challenging. Increase the distance and/or pace of your walk or run. Add more hills or stairs to your route, creating a more difficult course for yourself.

Of the activities you have added, which made your body feel the best? Which seemed to correspond to more healthy readings of your blood pressure? Is there another activity you have been interested in trying, but wonder if your health would support it? Now that you have gotten in better shape, these activities will become more and more accessible. Share your activity plans with your doctor and make sure he/she supports your participation in your chosen sport or activity.

The easy way to determine if you should limit the intensity of your exercise is to check your blood pressure at the peak of your workout. If it approaches 220/120, your intensity is too high and you need to take it down a notch.

CHOOSING AN ACTIVITY

If you are wondering which exercise is best, the answer is simple. The best exercise is the one you will stick with. Choose an activity that you will enjoy and look forward to so it becomes a habit. Be it an individual activity or a group sport, doing what you love and sticking to it are paramount. Here are some suggestions for activities that will boost your fitness:

Try a group sport. Increasing your interactions with other people is an important aspect of maintaining healthy blood pressure. Combining your quota of both physical activity and human interaction is an efficient way to heal your high blood pressure. Some adults enjoy playing tennis, racquetball, soccer, golf, or basketball.

Individual sports. These also are wonderful ways to improve your health. Some examples include skiing, rock climbing, hiking, walking, running, swimming, and cycling. Each of these offers opportunities to increase your activity level.

Sign up for an exercise class. Having guidance in your exercise routine can be helpful. Going to class and exercising with others can help your blood pressure continue to improve. It also has the benefit of helping you meet like-minded people who will encourage you on the road to better health. Taking a fitness class, such as spin, aerobics, or dance, might give you the opportunity to meet a new friend who can become a new exercise companion, or who will simply support your progress.

Include the kids. For those with small children, boosting your activity by joining in with them has a double benefit: It gets you both more active—and it brings you closer together. Instead of taking your kids or grandkids to the park and watching them play, get up and join them. Push them on the swings, boost them up to the monkey bars, and catch them at the end of the slide; try throwing or kicking a ball around. Some kids enjoy roughhousing and playing chase. Joining in will boost your activity level and strengthen your relationship.

Channel your "inner youth." Was there a sport or activity that you thoroughly enjoyed when you were younger? Getting involved in this activity again might be just the right type of activity for you. If you have a child, godchild, grandchild, niece or nephew in your life, consider including them.

Get a pet. Having a pet can help you increase your activity level, especially if you are willing to step out of your comfort zone. According to the American Heart Association, having a pet—particularly a dog—reduces a person's risk of heart disease. If you do not currently have a dog, consider getting one. Dog owners are 54% more likely to get the recommended level of physical activity compared with people without dogs. Studies also show that pets have a positive effect on your body's reaction to stress, including a decrease in heart rate and blood pressure when a pet is present.

If you do have a pet, assess the activity level you are currently giving your pet—and consider whether it can be increased. Try walking your dog farther than usual, or even jogging together. Prolong your playtime a little longer than usual; even grooming your dog counts as physical activity. All of this adds up to lower blood pressure and better health. Cat owners can also increase their level of activity through grooming and playing together. Try walking around the house dragging a string and watch your cat give chase. Buy a cat toy on a stick and bounce it around the room, keeping yourself moving the whole time. Consider yourself lucky if you have a horse, as this provides lots of opportunity to increase your activity in an enjoyable, companionable way.

Make an activity date. Try swapping "active dates" for sedentary standards such as dinner and a movie. Active date ideas include ice skating, flying a kite, taking a hike, strolling downtown, and dancing. You could even replace your sedentary dates for dancing lessons. Tango, salsa, merengue, and ballroom are all social dances that can help add movement to otherwise inactive date nights.

Turn chores into "exercise." Swap less active household chores for those that require large muscle movements. Negotiate with family members or housemates to take over those household chores that keep you moving from room to room. Try taking over chores like vacuuming, sweeping, and mopping.

Step up your activity by doing your own gardening. Mowing the lawn, pruning trees, and raking leaves are satisfying ways to add more activity to your life than before.

TODAY'S ACTION STEPS

- First, consult your doctor before increasing your activity level. Then, with his or her permission, increase your activity level by adding more distance and difficulty to your current routine.

- Choose a new activity to try. It may be an individual or group sport—or even an exercise class at the local gym.

- Assess your current activities and find ways to make them more physically intense. Turn date nights into opportunities for more physical movement. Turn routine trips to the park into opportunities to move alongside your children. Walk your dog farther and play harder. Look at routine chores around the house and yard as opportunities to increase your movement and focus on those chores that offer the most movement, such as vacuuming and mowing the lawn.

- Channel your youth by restarting an activity you once enjoyed as a youngster.

- If you have children or grandchildren in your life, include them in your new pursuits.

DAY 24: REDUCE YOUR EXPOSURE TO ENVIRONMENTAL TOXINS

"The best way to detoxify is to stop putting toxic things into the body and depend upon its own mechanisms."

~Andrew Weil, MD, author and wellness advocate

The time has come to better protect yourself from the absorption and accumulation of toxins in your body. Today, you will comb through your stock of cleaning supplies and personal care products, removing those that contain known toxic ingredients. Then, we will guide you in replacing these items with safe substitutes.

We are going to help you remove as many sources of these toxins as possible from your life. Set aside a big garbage bag in which to carry these toxin-laden products to the recycling center on a day it accepts toxic industrial chemicals.

POPs EXPLAINED

Persistent organic pollutants, or POPs, are defined by the EPA as "toxic chemicals that adversely affect human health and the global environment." Because they can be transported by wind and water, most POPs generated in one country affect people and wildlife far from where they are used and released. These POPs persist for long periods in the environment and can accumulate and pass from one species to the next through the food chain." [328] POPs are in our water, air, and in household cleaners, body care products such as shampoo and lotion, as well as in our food—as a result of its processing and packaging. Environmental POPs accumulate in body tissues. Over time, POPs stress the liver as it tries to eliminate them; cause cell mutations (cancer); cause disruption of all hormones in the endocrine system, upsetting blood sugar metabolism and the reproductive system; and depress the immune system, leaving you vulnerable to infections, disease and cancer. [329] Here are some common environmental toxins for you to be aware of:

- Antibiotics and growth hormones. These are routinely added to the grains eaten by factory feedlot animals. When animal products are consumed, antibiotics and growth hormones lodge in your body fat.

- Pesticides and fungicides are routinely sprayed on non-organic crops and absorbed by the plants themselves. [330] These have long been linked to the development of various cancers. [331]

- Genetically modified (GMO) crops. The effects of GMOs lack human testing, but the toxic effects in lab animals and the indirect evidence of improved human health when switching to a non-GMO diet provides ample reason for avoiding these crops. According to Martha Grout, MD, "Genetically modified foods create inflammation in the system." Inflammation, in turn, can lead to a wide variety of diseases, including allergies, autoimmune diseases, diabetes, and heart di`1sease.[332] Avoid GMOs by reading food labels and buying organic.

- PVC (polyvinyl chloride), BPA (bisphenol A), and styrene are common toxins found in plastic packaging materials. BPA is linked to a higher incidence of diabetes and other maladies, such as high blood pressure.[333] Most food cans are lined with BPA. Some hard plastic water bottles and baby bottles are also made of it. The plastic and Styrofoam packaging of meats and vegetables also contain these toxins.

- Dioxins and furans are produced during industrial processes. Bleaching, burning of medical and municipal trash also results in the production of these toxins. They're found in wood preservatives and garden and agricultural herbicides. These chemicals accumulate in animals, resulting in nearly 90% of human exposure coming from eating animal or dairy products. [334]

BEWARE YOUR PERSONAL CARE

Personal care products including shampoo and cosmetics are "the single largest source of risky chemicals that Americans are exposed to." This is largely because "companies are free to use almost any ingredient they choose in personal care products, with no proof of safety required." [335]

Shampoos are made with *sodium laureth* sulphate, a suspected carcinogen linked to kidney and liver damage. Parabens are known hormone disrupters, yet they remain in deodorant, cosmetics, and hair dyes. Hormone disrupting *phthalates*—in hair spray, nail polish, and products containing "fragrance"—are banned in Europe because of their link to birth defects and cancer, but are largely unregulated in the US.[336]

Go through all of your personal care items today and read labels carefully. Add any products containing toxic ingredients to your "toxic waste disposal" bag. A useful list of ingredients to avoid can be found at http://www.care2.com/greenliving/15-toxic-ingredients-in-personal-care-products.html?page=2. Remember that artificial fragrances are particularly harmful to your health.

TOXIC PLASTICS IN OUR FOOD

Plastic has become pervasive in our food supply, and its residue ends up in our bodies. BPA, one of the toxic compounds found in plastics, is particularly alarming. *The Journal of the American Medical Association* reported in 2008 that people with the plastic chemical BPA in their bloodstream have "an increased prevalence of cardiovascular disease, diabetes, and liver-enzyme abnormalities." [337]

Canned foods are considered the main cause of BPA exposure, because the chemical is known to transmigrate from the lining of cans into the liquids or foods they hold. Other studies show that BPA causes a variety of female reproductive organ disorders which women experience as ovarian cysts, fibroids, endometriosis, and cancers.

Here are some ways in which plastics come into contact with our food. Learn to look for these plastic components, and seek out food that is not exposed to plastic. Glass packaging is becoming more common, but it may be difficult to avoid some of these plastic containers.

- Packaged salad mixes, cold cuts, and bags of vegetables

- Milk jugs

- Yogurt tubs

- Bagged nuts and dried fruit snacks

TOP 10 ENVIRONMENTAL "TOXIN-ELIMINATORS"

Start reducing your exposure to environmental toxins by taking these steps:

Get a water filter. Buy a high-quality water filter to remove pesticides, pharmaceuticals, and other impurities from your drinking water (see Chapter Fifteen for suggestions). Use a glass bottle, glass-lined thermos, or stainless steel bottle to carry your drinking water with you.

Pitch the plastic. Replace plastic wrap, bags, and storage containers with good old-fashioned wax paper and aluminum foil. Wax-paper sandwich bags are available in natural foods stores, or just buy a roll of wax paper or foil. Wrap sandwiches with it and use it to cover glass bowls in the fridge. Then reuse it, reducing the amount of waste you produce and send to the landfill.

Go with glass. Look for Pyrex or other glass storage containers with rubber or plastic lids, in a variety of sizes. They are safer for your food, especially in the microwave. Remember to remove the lid before microwaving, as heated plastic gives off more toxins. Re-purpose all of your used plastic containers and yogurt tubs as containers for screws, nails, seeds, and small tools. Kids can play with them in the bathtub and sandbox, for craft projects, and to store collections. Or, simply recycle. Avoid buying products packaged in plastic in the future.

Check you city's approved plastics for recycling. For example, you city may only recycle plastics with codes 2, 4, and 5.

Avoid non-stick. Replace non-stick cookware with steel baking sheets, glass pans and casserole dishes, enamel cookware and cast iron or copper-clad skillets. Teflon and other non-stick coatings decompose at high heat—even if you don't cook at super-high temps. Teflon releases toxic gasses, including carcinogens, global pollutants, and other dangerous compounds.

No plastic utensils. There is no need for plastic serving and cooking utensils now that you've ditched your non-stick pans. Your cast iron skillet goes well with wooden spoons and metal spatulas. Replace plastic cups and plates with lightweight reusable bamboo ones when packing your lunches, snacks, or picnics. If you can't eliminate plastics entirely, at the very least keep them away from the dishwasher and other heat. Consider using silicone utensils instead, as silicone is not known to interact with foods and drinks or release toxins. As there are no conclusive studies that speak to its use over heat, so it would be prudent to avoid overheating it.

Avoid canned products, unless you're certain of their safety. While canned food products have made solid safety strides in recent years with improved composition and lining, and BPA leaching is not as prevalent as it was even five years ago, [338] it still can potentially be an issue with products made by the major food manufacturers. If you must purchase canned foods, check the safety record of a particular brand. Major manufacturers that have good track records with eliminating BPA include Hain Celestial, ConAgra and H.J. Heinz.

Cleaning supplies. Wean yourself off standard household cleaners with a trip to the natural foods store, where you'll find products made with naturally derived ingredients—and without phosphates and other environmental pollutants. Or go completely natural: Make your own cleaners from ingredients like baking soda, lemon juice, and white vinegar (see http://www. dummies.com/how-to/content/how-to-make-your-own-household-cleaners.navId-323630.html for tips). They'll leave your home clean and fresh with no toxic residue. Store these cleaners in glass spray bottles.

Avoid toxic body care products. Using chemical-laden makeup and other body products can mean your body is absorbing an astonishing five pounds of toxic chemicals each year. Look for skin products free of sodium laureth sulfate, parabens, and petroleum products. Parabens (para-hydroxybenzoic acids) are the most widely used preservatives in cosmetics. They're in everything from shampoo and soap to make-up, deodorant, and baby lotions. Parabens have even been detected in breast cancer tumors. [339] Start reading the labels on your shampoo, body lotion and cosmetics. The Environmental Working Group maintains an excellent database of body care products at http://www.ewg.org/skindeep/ where you can find how safe and healthy a particular product is. You can also see the highest-rated products in a particular category (such as shampoo, lip balm and toothpaste).

Forgo fragrances. Remove anything with a fake scent, including all air fresheners and scented dryer sheets, lotions, and candles. The Natural Resources Defense Council [340] released a study in 2007 which found that most air fresheners and other scented products contain chemicals called phthalates—known hormone disruptors that affect reproductive development. Especially harmful to young children and babies, many of the compounds used in fragrances are linked to cancer and problems with neurological, reproductive, and respiratory systems.

DETOXING WITH THE 30-DAY BLOOD PRESSURE CURE PLAN

By following *The 30-Day Blood Pressure Cure* plan, you've been reducing harmful ingredients and strengthening your health. This simple approach to detoxing will effectively reduce the amount of toxins present in the body.

By following our plan, you are helping your body's elimination system to rid the bloodstream and fat tissues of toxins accumulated over time. The liver is the body's "toxin filter," which neutralizes toxins and sends them to the kidneys for further processing before they are excreted via urine. The colon is involved in this detoxification process too. Its mucous membrane keeps bacteria and other toxins from entering the body, and also helps beneficial bacteria in the large intestine remove toxic wastes from consumed food. Here's how:

- Eliminate processed foods and factory meats, which are a major source of toxic chemicals.

- Load up on organic vegetables, fruits, and whole grains is providing extraordinary support to your digestive system—including your liver—in clearing toxins from your body.

- Fiber works in your favor, too, because fiber binds to wastes and moves them out of your system.

- Increase your activity level to stimulate your heart and lungs, which are natural detoxifiers.

- Lost weight is lost body fat—and body fat stores toxins.

- Quit sugary drinks and replacing them with pure water to help to flush toxins out of your body. Pure water is the best choice for flushing away impurities.

You also may want to give extra emphasis to the detox aspect of your high blood pressure-healing diet by following these ideas:

Strengthen your liver. As stated previously, your liver is your body's filter for toxins. Reducing the amount of toxins you consume allows the liver to be available for filtering other environmental toxins. You are already reducing your toxin exposure by following this plan.

Utilize your skin. Your body's largest organ is your skin, which releases toxins in perspiration and body oils. Sweat can remove heavy metals such as mercury and oil-based toxins like petroleum products. In keeping with the idea of a gentle detox, work up a light sweat through regular, vigorous exercise to stimulate perspiration and detoxing. Or, sweat in a sauna, steam room, or hot tub to open up pores and warm your body, mobilizing toxins for exit via the skin. Just a few minutes in any of these, drinking lots of fresh cool water afterward to replenish your liquid reserves, can be remarkably effective in releasing toxins through the skin.

Stay hydrated. Remember to drink a liberal amount of pure water throughout the day to support normal perspiration, which also eliminates unfriendly chemicals.

OUR TOXIC DRINKING WATER SUPPLY

Even our water supply is awash in toxic chemicals. Health officials stress that the levels are extremely low, but don't you believe it. Numerous studies have demonstrated that the occurrence of water contaminants is widespread and affects humans and wildlife at levels lower than the government says is safe.

In 2009, a comprehensive survey of US drinking water found widespread levels of pharmaceuticals and "hormonally active" chemicals nationwide. These included atrazine, *atenolol*, antidepressant drugs, estrogen hormones, the tranquilizer *meprobamate*, an epilepsy anticonvulsant, plus numerous antibiotics. [341] Even at concentrations that meet federal standards, atrazine (a widely used agricultural pesticide) is linked to low birth weight, birth defects, and menstrual problems. [342] Independent researchers are finding that children's reproductive and nervous systems suffer disproportionately from exposure, as does wildlife.

TODAY'S ACTION STEPS

Clear toxins from your body and from your immediate environment. Get rid of dangerous plastics in your food and cookware. Take toxic cleaning supplies and body care products to your local recycling center for proper disposal. Support your body's natural detox system by drinking lots of fresh water and working up a light sweat. Add liver-supporting spices, such as milk thistle and turmeric, to your food. Continue eating high-fiber foods.

DR. HEILBRON'S CASE STUDY: ROY SR.

"I am so proud of what my son has discovered."

Roy Sr. is Dr. Heilbron's father. Despite having a son who is a cardiologist and heart specialist, Roy Sr.'s blood pressure spiked as high as 202/83. Even with three blood pressure medications, his readings averaged out at 149/73.

It took a lot of counseling and persuasion to convince Roy Sr. to try *The 30-Day Blood Pressure Cure* plan—and to keep him compliant. Sometimes when a person has a doctor in the family, one feels "invulnerable" to any health problem, but of course this is wishful thinking.

Such denial can be dangerous. Tests showed that Roy Sr.'s cholesterol was high, and scans revealed that his heart muscle had thickened, placing him at risk for heart failure. Unless his blood pressure was controlled, his outlook was grim.

Roy Sr. also had elevated lead levels, no doubt caused by a career in the airline industry where he was exposed to the fumes of jet fuel and their exhaust.

After successfully sticking with *The 30-Day Blood Pressure Cure* plan, Roy Sr.'s blood pressure fell to 108/70 and his antihypertensive medications were withdrawn. In addition, his cholesterol level dropped significantly and his heart function and size normalized.

Lab Results	Before the 30-Day Plan	After the 30-Day Plan
Lead	102	1
Mercury	42	2
Total cholesterol	295	192
Triglycerides	315	88
HDL	90	58
LDL	212	98

DAY 25: ADD VITAMINS AND SUPPLEMENTS

"Take care of your body. It's the only place you have to live."

~Jim Rohn, author and business philosopher, 1930–2009

Add these vitamins, minerals, and herbal supplements to help lower your blood pressure and improve your health. Here is a basic regimen to start with. For additional supplement recommendations, be sure to re-read Chapter Thirteen in Part One of this book.

WHY YOU NEED SUPPLEMENTS

Even the most balanced of diets does not deliver all of the vitamins and minerals necessary for optimal health. This is because modern agricultural methods have leached the soil of many essential minerals and nutrients—and if the soil is lacking in vitamins and minerals, the food grown in it will be lacking too. Studies show that much of today's produce has significantly lower nutrient content than the crops grown just 50 years ago. So, even if you consumed a "perfect" diet of fresh whole foods, it is no guarantee that your body will receive optimal levels of the vitamins and minerals necessary to support healthy blood pressure. The good news is that additional nutrients, taken in supplement form, can help lower blood pressure and support your general health.

THE BLOOD PRESSURE "SUPER-STAR" SUPPLEMENTS

The super-star supplements that support healthy blood pressure are magnesium, L-arginine, coenzyme Q10, fish oil, and vitamin C. These nutrients work especially well—and can help to reverse much of the damage done to arteries by uncontrolled hypertension. In this section we'll take a look at how each of these nutrients helps to normalize blood pressure. The recommended amount provided for each nutrient is the total suggested daily intake.

Magnesium. This essential mineral helps to lower blood pressure by relaxing the tiny muscles in the walls of your arteries so blood can circulate with greater ease. [343] We recommend at least 600 mg of magnesium daily. Magnesium is also found in spinach, almonds, cashews, soybeans, lentils, and whole grains.

L-arginine. This important amino acid has been shown to decrease blood pressure levels when taken in supplement form, either as a powder or capsule. [344] A common arginine dose is 2 to 3 grams taken three times daily. L-arginine is the building block for nitric oxide, a naturally occurring gas, which widens (dilates) arteries so that more blood can flow with less pressure. Foods high in L-arginine include poultry, fish, and dairy products. [345]

Coenzyme Q10 (CoQ10). When it comes to blood pressure, this humble enzyme plays an important role. It acts as a spark plug for the mitochondria, the energy-producing "furnace" in your cells. [346] It also is a powerful antioxidant that helps arteries manage blood flow. Both of these functions explain why it is so superb for heart health. Taking a CoQ10 supplement daily has been found to lower both systolic and diastolic blood pressure in people suffering from hypertension. [347] In one study, a daily dose of 100 mg given to hypertensives for 10 weeks resulted in a 10% reduction in blood pressure. [348] We recommend taking 100 mg of CoQ10 with breakfast and with lunch. Some people prefer *not* to take it in the evening because it can have an energizing effect.

Fish Oil. Omega-3 fatty acids found in fish oil can expand blood vessels, improving high blood pressure in the process. Eicosapentaenoic (EPA) and docosahexaenoic acids (DHA) are found in fish oil and are associated with lower blood pressure. We recommend a daily dose of between 3 g (3,000 mg) and 10 g (10,000 mg) of high-quality fish oil daily. Note: People with diabetes should consult their physicians before taking this much fish oil because of its effect on blood sugar. Diabetics can safely consume 1 g (1,000 mg) of fish oil every day.

Vitamin C. An invaluable antioxidant, vitamin C fights and neutralizes free radicals, those rogue molecules that bind with oxygen and destroy cells. Researchers at Boston University School of Medicine found that one large dose of 2,000 mg followed by daily doses of 500 mg of vitamin C over one month resulted in lower blood pressure. [349] Up to 12 g (12,000 mg) of vitamin C can be consumed daily.

WHY YOUR ARTERIES NEED EXTRA ANTIOXIDANTS

Antioxidants provide your body with an insurance policy against free radical damage, which can contribute to high blood pressure. Free radical molecules harm the delicate endothelial lining of blood vessels, causing them to become inflamed and plaque-ridden. Antioxidants have been shown to prevent this damage.

MINERAL BALANCE IS ESSENTIAL

Researchers publishing in the *Archives of Internal Medicine* found that the imbalance of potassium to sodium in the diet is a significant factor driving high blood pressure. Potassium helps the body excrete sodium and dilate arteries, both of which help lower blood pressure. Maintaining an optimized ratio of 2:1 (potassium to sodium) by increasing natural fruits and vegetables is shown to significantly lower out of control blood pressure readings. Bananas, papaya, cantaloupe, carrots, celery, turkey, beans, squash, and leafy greens all contain high levels of potassium. It is generally not necessary to take potassium in supplement form.

OTHER HELPFUL SUPPLEMENTS

Chlorella. This green algae powder contains protein and vitamins C, K, B-12, beta-carotene, iron, and several amino acids. This powerful superfood is a natural detoxifier.

Coleus Forskohlii. Used in the Ayurvedic tradition for thousands of years to treat heart-related illnesses, coleus forskohlii is gaining attention from Western health practitioners for its ability to reduce blood pressure. Coleus Forskohlii has anti-inflammatory properties and since inflammation is the root of hypertension, this herb is extremely beneficial to those with high blood pressure. A common supplement dosage includes 125 mg Coleus forskohlii standardized for 10% forskolin.

Cordyceps. These mushrooms are a powerful Chinese herb that not only reduce blood pressure and heart rate, but also increase blood supply to arteries and the heart. Take cordyceps in tablet form, 3 to 6 grams a day.

TODAY'S ACTION STEPS

- Continue to eat blood pressure-healing foods, but give your body a healing boost with supplements. Maintain this regimen at least until your blood pressure normalizes.

- Focus first on adding magnesium, L-arginine and vitamin C in the doses recommended above.

- Then, as you are ready, expand this basic supplement program according to your specific needs and the information provided in Chapter 13. (Of course, seek your physicians approval on all new supplements.)

DAY 26: RESPOND, INSTEAD OF REACT

"How people treat you is their karma; how you react is yours."

~Wayne Dyer, self-development guru

In order to control your emotions and to reduce the stress in your life, it is important to train your mind to respond thoughtfully, instead of reacting out of anger or frustration. The practice of controlling your temper and emotions will keep your blood pressure steady. Today you are going to learn effective "hesitation techniques" that can help you collect yourself before you speak or act. This is not easy, so don't be afraid to ask for professional help if you think you need it.

RESIST THE IMPULSE TO REACT

When faced with challenges and stressors in life, it is common for people to react rather than to respond. Reactive habits are usually associated with anger, but anxiety and fear can also make blood pressure rise. Many psychologists believe that anger is actually just another manifestation of anxiety and fear. To react is the first instinct—the first line of psychological defense. But if reacting, rather than responding, becomes a habitual way of responding to the challenges of life, our relationships and physical and emotional health suffer.

TRY TO RESPOND INSTEAD

When we respond to life, we are steering our own course. When we become reactionary, we are allowing other people and circumstances to control us.

The legendary Zig Ziglar tells this story to illustrate the difference between reacting and responding:

"Imagine you are ill, and your physician gives you a prescription and asks you to return in a week. If, when you walk back in the door, the doctor starts shaking her head and says, 'It looks like your body is reacting to the medicine; we're going to have to change it,' you probably would get a little nervous.

"However, if the doctor smiles and says, 'You're looking great! Your body is responding to the medication,' you would feel relieved. Yes, responding to life is good."

TOOLS TO HELP YOU RESPOND

Breathe. It is very rare that you actually have to give someone an immediate answer. We've all heard the advice to take a deep breath and count to 10 before we speak or act. It really is a good practice.

Place the situation in context. What a reactionary person may take as a personal affront, a more self-directed person may view as having nothing to do with him. In dealing with the struggles of his own life, he very well may not even be considering or even noticing you.

Blend logic and emotion. The goal is not to deny your emotions, but to balance those immediate reactive emotions with rational thoughts, choice, and facts to fill in the blanks. This is the essence of responding.

Ask yourself important questions. The key question is: "Am I reacting?" Simply asking yourself that question can calm you and interrupt the reactive cycle, giving you enough of a mental break that you can choose differently. Other helpful questions include: "What am I so afraid of?" "Why am I allowing this situation to upset me?" "Am I safe now?" "How would an impartial third party describe this situation?"

When someone swerves into our lane in traffic, we may fear for our safety, or we may be upset that not everything is under our control. Reacting might mean cursing or yelling at the inattentive driver. Responding might mean slowing down and avoiding being in close proximity to that other driver.

Recognize that you always have choices. Reactive emotions interfere with the ability to think clearly. When you realize that you always have choices, you can remember to consider them *and the consequences* they bring before moving forward with any words or actions.

Improve your internal vision. Hindsight is 20/20. If you have had a reactive emotional episode, review it afterward when you are feeling calm. By seeing exactly how and when you chose to let fear or anger control you, you can learn from your experience and imagine other more peaceful ways you could deal with a similar situation in the future. This mental rehearsal of other possible options helps change your past reactions into healthier responses in the future.

Remain calm. The best crisis managers (emergency management officials, firefighters, emergency room personnel) are trained by practicing a variety of scenarios precisely so they can respond rather than react. Mental rehearsal helps these trained professionals stay cool and calm under pressure. They learn to be in charge of themselves so that they can also help others.

WHEN TO ASK FOR HELP

Reactionary emotions produce adrenaline. In this way, emotional outbursts actually give our bodies a chemical "rush." Some people can become addicted to the drug of adrenaline produced by emotional outbursts.

If you find yourself frequently in conflict, experiencing dramatic mood swings, blaming others for your experiences, slamming doors, crying, yelling, or otherwise creating drama; or, if you have difficulty maintaining friendships, you might benefit from having a professional help you learn to respond rather than react.

CHANGE IS POSSIBLE

A study of high school students in Georgia demonstrated three important points:

1. Emotional habits can be changed.

2. Working with a professional can help a person learn to respond, rather than react.

3. Learning to respond lowers blood pressure.

The study involved ninth graders in Augusta. The teens were taught anger and stress management techniques by health and physical education teachers. A separate group of their peers received no intervention.

Vernon A. Barnes, PhD, physiologist at the Institute of Public and Preventive Health at Georgia Health Sciences University, said the 10-week program could fit easily into the high school curriculum and give students a lifetime of less anger and lower blood pressure.

The study, published in the journal *Translational Behavioral Medicine,* found that there was a lowering of overall blood pressure among the group of students who learned anger management and stress management tools. [350]

Of course, anger and anxiety are not the only causes of high blood pressure. However, young or old, you want to use every possible tool available to reverse your hypertension. If learning to manage your emotions can help lower your blood pressure, it just makes sense to acquire this skill.

TODAY'S ACTION STEPS

- Imagine a situation that upsets you. Now think of at least five ways you could respond rather than react to this situation.

- Train your mind to respond thoughtfully instead of reacting out of instinct. Try to control your temper and emotions.

- Practice techniques that help you slow down and collect yourself before you speak. Learn to buy yourself time to cool down by counting, observing, and breathing.

- Ask for help when you feel you need it.

DAY 27: CONQUER SELF-SABOTAGE

"The only proper way to eliminate bad habits is to replace them with good ones."

~Jerome Hines, American opera singer, 1921–2003

Humans are creatures of habit. This includes eating habits and activity habits, but it also includes the way we talk to ourselves subconsciously. If you repeatedly find yourself falling back into old dietary habits, do not berate yourself. Instead, recognize these instances as opportunities for further improvement. Rather than tell yourself that change is impossible, or that what you are attempting is too hard, think about the progress you have made and feel proud of it. Be conscious of the choices you are making, as many of them may be unconscious.

It is absolutely possible to transform negative thoughts and feelings into positive ones—and our emotional and spiritual growth depend upon our ability to do so. Be patient with yourself, and don't let small lapses or forgetfulness discourage you. Choose to feel good about the progress you have made and do your best to change your more ingrained habits today.

The 30-Day Blood Pressure Cure provides you with a plan to kick-start a new lifestyle. This means you are learning to increase the healthfulness of your diet, increase your fitness level, and increase your interaction with your community. In addition to all this, we want to help you improve your attitudes and self-talk.

THE TOP 10 SELF-SABOTOGES

There will be times when you want to make an exception to your diet, but all these exceptions add up to habits that sabotage your blood pressure. Here are the top 10 most common "cheats" and how you can keep yourself on track when these situations arise:

1. Sneaking treats. Do not justify "I will have just one" snack. Make sure you have removed all processed snacks from your home and office, and wherever else you may have been in the habit of indulging. Remember that one square of a chocolate bar that is at least 70% pure *cocao*—as opposed to the cocoa drink mix [351]—is a healthy way to get a fix for your sweet tooth. Plan ahead and have high-fiber and protein snacks easily accessible.

2. Special food rules. Allowing yourself to deviate from *The 30-Day Blood Pressure Cure Plan* when at a party or your friends' house is a common temptation. You are working hard to reset your metabolism and stabilize your glucose levels. Remember how important it is to your health that you heal your high blood pressure—and stick to eating foods and drinks that support your decision, no matter where you are.

3. Peer pressure. Do not let others "guilt or pressure" you into trying the super-sweet dessert they just made for the first time. Your co-workers may all be getting free donuts today, but you know that your healthful snack of carrot sticks and almond butter is satisfying and healing to your body. Bring extra veggies and nut butter to share with friends and coworkers who want to increase their health and become an advocate for everyone's health.

4. Unconscious "stress eating." If you have been in the habit of finding comfort from stress, loneliness, or anxiety in unhealthy snacks, it will be especially important for you to make sure you do not have them anywhere in your home. Changing your routine will help you change your eating habits. Making the conscious decision to eat a high blood pressure healing snack, instead of an unhealthy one, will help you change these dietary habits for good. The best defense is to correct the source of your stress—or find a more healthful way to relieve its effects.

5. Doubting your knowledge. If your friends or family ridicule your new dietary habits, remember that they may be stuck in the mainstream way of dealing with health issues—namely, that medications are the ideal answer. However, you have learned that pharmaceutical drugs do not address the *causes* of hypertension, nor do they heal it. Remind yourself of why you are changing your lifestyle and perhaps figure out ways to share this knowledge in a non-confrontational manner.

6. "Lack of time." It is no secret that our modern lifestyle is fast-paced and packed with tasks to complete. Just remember: You are the manager of your time. If you fail to make time for preparing healthy meals and snacks, it won't happen. Likewise, schedule sufficient time for walks and other regular exercise routines. Prioritize these activities over others that do not improve your health.

7. Not asking for support. Do not isolate yourself, even in your diet and lifestyle changes. Having a support system of family and friends will make these changes easier and more rewarding. Learn how to tell others what you need from them; you might be surprised by how eager your loved ones are to show you support. Someone might want to walk regularly with you, take shopping trips together, or even just listen to your thoughts and ideas on this new undertaking.

8. Forgetting to carry healthful snacks with you. Getting hungry while away from your healthfully stocked fridge is a major temptation for fast-carb snacking. Forgetting to provide your body with healthy snacks in between meals can be just as detrimental. Remember to bring snacks and water with you whenever you leave the house, and remember that having foods prepared for snacking while at home will also help you stay on track.

9. Giving in to sugary drinks. If you are still drinking any beverages that contain sugar, switch them out for water, herbal tea, or another healthful option from Day 3. Remember that Americans obtain an exorbitant amount of refined carbohydrates from soda pop and other sugary beverages, so change this habit today.

10. Not getting enough sleep. Your body rejuvenates itself during sleep. Give your body restful, deep sleep in order to support your high blood pressure-healing regimen of diet and lifestyle changes.

REPROGRAMMING YOUR OLD HABITS

Forming new habits, be they around eating, exercise, or social interaction, is key to healing your high blood pressure. Success is entirely in your own hands. Continually remind yourself that you are fully capable of making healthy choices and following through.

One way to break unhealthful habits is to alter the times and locations that your daily activities are carried out. As demonstrated in a study at Duke University, nearly half of all daily activities occur at the same location every day. [352] This means that time and location serve as triggers for habits, be they healthful or detrimental.

There are many ways you can have built-in support for your new lifestyle and remind yourself to stay on track. Here are some ideas to keep in mind:

Re-motivate yourself regularly. You are truly the only person who can heal your high blood pressure and improve your health. Remind yourself that following this plan is increasing your health and vitality. Review the information pertinent to areas of the plan you might be having more difficulty following, and recommit to healthful changes.

Menu and meal planning. If you know exactly what you want to eat throughout the week, you can purchase the proper ingredients, prepare meals and snacks ahead of time, and avoid being caught in situations that encourage old habits of fast-carb, high-sugar eating. Cooking double batches will save you time and provide leftovers to be eaten for lunch the next day or when you are in a hurry.

Become accountable to someone. Tell a close friend or relative about your new diet and lifestyle, and ask him or her to remind you to stick with it if he or she notices you reverting to an old, unhealthful habit. This could be another person you know who has also healed his body by changing his habits, or simply be someone you know to be supportive. Having encouraging support could make that extra difference in sticking with the plan.

Record your progress. Look back at all the entries you have made in your Success Planner about your diet and lifestyle changes. You will find encouragement in your progress. Notice how your blood pressure readings have improved. Remind yourself of all the new knowledge that is yours to wield. Continue to log your progress. Think positively about your successes and learn from your lapses.

Recognize problem habits and triggers. Be conscious of those times when and places where you have had a hard time sticking to the plan. Avoid or alter these situations so that the formation of healthful new habits will be easier.

Be present. Choose to make the right choice right *now*. Do not dwell on past mistakes. Instead, recognize that certain habits are more difficult, but that you are changing them a little at a time. Consider "slip-ups" opportunities to notice where you need to be stronger and more committed. Keep your eyes on the prize.

DEVELOP POSITIVE SELF-TALK

Whenever you realize you are telling yourself this plan is too hard, or that you can't stick to it, replace this negative thought with a positive one. Tell yourself, "I can do it!" We live up to our inner mantras according to the psychological concept of self-fulfilling prophecy. Our thoughts and attitudes guide our actions, whether we are conscious of them or not. Therefore, if you praise yourself for your progress and tell yourself you are healing your high blood pressure, you will.

Replace negative thoughts with positive ones. The more you practice positive affirmations, the easier it gets to accomplish your goals. Try these positive self-talk tips:

- When you feel yourself thinking or saying something negative, say "stop" out loud and affirm the opposite. "I can't eat a healing dinner because I didn't shop for food" becomes "I have a can of beans in the pantry, olive oil, and an onion, so I can make a yummy meal."

- Modify your wording to use less powerful phrases. "I can't" find a way to stay on the eating plan changes to "it's challenging to stay on the eating plan." Then, explore ways to make it less challenging and you'll be able to add "…but I'm getting better at it."

- "This will never work" becomes "how can I make this work"? Imagine the possibilities when you shift your mindset.

- Be optimistic—even if you're not! Count your successes every day and record them in your journal. Healing breakfast? *Check.* Healing snack? *Check!* Walked at lunch? *Double check!* You're on your way to being more optimistic already.

- Draft a few positive affirmations and repeat them aloud or to yourself daily. Repetition is key. Create sentences phrased as if they're true right now. You can use these or write your own: "I'm healing my blood pressure with every step I walk." "I'm healthier with every sip of this delicious fruit and yogurt smoothie." "I feel peaceful and happy with my decision to stick with this plan."

- Jot down your affirmations and post them strategically on the bathroom mirror, home refrigerator, and workplace drawer.

TODAY'S ACTION STEPS

- Practice positive self-talk today by affirming your commitment and capability in this high blood pressure healing diet.

- Put sticky notes on your mirror and other strategic spots to remind yourself of your goals each morning and throughout the day.

- Slightly change your routine to break unhealthful habits. Remind yourself that you always have ample time to take care of your health.

- Keep yourself motivated by tracking your progress and planning your week. Include friends and family in your journey to help make these healthful habits stick.

DR. HEILBRON'S CASE STUDY: CHARLENE

"Dr. Heilbron has given my peace of mind back."

Charlene's blood pressure became a problem after her open-heart surgery. Despite taking several medications and numerous nutritional supplements to bring it down, her readings were stuck at 139/90, on average. She came to see me because she had heard I was one of the very few holistic cardiologists in the world seeing patients.

Our tests also revealed that Charlene had high levels of lead in her body. As with other patients, this could explain why her arteries were inflamed, stiffened, and calcified, thus leading to her hypertension.

We immediately started Charlene on *The 30-Day Blood Pressure Cure* plan and her body responded beautifully. Her blood pressure levels fell steadily—and by the end of the program, her readings were 115/75. By then I had completely withdrawn her antihypertensive medications.

Lab Results	Before the 30-Day Plan	After the 30-Day Plan
Lead	34	6
Mercury	17	2
Arsenic	67	26
Cholesterol	272	201
HDL	27	58
LDL	182	91
Triglycerides	424	106
Blood Sugar (fasting)	112	84

The chelation treatments also dropped her lead levels into the normal zone. Relieved, Charlene told her friends: " Dr. Heilbron has given my peace of mind back."

DAY 28: VOLUNTEER

*"What is important is family, friends, giving back to your community
and finding meaning in life."*

~Adrian Grenier, American actor

Helping others improves your own self-esteem and helps to conquer loneliness, anger, and the other negative emotions that can lead to high blood pressure—or make it worse. As a volunteer, you will reap a variety of benefits, including pleasure, feeling connected, and developing enhanced people skills. There is no shortage of need in today's world. Here are some ways to make a difference in others' lives—including your own.

VOLUNTEERING FEELS GOOD

The funny thing about volunteering is that you often benefit as much—or more—than those you help. Studies show that giving back to society or to nature can make you feel as good as eating a fantastic meal or some other pleasurable activity. *Helping others may be one of the best things you can do to help yourself.* [353]

Volunteering makes you feel good. Scientists have long theorized that the antidepressant boost people get from volunteering is triggered by positive social interaction. People are always happy to see a volunteer, and this positive feedback and interaction stimulates good feelings for both parties involved. Research has clearly found that volunteer work conquers depression, boredom and anxiety—and it is effective at any age. [354] Studies show that being a Good Samaritan lights up the pleasure centers in the brain. This warm, happy feeling in the brain decreases stress and elevates mood, which can help lower blood pressure.

CONNECT WITH YOUR COMMUNITY

Volunteering connects you with your community. Having a sense of connection to the world outside your door is one of the contributing factors to good mental, emotional, and physical health. Volunteering helps you see how important your time and energy can be in the lives of others or toward the advancement of a noble cause. It also exposes you to new people and helps widen your circle of friends. Volunteering increases your confidence, which in turn makes it easier for you to accomplish your goals in other areas of your life.

KEEPS YOUR MIND SHARP

In addition, volunteering keeps your mind sharp, because you are usually learning new skills in the process. These skills can then be used to enhance your career and enrich your personal life. Volunteering is an easy way to explore new interests and add more fulfillment to your life.

CLARIFY YOUR GOALS AND INTERESTS

Before you begin, take time to clarify your goals and interests. Which causes are you passionate about? In what environments do you prefer to spend your time? Do you like to be outdoors or indoors? Do you prefer to work with children, teens, adults, animals, or plants? Do you prefer group activities or would you be happier in a one-on-one situation? Are you better behind the scenes in a support capacity, or are you comfortable in the spotlight? What skills and abilities do you bring to the table? How much time can you realistically commit?

VOLUNTEERING OPPORTUNITES

Volunteering opportunities are everywhere. Many local newspapers even have a section where local organizations can put out their calls for volunteer help.

Pick an organization that is a good match for you. Start off slowly, enjoy yourself, and you can create a win-win situation for all involved. Ponder how your loving assistance and attention might change the lives of those in great need…

■   Teach an adult to read.

■   Visit an elderly person stuck in a nursing home with no one to talk to.

■   Do something to help a veteran whose psyche and body is shattered.

■   Help kids in foster care by becoming a foster parent or donating toys or clothes during the holidays.

■   Volunteer to help women and children who have been abused.

■   Walk dogs or play with cats at the animal shelter.

■   Remember members of your own family who may feel forgotten.

HELP OTHERS AS YOU HELP YOURSELF

You are not the same person who began this journey 29 days ago. You are very different. You have developed a more mindful approach to life by paying attention, being calm, and choosing the path of healing and helping. You are developing the wisdom and personal power to improve your life and our world. You are accomplishing something that very few people are able to: You are transforming your life. What a miracle!

But there is an even bigger miracle in store for you—and that's by helping others to transform their lives. We urge you to step out into the world and lend a helping hand.

Be conservative and start small. Don't over-commit yourself or you could lose the positive benefits of volunteering. Here are a few suggestions:

Spend one hour a week or one day a month—whatever you can fit in—to volunteer in your community. Visit the sick. Serve food to the hungry or homeless. Be a shoulder for someone's tears. Write a letter to a relative. Become a mentor in a support group. Share your wisdom and experience. Inspire someone who feels powerless. Support a cause you believe in. Register people to vote. Donate your old belongings. You get the idea. Just look around—there are hundreds of ways you can be of service.

TODAY'S ACTION STEPS

- Which of the volunteer categories we mentioned appeal to you most? Do you have a particular new interest or skill you would like to develop? Is there a worthy cause you would like to support? Record your ideas for volunteering in your Success Planner.

- Set aside some time today to investigate volunteer opportunities in your area, and make an appointment to meet the people involved.

- Start small by volunteering a little of your time in the beginning and then expand it as you feel more comfortable. The goal is to reap the benefits of volunteering without feeling stress from having taken on too much.

DAY 29: ADD TRAVEL, RESTAURANTS, AND PARTIES

"Certainly, travel is more than the seeing of sights; it is a change that goes on, deep and permanent, in the ideas of living."

~Miriam Beard, American historian, 1876–1958

For the past month, you have prepared your own home-cooked meals so you would get accustomed to eating foods that are whole, natural, and nutritious. Now that you are accomplished at this, it's time to extend your healthy new habits to the challenges of travel, restaurants and parties.

Unless you live in a cave, there is no escaping social occasions where you almost surely will be tempted by foods that can increase your weight, raise your blood pressure, and spike your blood sugar. No worries, because today you are going to learn how to enjoy restaurants and social gatherings without giving in.

MASTERING HEALTHFUL RESTAURANT DINING

The biggest key to healthful dining out is your choice of restaurant. For instance, it is difficult to find a healthful meal in a fast food joint—but it is very easy to be tempted. So, be smart and steer clear of any establishment that threatens your resolve. Just as it took time to develop good eating habits at home, you will need to take extreme care as you venture out into the food court. If there is a restaurant that represents your old life, it is smart to avoid it all together. Discover new places to dine that support your new, healthy lifestyle. Familiarize yourself with restaurants in your area that take pride in serving nutritious meals, especially those that serve locally grown organic produce, pasture-raised meats, and wild-caught fish.

If friends invite you to a restaurant that you are not familiar with, go online and check out their menu. If you fail to spot items that fit your new eating style, ask your friends if it would be okay to change restaurants. If they balk, it is better to graciously decline their invitation rather than forcing yourself to eat a meal that you know will not be good for you.

NAVIGATING THE MENU

Once you've selected a restaurant, spend some time with the menu. (*Tip:* Check out its menu online beforehand.) Look for the healthiest, cleanest protein options. Which fresh vegetables are available?

Most restaurant kitchens contain everything you need for a healthy, nutritious meal. However, not all of these options are packaged together on the menu. Once you discover the menu items you prefer, you can order them individually and ask that they be prepared in a way that supports your good health. For example, if the menu offers salmon in a cream sauce with a side of fried potatoes, you can ask that your salmon come lightly grilled without the sauce. Substitute a salad or fresh vegetable for the potatoes. Most restaurants are happy to accommodate simple requests. Do not patronize inflexible restaurants.

WHAT TO ORDER

Start with soup *and* salad. Soup is an excellent way to start your meal—just as long as it is not cream-based. Soup will fill you up with a minimum of calories. Then, follow the soup with a salad. Choose extra virgin olive oil vinaigrette dressing and ask for it "on the side," so you are in control of how much dressing is on your salad.

Choosing the entrée. Select some type of lean protein and surround it with lots of steamed or sautéed vegetables. When your entrée arrives, assess the portion size. Many restaurants serve entrées that are big enough for two. If this is the case, divide the food on your plate into a normal portion and ask the waiter to immediately remove the rest so you will not be tempted to overeat. You can request a "doggie bag" immediately if you feel you might be tempted to eat too much—or just push the extra food to the side of your plate to be bagged after you finish your meal.

What about dessert? If your dining companions are having sweet treats, allow yourself a taste, but set your limits. One small bite of Chocolate Decadence tastes exactly the same as an entire, heaping serving. (Studies show that the taste buds on your tongue do not even register the third bite of dessert.) So savor the taste—and remember that good health is the sweetest treat of all.

WHEN YOU NEED FOOD—FAST

There may be times when you need to eat, but do not have time for a sit-down restaurant meal. Instead of giving into the call of fast food and heading for the drive-thru, make a path to the nearest grocery store instead. Use your new knowledge of healthy food choices and grab something nutritious. A piece of fruit, a bag of unsalted mixed nuts or a small veggie platter, and a bottle of water might be just enough to keep you going until you can get home and cook something healthy.

PARTY ON!

Social events are a time for celebrating with family or friends and meeting new people. Remember that food and drinks are the backdrop of such situations, but the main focus should be people. Make it a point at social gatherings to introduce yourself to interesting strangers and to enjoy the people you already know. When you focus on socializing, food and drink become less important.

If you know you will be attending a party, eat before you go. When your body has been nutritionally satisfied with quality protein and vibrant vegetables, you are less likely to be tempted by "trouble foods." If there are raw vegetables at the party, enjoy them—but skip the creamy dips, preferring salsa or hummus instead.

At cocktail parties, ask for sparkling water. If you truly want to have alcohol, then limit yourself to one drink. Sip that drink slowly throughout the event and switch to sparkling water after it is gone.

For parties at work, reach for the nutritious snacks in your lunch bag. You can celebrate a co-workers birthday without eating cake. Again, if you really want a taste, have one bite and savor it. One trick we recently heard from a health-conscious actress is quite clever. She was working in the theatre in a successful long-running production with a large cast and crew. It seemed there was a birthday cake and celebration almost every other day. She learned that if she simply put a used plate in front of her at the table, no one would try to push her to have "just a small piece" of cake. Smart.

EATING ON THE GO

When travelling, eating well might be easier than you think. Natural foods stores can be found almost everywhere now. You only need to make the effort to go shopping. Employees at these stores can also give you tips on which local restaurants have the most healthful food. Your smart phone or GPS is a powerful tool in your search for healthy restaurants.

Always travel with a food supply. Airport food courts are a nutrition wasteland. There is something about sitting for long periods of time, such as in an airplane, that triggers hunger. Be prepared for this with a stash of fruit, raw veggie slices, nuts, and some clean proteins such as a hard-boiled egg or grilled chicken breast. Snack leisurely and say "no thanks" to the flight attendants passing out junkie snacks. Have bottled water or seltzer instead of juice or soda pop.

Always carry a bottle of clean water or herbal tea. This is a must when you are traveling. Remember that delays can happen, so be prepared. Being able to take care of your own nutritional needs will help you stay calm if you are snowed in at the airport (of course, bear in mind that it's not possible to bring liquids past security) or your tour bus breaks down on the side of the road. You can also bring your own insulated lunch bag or cooler packed full of healthful foods and beverages.

CRUISE SHIPS

Cruise ships are a world unto themselves. Some people call them floating buffets, and not without reason. Food and alcohol are waiting around every corner any time of the day or night. You can almost always find something healthful to eat at these lavish buffets. Sometimes just looking at the dessert table is enough to satisfy your desire. If not, go ahead and have a bite or two. Just be sure you can stop yourself.

Plan ahead with your traveling companion to set healthy limits for yourself. Go ahead and have one of those strawberries from the three-foot-tall chocolate fountain. Just have one. Then enjoy the rest of your strawberries in their own natural goodness. Realize that not only is an abundance of food on a cruise ship, there are also plenty of opportunities to be active. Most boats have a gym and nightly dancing. Many also have climbing walls, fitness classes, and swimming pools. And you can always walk around the deck in the sunshine (or moonlight) in the fresh ocean air. Use the stairs instead of the elevator. Bring back photos and memories, instead of an extra 10 pounds of body weight. There are plenty of ways to have fun on a cruise without going overboard.

TODAY'S ACTION STEPS

- Research local restaurants and make a list of those that specialize in healthful fare. Plan to dine at one of these this week as a "practice session." Dine alone or with a supportive companion to make it easier.

- Healthful dining is a skill that you must learn—so use this opportunity to discover your strong and weak points. Do not beat yourself up if you slip up somewhere. Just notice that this is a trouble point for you, so you can be more careful at your next outing. After the meal, be honest with yourself about what was easy and difficult.

- Make notes in your Success Planner afterward so you will not have unrealistic expectations of yourself the next time you dine out.

- Most of all, enjoy yourself. Take pleasure in your surroundings. Delight in the camaraderie and conversation with your dining companion. Feel gratitude for being alive.

DAY 30: CELEBRATE!

"The more you praise and celebrate your life,
the more there is in life to celebrate."

~Oprah Winfrey

It's time to celebrate! You made it through the program—and day after day you saw your blood pressure drop and stabilize. Along the way, you may have discovered some serendipitous bonuses. You probably lost weight and added muscle. No doubt, you have more energy and get up and go. And, we are betting that your moods have brightened and you have a more positive mental outlook on life. All in all, you are probably feeling better than you have in many years—perhaps even decades. So today it is time to celebrate your many accomplishments and your new found health. Today is just for you: a day to relax, reflect, and rejoice. You certainly deserve it!

REVIEW YOUR ACCOMPLISHMENTS

You have come so far in these past 30 days. Take a look back over your Success Planner and notice how you have taken charge of your health and your life. You are monitoring your blood pressure daily. You have become more physically active—and are enjoying your newfound strength and stamina. You are learning to cook new recipes made from foods that strengthen and support you. Way to go!

You now have the knowledge and habits that will help you to lead a healthy, active, and vibrant lifestyle. Today is a day to rejoice in all the wonderful new things you've done for yourself. And you're just getting started…

CELEBRATE YOURSELF TODAY

Please don't allow your accomplishments and progress to go unacknowledged. Even though you will stay with this new healthful living plan for the rest of your life, this is a watershed moment. You should take time to congratulate yourself for your determination to succeed—and your commitment to good health and a more hopeful future. Here are a few suggestions for making today truly special:

Arise early. Arise earlier than usual to give yourself extra time to appreciate this day and your accomplishments. Spend 20 to 30 minutes quietly contemplating or meditating. (See suggestions below.)

Meditate. Go to a quiet spot and do a simple meditation. You may want to have some soft music playing in the background, or you may prefer silence, or the sounds of the birds singing their morning songs.

Sit comfortably. Let your eyes gently close. Breathe deeply. Now begin to count your blessings. With each in-breath, think of something or someone for which or for whom you are especially grateful. With each out-breath, whisper, say or sing "Thank You." Allow your face to smile. Are you thankful for a new day? "Thank you." Are you grateful for a special friend? "Thank you." Are you happy that your body is healing? "Thank you."

Just sit and breathe and smile and bask in the healing power of gratitude.

When you feel complete, stand and stretch and start your day.

Take a walk. Put on your walking shoes and go outdoors. Hold your head high. You've accomplished a great deal. You may enjoy continuing to look at the world with eyes of gratitude while you walk. Notice the trees, the sky, how much stronger your legs are than they were just a month ago. "Thank you."

Dress up. Once you're back home and have showered, dress in clothes that make you feel really good about yourself. You have a date with yourself today. Take a little extra time to dress up.

Eat well. Make yourself a delicious and healthy breakfast. Pack a healing lunch and some natural snacks that will fuel your day. There are recipes scattered throughout this book, in the appendix, and even more online at www.myhealingkitchen.com and www.bottomlinepublications.com.

Do something "just for you." Whether you work today or not, plan to do something special just for you, either during the day, on your lunch break, or after work. Treat yourself to a massage or visit a museum or an art gallery. Be extra-nice to yourself. Buy yourself some fresh flowers, or something you may have been wanting for some time. Plan on treating yourself to a delicious (but healthful!) dinner.

Remind yourself again. Remember that you are living differently now. You have given yourself the gift of a brighter future. You have learned skills and tools that will continue to improve the quality of your life. Be grateful to yourself for choosing a better life and taking action to heal. Write a little in your journal or Success Planner about how much you appreciate yourself and your life. Write about what inspires you.

Relax before bedtime. Do a little yoga or Tai Chi. Prepare healthy meals for tomorrow. Then, put on your pajamas and rest.

This is just the beginning...

TODAY'S ACTION STEPS

- You have surely inspired your friends and family, who have observed your "health trans-formation." You're a hero to them and have set a wonderful example for them to follow!

- To celebrate, plan a movie night with someone very special and view the moving true story of another person's determination and passion.

- The film we would like you to watch is *A Man Named Pearl*. This documentary follows Pearl Fryar, son of a poor sharecropper, as he creates a stunning 3.5-acre topiary garden from plants other people have discarded. In the process, Fryar rises to international prominence as an acclaimed topiary artist and brings together one of the poorest communities in South Carolina. Pearl will make your heart sing as you set a course for your future. (The film is available through Netflix or see if your local library has a DVD copy you can check out.)

A SAMPLE DAY IN THE 30-DAY BLOOD PRESSURE CURE PLAN

Time	Food	Drink	Exercise
Breakfast	Veggie omelet, whole grain gluten-free bread. Take vitamins and supplements	Tea or coffee substitute	Stretch/meditate/ breathe deeply, take a walk
Snack	Veggie sticks dipped in almond butter	Filtered water in a glass or stainless steel bottle	Get up and move every hour
Lunch	Salad drizzled with vinaigrette (made with cold-pressed olive oil) and topped with grilled, organic chicken breast or wild-caught salmon	Filtered water in a glass or stainless steel bottle	Take short walk
Snack	Vegetable juice with side of sharp cheddar cheese	Tea or coffee substitute	Get up and move every hour
Dinner	Bean soup with berries for dessert. Take vitamins and supplements	Sparkling water with a twist of lemon	Step up your activity level by walking longer or faster or participating in an activity of your choice
Bedtime			Stretch/meditate/breathe deeply. Give yourself a full night's sleep

DR. HEILBRON'S CASE STUDY: OFFICER JAMES

"I feel like a man again."

James is a police officer with a history of high blood pressure. He came to our clinic because he was unhappy with the side effects of his antihypertensive medications and was hoping to get off them. He had also suffered a heart attack and was not pleased with the sexual side effects of these medications. (Neither was his wife.)

He asked me to write him a prescription for Viagra. (I should mention that Officer James is about 6 feet 4 inches tall, and 245 lbs of solid muscle.) He was on a statin and three different anti-hypertensive medicines, and we had to get him off these medications. "I don't feel like much of a man," he confided to me.

His blood pressure readings, even with medication, averaged at 142/84, with peak systolic pressure rising as high as 223. I immediately started him on *The 30-Day Blood Pressure Cure* plan.

When we tested his lead levels, they were very high—no doubt from years of pistol shooting and inhaling the exhaust from his ammunition. So I also started him on a program of intravenous and oral chelation treatments.

Lab Results	Before the 30-Day Plan	After the 30-Day Plan
Lead	90	15
Mercury	12	4
Arsenic	42	11
Total cholesterol	211 (on a statin)	57 (off medication)

By the end of *The 30-Day Blood Pressure Cure Plan*, James' blood pressure had fallen to a healthy 110/70—allowing me to withdraw all of his antihypertensive medications.

The chelation treatments dropped his lead levels into the normal range. He and his wife are very pleased. "I thank Dr. Heilbron for his holistic approach. I don't need Viagra anymore—and I feel like a man again."

THE 30-DAY BLOOD PRESSURE CURE PLAN

APPENDICES

APPENDIX A

HIGH BLOOD PRESSURE MEDICATIONS

The following is a list of commonly prescribed blood pressure medications with explanations of how they work. Depending on what other conditions you might have, some of these medications are more effective than others. As we have said previously, we believe medications should be used in the short-term for emergency situations only. Once your blood pressure is out of the danger zone, it is our belief, as we have explained in this book, that other approaches addressing the causes behind hypertension, rather than just the numbers themselves, are safer and far more effective.

Thiazide diuretics. Diuretics, also referred to as "water pills," increase the kidneys' excretion of sodium and water,. This causes frequent urination, thus decreasing the volume of fluid in the bloodstream and the pressure in the arteries. Frequent urination also results in a loss of vitamins and minerals, especially magnesium and potassium, which are valuable in the body's natural regulation of blood pressure. Because of this, some doctors monitor blood potassium levels (and magnesium, though this isn't as common) during therapy. Patients who have low potassium levels are encouraged to eat foods rich in potassium, such as bananas, Swiss chard, and yams, or may be prescribed a potassium supplement.

Diuretics are one of the oldest and best-studied classes of anti-hypertensive agents. Thiazide diuretics are often the first—but not the only—choice in high blood pressure medications. They are also the least expensive. If you're not taking a diuretic and your blood pressure remains high after trying other measures, ask your doctor about adding one, or replacing a drug you currently take with a diuretic.

One of the most commonly used diuretic agents is hydrochlorothiazide (HydroDiuril, Microzide). Other diuretics used to treat hypertension include the following:

- *Acetazolamide* (Diamox)
- *Furosemide* (Lasix)
- *Indapamide* (Lozol)
- *Metolazone* (Zaroxolyn)
- *Spirnolactone* (Aldactone)
- *Torsemide* (Demadex)
- *Triamterene* (Dyrenium)

Combination medications, which contain both a diuretic and a different class of anti-hypertensive agent, are now being produced and prescribed. The main side effects of these combined treatments are fatigue and dizziness.

Beta blockers. These drugs reduce blood pressure by decreasing the force of a heartbeat, the heart rate, and the amount of blood the heart pumps out. When prescribed alone, beta blockers are not as effective in the elderly and people of African descent, unless combined with a thiazide diuretic. In addition to lowering blood pressure, beta blockers have additional benefits, which include prolonging the lives of patients with coronary artery disease, patients who have suffered a heart attack, and those with congestive heart failure (CHF). Commonly used beta blockers include the following:

- *Acebutolol* (Sectral, Prent)
- *Atenolol* (Tenormin)
- *Bisoprolol* (Zebeta)
- *Carvedilol* (Coreg)
- *Metoprolol* (Lopressor, Toprol XL)
- *Timolol* (Blockadren)

Another beta blocker, *labetolol* (Normodyne, Trandate), possesses alpha blocker properties. Alpha blockers dilate the arteries in order to lower blood pressure.

Potential side effects of the beta blockers include slowing the heart rate excessively; worsening heart failure; and contributing to mental confusion, depression, and impotence (erectile dysfunction).

Calcium channel blockers. These medications help relax the muscles inside your blood vessels so they expand (dilate) more readily. Some also slow the heart rate. Calcium channel blockers seem to work better for the elderly and people of African descent, compared with ACE inhibitors or beta blockers alone. A word of caution: Grapefruit juice interacts with some calcium channel blockers, increasing blood levels of the medication and putting you at higher risk for side effects. Talk to your doctor or pharmacist if you're concerned about these interactions.

Two popular drugs, *diltiazem* (Cardizem) and *verapamil* (Calan, Covera HS, Isoptin, Veralan), act, in part, like the beta blockers, decreasing the strength of the heartbeat, thus decreasing blood pressure by reducing the force with which blood is pumped into the arteries. These agents also dilate (open up) arteries, decreasing the resistance to blood flow, thereby decreasing blood pressure.

The newer calcium channel blockers primarily dilate the arteries and have little effect on the forcefulness of the heart's contractions. These include:

- Amlodipine (Norvasc)
- Felodipine (Plendil)
- Isradipine (DynaCirc)
- Nicardipine (Cardene)
- Nisoldipine (Sular)

Norvasc has been combined with the cholesterol-lowering drug Lipitor to treat patients with high blood pressure and high cholesterol. This combination drug, branded as Caduet, appeals to physicians who like the convenience of one medication that supposedly controls both conditions.

Calcium channel blockers may have serious side effects and should be used with caution in patients with pulmonary arterial hypertension (PAH). PAH, which is life-threatening, is high blood pressure in the arteries that supply blood to the lungs (the pulmonary arteries).

In some cases, diltiazem and verapamil, which weaken the force of the heart's contractions, can worsen congestive heart failure symptoms. Verapamil may occasionally cause constipation, especially in elderly patients. Many of the calcium channel blockers routinely cause headache and edema (swelling) in the ankles and feet.

Angiotensin-converting enzyme (ACE) inhibitors. These medications help dilate the arteries by blocking the formation of a natural chemical that narrows blood vessels. This action allows arteries to expand when blood pressure typically rises, as with exertion or stress. These drugs also produce other beneficial cardiovascular effects and are commonly used to treat patients with congestive heart failure. Studies show that treatment of heart failure patients with ACE inhibitors can improve heart failure symptoms, decrease the chance of future hospitalizations, reduce the risk for future heart attack, and lower the risk of death from heart failure. There are many ACE inhibitors available, including the following:

- Benazepril (Lotensin)
- Captopril (Capoten)
- Enalapril (Vasotec)
- Fosinopril (Monopril)
- Lisinopril (Prinivil, Zestril)
- Quinapril (Accupril)
- Ramipril (Altace)
- Trandolapril (Mavik)

ACE inhibitors are usually tolerated well, but have potential side effects. Approximately 10% of patients develop a chronic cough. Occasionally, ACE inhibitors can produce a sudden swelling of the lips, face, and cheek areas, which is an allergic reaction that can occur at any time during therapy. If an allergic reaction occurs, medical attention should be sought immediately. Because ACE inhibitors can affect kidney function and raise potassium levels, doctors monitor these during the first several weeks of therapy and periodically thereafter.

Angiotensin II receptor blockers (ARBs). Also simply called angiotensin-receptor blockers, this class of medications is similar to ACE inhibitors in that they lower blood pressure by dilating arteries, thus making it easier for the heart to pump blood throughout the body. Also, like ACE inhibitors, they seem to improve the symptoms of congestive heart failure and have been shown to prolong life. ARBs, like all of the medications listed below, are generally taken once a day and are generally well-tolerated, producing few significant side effects (although they have been observed to interfere with or worsen kidney function). Currently prescribed ARBs include:

- *Azilsartan medoxomil* (Edarbi)
- *Candesartan* (Atacand)
- *Irbesartan* (Avapro)
- *Losartan* (Cozaar)
- *Telmisartan* (Micardis)
- *Valsartan* (Diovan)

Renin inhibitors. Direct renin inhibitors are the newest type of medicine for high blood pressure. Drugs in this class, such as *aliskiren*, work by blocking enzymes (renin) that cause blood vessels to tighten up. As a result, the vessels relax and widen, making it easier for blood to flow, which lowers blood pressure. Commonly prescribed renin inhibitors include Tekturna.

However, not everyone agrees that this new drug is effective. In a review of six large-scale clinical trials of aliskiren, published in the *American Journal of Hypertension*, researchers report that it is no more effective than those already widely available to control hypertension. Although aliskiren lowered blood pressure to a greater extent when combined with a converting enzyme inhibitor (CEI), an ARB or a diuretic, fewer than half of the patients achieved blood pressure control. [355]

The most common side effect of renin inhibitors is diarrhea. Stomach and abdominal pain also frequently occur, but they're not considered serious unless they become severe. Pregnant women should not use renin inhibitors. If you become pregnant, stop taking this medicine and call your doctor. Before taking a renin inhibitor, tell your doctor if you have kidney problems. People with kidney problems may need to have regular blood tests to make sure this medicine does not reduce kidney function.

The website www.drugs.com notes that renin inhibitors can cause extremely low blood pressure (hypotension). Symptoms of low blood pressure include feeling light-headed or faint, having a weak pulse or developing an uneven heart rate, which can be quite dangerous. [356]

When Your Blood Pressure Needs Extra Help

If you're having trouble reaching your blood pressure goal with any of the above medications (or combinations), your doctor may choose to prescribe:

Alpha blockers. These medications, which include *doxazosin* and Flomax, reduce nerve impulses to blood vessels, reducing the effects of natural biochemicals that narrow blood vessels. Side effects can range from sudden drops in blood pressure upon standing and fainting.

Alpha-beta blockers. In addition to reducing nerve impulses to blood vessels, alpha-beta blockers also slow the heartbeat to reduce force of the blood pumped through the vessels. Similar side effects as those produced by Alpha blockers are typical, as well as diarrhea and depression. Brand names in this class include Normodyne and Coreg.

Central-acting agents. These medications prevent your brain from signaling your nervous system to increase your heart rate and narrow your blood vessels. Such medications include *clonidine* (Catapres) and *methyldopa* (Aldomet). Because these drugs act directly on the brain, they occasionally cause drowsiness, depression, and other symptoms.

Direct-acting vasodilators. These directly dilate the arteries, opening them wider to allow for easier blood flow. The most important of these drugs is *hydralazine*, which has been largely replaced by newer drugs, though it still plays an important role with certain types of patients, especially those with newly diagnosed gestational hypertension.

Hydralazine works by causing the muscles that line and surround arteries to relax, resulting in dilation and lowered blood pressure. Along with this relaxation, hydralazine also causes a rise in the heart rate and an increase in the total amount of blood being pumped by the heart. Though typically dispensed as a generic drug, hydralazine may sometimes still be found as the brand-name drug, Apresoline.

Hydralazine tends to increase heart rate and may cause fluid retention through its action on the kidneys. These effects are usually countered by giving hydralazine along with other medicines such as beta blockers and diuretics, though this is not always possible in pregnant patients.

Hydralazine is sometimes used in combination with isosorbide dinitrate to treat patients with congestive heart failure.

APPENDIX B

THE GLYCEMIC INDEX AND GLYCEMIC LOAD FOR 100+ FOODS

The glycemic index and glycemic load offer information about how foods affect blood sugar and insulin. The lower a food's glycemic index or glycemic load, the less it affects blood sugar and insulin levels. For more information on glycemic index and glycemic load, see Chapter Nine.

On the following pages a list of the glycemic index and glycemic load for more than 100 common foods created by Harvard Medical School's *Harvard Health Publications*. For additional details, please visit http://www.health.harvard.edu/newsweek/Glycemic_index_and_glycemic_load_for_100_foods.htm.

FOOD	Glycemic index (glucose = 100)	Serving size (grams)	Glycemic load per serving
BAKERY PRODUCTS AND BREADS			
Banana cake, made with sugar	47	60	14
Banana cake, made without sugar	55	60	12
Sponge cake, plain	46	63	17
Vanilla cake made from packaged mix with vanilla frosting (Betty Crocker)	42	111	24
Apple, made with sugar	44	60	13
Apple, made without sugar	48	60	9
Waffles, Aunt Jemima (Quaker Oats)	76	35	10
Bagel, white, frozen	72	70	25
Baguette, white, plain	95	30	15
Coarse barley bread, 75% to 80% kernels, average	34	30	7
Hamburger bun	61	30	9
Kaiser roll	73	30	12
Pumpernickel bread	56	30	7
50% cracked wheat kernel bread	58	30	12
White wheat flour bread	71	30	10
Wonder bread, average	73	30	10
Whole wheat bread, average	71	30	9
100% Whole Grain bread (Natural Ovens)	51	30	7
Pita bread, white	68	30	10
Corn tortilla	52	50	12
Wheat tortilla	30	50	8

50% cracked wheat kernel bread	58	30	12
White wheat flour bread	71	30	10
Wonder bread, average	73	30	10
Whole wheat bread, average	71	30	9
100% Whole Grain bread (Natural Ovens)	51	30	7
Pita bread, white	68	30	10
Corn tortilla	52	50	12
Wheat tortilla	30	50	8
BEVERAGES			
Coca Cola, average	63	250 mL	16
Fanta, orange soft drink	68	250 mL	23
Lucozade, original (sparkling glucose drink)	95±10	250 mL	40
Apple juice, unsweetened, average	44	250 mL	30
Cranberry juice cocktail (Ocean Spray)	68	250 mL	24
Gatorade	78	250 mL	12
Orange juice, unsweetened	50	250 mL	12
Tomato juice, canned	38	250 mL	4
BREAKFAST CEREALS AND RELATED PRODUCTS			
All-Bran, average	55	30	12
Coco Pops, average	77	30	20
Cornflakes, average	93	30	23
Cream of Wheat (Nabisco)	66	250	17
Cream of Wheat, Instant (Nabisco)	74	250	22
Grapenuts, average	75	30	16
Muesli, average	66	30	16
Oatmeal, average	55	250	13
Instant oatmeal, average	83	250	30
Puffed wheat, average	80	30	17
Raisin Bran (Kellogg's)	61	30	12
Special K (Kellogg's)	69	30	14

GRAINS			
Pearled barley, average	28	150	12
Sweet corn on the cob, average	60	150	20
Couscous, average	65	150	9
Quinoa	53	150	13
White rice, average	89	150	43
Quick cooking white basmati	67	150	28
Brown rice, average	50	150	16
Converted white rice (Uncle Bens)	38	150	14
Whole wheat kernels, average	30	50	11
Bulgur, average	48	150	12
COOKIES AND CRACKERS			
Graham crackers	74	25	14
Vanilla wafers	77	25	14
Shortbread	64	25	10
Rice cakes, average	82	25	17
Rye crisps, average	64	25	11
Soda crackers	74	25	12
DAIRY PRODUCTS AND ALTERNATIVES			
Ice cream, regular	57	50	6
Ice cream, premium	38	50	3
Milk, full fat	41	250mL	5
Milk, skim	32	250 mL	4
Reduced-fat yogurt with fruit, average	33	200	11
FRUITS			
Apple, average	39	120	6
Banana, ripe	62	120	16
Dates, dried	42	60	18
Grapefruit	25	120	3
Grapes, average	59	120	11
Orange, average	40	120	4
Peach, average	42	120	5

Peach, canned in light syrup	40	120	5
Pear, average	38	120	4
Pear, canned in pear juice	43	120	5
Prunes, pitted	29	60	10
Raisins	64	60	28
Watermelon	72	120	4
BEANS AND NUTS			
Baked beans, average	40	150	6
Black-eyed peas, average	33	150	10
Black beans	30	150	7
Chickpeas, average	10	150	3
Chickpeas, canned in brine	38	150	9
Navy beans, average	31	150	9
Kidney beans, average	29	150	7
Lentils, average	29	150	5
Soy beans, average	15	150	1
Cashews, salted	27	50	3
Peanuts, average	7	50	0
PASTA and NOODLES			
Fettucini, average	32	180	15
Macaroni, average	47	180	23
Macaroni & Cheese (Kraft)	64	180	32
Spaghetti, white, boiled, average	46	180	22
Spaghetti, white, boiled 20 min, average	58	180	26
Spaghetti, wholemeal, boiled, average	42	180	17
SNACK FOODS			
Corn chips, plain, salted, average	42	50	11
Fruit Roll-Ups	99	30	24
M & Ms, peanut	33	30	6
Microwave popcorn, plain, average	55	20	6
Potato chips, average	51	50	12
Pretzels, oven-baked	83	30	16

Snickers Bar	51	60	18
VEGETABLES			
Green peas, average	51	80	4
Carrots, average	35	80	2
Parsnips	52	80	4
Baked russet potato, average	111	150	33
Boiled white potato, average	82	150	21
Instant mashed potato, average	87	150	17
Sweet potato, average	70	150	22
Yam, average	54	150	20
MISCELLANEOUS			
Hummus (chickpea salad dip)	6	30	0
Chicken nuggets, frozen, reheated in microwave oven 5 min	46	100	7
Pizza, plain baked dough, served with parmesan cheese and tomato sauce	80	100	22
Pizza, Super Supreme (Pizza Hut)	36	100	9
Honey, average	61	25	12

APPENDIX C

HYPERTENSION-HEALING MEAL SUGGESTIONS

All meals and snacks should combine a protein food, a healthful fat source and low-glycemic carbohydrates such as vegetables or whole grains. Some suggested meals might include:

Breakfast

Protein source: Eggs and/or meat.

Fat source: This may already be included in your protein (both bacon and eggs contain fat). You may also add butter, cream (in coffee) or cheese.

Carbohydrate source: Low GI vegetables, including beans or sautéed vegetables in an omelet or breakfast quiche.

Lunch

Protein source: Hard-boiled eggs, meat or fish, beans, or a whole grain such as quinoa.

Fat source: Extra virgin olive oil as a dressing for steamed vegetables or a salad. Cheese and avocado are other good sources of healthful fats.

Carbohydrate source: Salad greens, vegetables (steamed, sautéed, or stir-fried), soup.

Snack

Include two between-meal snacks ever day. The ideal snack contains 100–150 calories and combines either fat or protein with a low-glycemic carbohydrate. Examples: Cheese and raw vegetables, peanut butter on celery sticks, unsweetened yogurt and fruit, nuts and fresh fruit.

Dinner

Protein source: Meat or fish, beans, or whole grain.

Fat source: Extra virgin olive oil as a dressing for steamed vegetables or a salad, butter, or avocado.

Carbohydrate source: Salad greens, cooked greens, or whole grain.

SAMPLE MEAL AND SNACK SUGGESTIONS

Breakfast: Vegetable omelet, black beans, side of avocado, coffee or tea.

Mid-morning snack: 3–4 small celery sticks filled with a thin layer of chunky peanut butter.

Lunch: Hearty vegetable soup, salad with grilled chicken or fish, dressing of extra virgin olive oil and balsamic vinegar, unsweetened ice tea or mineral water.

Mid-afternoon snack: Small handful of almonds, walnuts, or cashews with ½ cup Greek-style yogurt topped with cinnamon.

Dinner: Three-bean chili, half-sweet potato with tangy Greek-yogurt topping, small veggie salad with tangy garlic vinaigrette dressing, hot herbal tea.

ADDITIONAL SUGGESTIONS

Breakfast: Bowl of steel-cut oatmeal topped with fresh berries, soy yogurt, and flax meal, side of bacon (optional), coffee or tea.

Mid-morning snack: Crunchy apple with small piece of cheddar cheese.

Lunch: Quinoa and babaganoush (roasted eggplant dip) with raw celery and carrot sticks, pickled onions and olives, fresh cherry tomatoes.

Mid-afternoon snack: Hard-boiled egg with leftover celery and carrot sticks from lunch.

Dinner: Free-range steak, roast chicken, or grilled fish, steamed broccoli or green beans (drizzled with melted butter or extra virgin olive oil), quinoa and mushroom ragout, glass of white wine.

APPENDIX D

THE HYPERTENSION-HEALING KITCHEN MAKEOVER

In order to heal your hypertension, your kitchen will need a makeover to get rid of all foods, beverages, and ingredients that aren't beneficial to your blood pressure. Go through your kitchen and remove all the foods and ingredients in the left column below and replace them with the more healthful versions on the right.

REFRIGERATOR

REMOVE	REPLACE (with organic, when possible)
Margarine	dairy butter, coconut butter
Low fat, nonfat cheese	full-fat cheese
Mayonnaise	plain Greek yogurt
Skim milk, coffee creamer	whole milk, half and half, unsweetened soy milk
Sweetened yogurt	plain Greek or homemade yogurt
Conventional produce	organic produce
Factory-farm eggs	omega-3 eggs
Store-bought salad dressings	homemade vinaigrette
Condiments containing high fructose corn syrup	HFCS-free condiments
Unhealthful dips	salsa and hummus
Soda	sparkling water
Most juices	fresh fruit, unsweetened pomegranate juice or water
Whole wheat or processed bread	100% whole grain, gluten-free bread
Nitrate/nitrite-containing breakfast/lunch meats	nitrate- and nitrite-free lunch meat

FREEZER

Artificially sweetened frozen desserts	frozen fruit for yogurt smoothies
Ice cream (full-fat, low-fat, nonfat)	frozen fruit for yogurt smoothies
Frozen juice concentrate	frozen fruit
TV dinners and frozen packaged meals	healthful leftovers in one portion servings
Frozen vegetables in cheese and other sauces	plain frozen vegetables
Breaded/farmed fish	plain wild-caught fish
Breaded/conventional chicken	free-range, organic chicken
Factory-farmed beef	organic, grass-fed and finished beef

PANTRY AND CABINETS

Sweetened applesauce	unsweetened applesauce
Sweetened cocoa	unsweetened cocoa
Flavored/canned coffee	green teabags and whole coffee beans (store in freezer)
Rice-a-Roni	whole-grain pilaf
Macaroni and cheese	whole-grain, gluten-free pasta
White flour pasta	whole-grain, gluten-free pasta
White rice	brown rice, quinoa, amaranth, barley, etc.
Canned beans	dry beans
BPA-containing canned goods	BPA-free canned goods, jarred goods, homemade
Canned soups	homemade soups
Chips and crackers	nuts and seeds
Instant oatmeal	steel-cut oats
Cold cereal	unsweetened whole grain hot cereal

White flour	whole grain, high-fiber, gluten-free flour
Crisco	lard (store in fridge)
Canola oil	grape seed, coconut, sesame, peanut oil
Poor-quality olive oil	fresh, reputable extra virgin olive oil
Sugary liqueurs and mixers	red and white wines
Sugar-added tomato sauce	unsweetened tomato sauce
Bottled salad dressing	Homemade dressing from extra virgin olive oil and balsamic or other vinegars

APPENDIX E

EVALUATING THE MOST POPULAR HYPERTENSION-FIGHTING DIETS

There are numerous diets that promote their ability to fight hypertension. What follows is a list of some of the more popular ones. While these diets can, to varying degrees, succeed at managing hypertension, they will not reverse the condition—or at least not as effectively as the diet and lifestyle changes we outline in *The 30-Day Blood Pressure Cure Plan.*

The DASH Diet. One of the most common diets prescribed to people with high blood pressure is the DASH diet, developed by the National Heart, Lung and Blood Institute (NHLBI). DASH, which stands for Dietary Approaches to Stop Hypertension, emphasizes eating more fruits, vegetables and non- or low-fat dairy products, poultry and fish, and fewer portions of red meat, sugars, and salt. It seems to provide adequate amounts of potassium, calcium, magnesium, protein, and fiber and calls for a reduced sodium consumption of between 1,500 to 2,300 milligrams per day.

We don't believe the reduction in sodium is necessary, but the diet's general approach does seem to help reduce hypertension. In one clinical study, DASH lowered systolic blood pressure by 11 mmHg and diastolic blood pressure 5.5 mmHg on average. In fact, multiple studies funded by the National Heart, Lung and Blood Institute have found that the DASH diet improves blood pressure as well as or better than any of the expensive (and sometimes dangerous) medications now in use.

However, DASH is far from perfect. According to researchers at Johns Hopkins University,[357] although following this diet can help lower blood pressure and LDL cholesterol, it doesn't do much for other blood lipids. It actually reduces levels of protective HDL cholesterol and has no effect whatsoever on triglycerides, another lipid that signals an increased risk for strokes and heart attacks. When lead researcher, Lawrence Appel, MD, and his team added monounsaturated fats and more protein back into the diet, however, they saw participants' triglycerides go down and HDL cholesterol go up.

A lack of healthful fats and proteins isn't DASH's only problem. A study published by the Department of Nutritional Research and Education at Calton Nutrition in North Venice, Florida,[358] found that DASH, as with The South Beach Diet and Atkins for Life Diet, is deficient in a number of essential micronutrients, including vitamin B7, vitamin D, vitamin E, chromium, iodine, and molybdenum.

Clearly, the DASH diet, as currently constituted, isn't adequate to promote all aspects of good cardiac health.

Mediterranean Diet. People in the Mediterranean love their olive oil. Since cold-pressed extra-virgin olive oil is rich in monounsaturated and polyunsaturated fat, their cardiovascular systems love it, too. Like DASH, this diet goes heavy on the fruits, vegetables, and low/

nonfat dairy and light on red meat and poultry. But the Mediterranean Diet makes a distinction between fats, noting that not all fats are created equal and that monounsaturated and polyunsaturated fats—as opposed to saturated fats—are actually *good* for you. So instead of butter, drizzle olive oil onto your Italian bread. An added benefit: On this diet, you can even savor up to one glass of red wine a day. Eating healthfully can feel decadent.

Now, a recent study[359] has found that eating a Mediterranean diet can slash your risk of first-time heart attack, stroke, or cardiovascular death by a whopping 30%, compared with the official low-fat diet recommended by the American Heart Association, the American Diabetes Association and the American Medical Association.

The five-year study, called PREDIMED, included 7,447 people at high risk for heart attack or stroke with major cardiovascular risk factors, such as being overweight, cigarette smoking and having hypertension, diabetes and/or metabolic syndrome.

Participants were divided into a group that ate the standard, doctor-recommended low-fat diet compared with those who ate a typical Mediterranean diet defined as including…

- Fruits—3 servings daily
- Vegetables—2 servings daily
- Fish—3 or more servings weekly; preferably fatty fish
- Beans—3 or more servings weekly
- Sofrito—2 or more servings weekly*
- Poultry (in place of habitual red meat)
- Extra virgin olive oil (EVOO)—4 tbsp daily; or nuts—3 servings weekly (walnuts, almonds, and hazelnuts)
- Glass of wine at dinner (optional)

*Sofrito is a traditional Mediterranean sauce of tomato, onion, garlic, EVOO, and herbs.

The Mediterranean diet groups were asked to limit dairy foods, red meats, processed meats and avoid soda and commercial baked goods (cookies, cakes, and pastries).

After five years, the participants who followed either of the Mediterranean diets (more EVOO vs. more nuts) showed a substantial 30% reduction in heart attacks, strokes, and cardiovascular deaths, compared with the low-fat group. In other words, the Mediterranean diet saved 30% more lives among the high-risk patients.

Ornish Diet. Dr. Dean Ornish made a name for himself with this vegetarian diet, which emphasizes complex carbohydrates and a minimum of fat with some protein. Only 10% of calories are allowed from fat. This was combined with a regular program of meditation, relaxation, physical activity, and group interaction.

Whole grains, vegetables, and legumes can be consumed in unlimited quantities, but meat is excluded. To keep cholesterol consumption down to 5 milligrams per day, the 15% to 20% protein called for in this diet comes mostly from egg whites and non- or low-fat dairy products. Caffeine is completely forbidden. Sugar, salt, and alcohol are allowed only in moderation.

Paleolithic Diet. The Paleo Diet (also called the Paleolithic or Caveman Diet) is extremely healthful. It emphasizes:

- High protein, from wild game (mammals, fish, and birds), if possible, or from grass-fed animals
- High fiber
- Low fat
- Foods that are gathered in the wild, such as fruit, honey, vegetables, eggs, berries, and roots; or at least fruits and vegetables that are organic
- Beverages should include only coconut milk, organic green tea, or water
- None of the following foods: Dairy, grains, sugar, potatoes, and processed oils (some versions of the diet allow for olive oil and flaxseed oil)

Researchers at the University of California San Francisco did the most important study on this type of diet in 2009.[360] Participants ate their usual diet for three days, three "ramp-up diets" of increasing potassium and fiber for seven days and then a Paleolithic-type diet, consisting of lean meat, fruits, vegetables, and nuts for 10 days. Consuming the Paleo diet resulted in significant reductions in blood pressure, blood insulin levels, total cholesterol, LDL cholesterol, and triglycerides. The results, in brief, were remarkable.

Pritikin Program. The Pritikin Program, created by diet and exercise guru Nathan Pritikin in the 1970s, is very similar to the DASH (Dietary Approaches to Stop Hypertension) diet. It focuses on vegetables, fruits, whole grains, beans, peas, and potatoes, along with small amounts of nonfat dairy foods and fish. More than 100 peer-reviewed studies have concluded that Pritikin's approach can substantially lower risk for heart disease, stroke, and diabetes.

In fact, many of the participants in these studies were able to get off anti-hypertensive drugs completely. According to a new meta-analysis of more than 1,000 hypertensive patients who attended the Pritikin Longevity Center, 55% went home with their blood pressure returned to normal levels. You can learn more about the Pritikin Program at http://www.pritikin.com.

The Rice Diet. The premise of the rice diet is that people in cultures where rice is a staple food often enjoy healthy cardiovascular systems. High blood pressure is not a problem, so why not emulate them? "Rice diet" sounds pretty austere, but actually the diet plan features more than 30 different foods, including fruits, vegetables, fish, beans, and dairy products and, oh yes, several kinds of rice. Low in fat and sodium, the rice diet has been used since the 1930s to treat thousands of people with hypertension with great results. It should be called the non-white-rice diet, though, because rice is only helpful if it's the whole grain kind. White rice will cause harmful spikes in your insulin levels.

South Beach Diet. Cardiologist Arthur Agatston, MD, originated this diet with his medical team which included this book's coauthor, Roy Heilbron, MD. The South Beach Diet is implemented in three phases. Phase One is two weeks long and is meant to stabilize blood pressure, eliminate cravings for sugar and refined starches, and kick start weight loss by including high-fiber, low-glycemic vegetables, reduced-fat dairy products, lean meats and poultry, and fish. It excludes sugar, fruit, and starches such as pasta. Phase Two adds more complex carbs such as rice; and phase three is about maintaining weight. Alcohol is a no-no in every phase of the diet.

The 30-Day Diabetes Cure Diet. Though this diet, explained in our earlier book, *The 30-Day Diabetes Cure*, is meant for diabetics, it's also great for people with hypertension as well. Why? Insulin resistance is an issue for both conditions. And the remedy for insulin resistance—a low-carbohydrate/high-protein diet that is low in "bad" polyunsaturated vegetable oils—is just what *The 30-Day Diabetes Cure* diet plan offers. Similar to Atkins, the Mediterranean Diet (above) and the Paleo Diet (above), *The 30-Day Diabetes Cure* diet plan focuses on healthy fats, clean protein foods, and a wide variety of non-starchy plant foods. Whole grains are minimized and all foods, and beverages that stimulate the body's insulin response are eliminated.

APPENDIX F

BLOOD PRESSURE–HEALING BREAKFAST SUGGESTIONS

Breakfast is the most important meal of the day, especially if you are among the approximately 67 million Americans who suffer from high blood pressure (hypertension)—or who have symptoms but haven't been formally diagnosed yet.

The typical American breakfast options need to be avoided at all costs. Most processed breakfast foods only add excess calories and excess pounds without any nutritional value. Plus, they are a *major factor* contributing to your blood pressure problems and increasing your risk for other related conditions such as artery disease, stroke, heart attack, Type 2 diabetes, poor circulation, and others.

A donut and candy-cane flavored coffee. A bowl of cold cereal and packaged orange juice. The remains of last night's take-out pizza. Something wrapped in paper that vaguely resembles an old-fashioned bacon-and-egg sandwich obtained from a drive-through window and eaten with your fingers while also juggling a cell phone and a steering wheel. Sound familiar? Breakfast has gone from being the most important meal of the day—the one that not only "breaks the fast" of the long night of sleep, but also sets up your energy level for the day to come—to something that offers convenience, as well as lots of sugar, refined carbohydrates, bad fats, and heaps of sodium that are devoid of nutritive benefit, inflame your arteries, cause your body to retain fluid, and drive up you blood pressure (as well as your weight).

So if you truly want to take control of your blood pressure, the first place to start begin is with the first meal of the day. We urge you to commit yourself to start every day with a Blood Pressure-Healing Breakfast.

BASIC INGREDIENTS OF A
BLOOD PRESSURE–HEALING BREAKFAST

In this Appendix, you'll find 10 Blood Pressure-Healing Breakfast recipes designed to your day feeling satisfied, energized, and sustained. These meals are designed to lower your blood sugar, reduce inflammation, cut excess calories, increase your energy, help you shed fluid and weight, and lower your blood pressure.

The elements of the ideal breakfast are pretty simple. You want to build your meal around high-quality, "clean" protein. Then you want to add healthful fats. Finally, your breakfast will include complex carbohydrates (fruits and vegetables) that pack in as much fiber as possible. Let's look at each element individually:

Protein. Healthful sources of protein such as omega-3-rich eggs, cheese, dairy products, and non-processed meats represent the most important part of breakfast. They build muscle, promote tissue repair and provide sustained energy throughout the morning. They also satiate your hunger longer than carbohydrate-based meals, so you will be less likely to need a midmorning snack or pick-me-up. This also helps to control your weight.

Fats. The key here is to select healthful fats that will not inflame your arteries or oxidize your bloodstream. Generally speaking, you want to choose fats that are either monounsaturated or saturated, and non-refined polyunsaturated fats (PUFAs). Omega-3 fats found in fish and pasture-raised meat and poultry represent healthful PUFAs. Meat, butter, and other organic dairy products and coconut oil are healthful sources of saturated fats. Avocado, nuts, and seeds are good sources of healthful monounsaturated fats. Avoid refined vegetable oils and all food products containing trans fats.

Carbohydrates. Vegetables, fruits, beans and legumes, nuts and seeds, plus whole grains in their natural state are good examples of complex carbohydrates. These also provide the greatest volume of fiber, which helps normalize blood pressure. Shoot for 50 g of fiber per day—or more.

That said, what follows are recipes for delicious breakfasts that will satisfy your taste buds and help to normalize your blood pressure.

10 BLOOD PRESSURE-HEALING BREAKFASTS

BLT Breakfast Wrap with Avocado Spread

Serves: 2

Total Time: 15 minutes

This is a quick on-the-go breakfast that will make you feel like you sat down to a full meal. Classic BLT flavors combine with creamy avocado to give you an all-day energy boost in the palm of your hand. And it is protein-rich for steady energy throughout your morning.

Ingredients:

4 slices low sodium all natural turkey bacon

2 teaspoons pure olive oil

2 omega-3 eggs, beaten

½ large tomato, diced

1 cup fresh spinach leaves

1 small avocado, pit and skin removed

2 tablespoons low-fat cream cheese, softened

2 quinoa or other gluten-free tortillas

Instructions:

In a small bowl, combine the avocado flesh and cream cheese and stir until creamy and smooth. In a medium sauté pan, cook the bacon until crispy. Drain the fat and rinse the pan. In the same pan, heat the olive oil and scramble the eggs to desired doneness. Heat the tortillas for a minute over a glass flame or in the oven and spread with the avocado spread. Add the tomato, spinach, bacon and eggs and wrap together.

Tips and Notes:

If you like a spicy breakfast, add some jalapenos or hot sauce to your wrap. Sliced black olives are also a nice addition.

Nutrition Facts:

Serving Size 204g, Calories 245, Total Fat 13g, Sat. Fat 4g, Cholesterol 190mg, Sodium 347mg, Carbs 32g, Fiber 6g, Sugars 3g, Protein 14g

Crunchy Blueberry Walnut Granola

Serves: 6–8

Total Time: 1 hour

Serve this super blood pressure-healing granola with a dollop of plain yogurt and a sprinkling of fresh fruit and your family will be jumping out of bed in the morning to get to the breakfast table. With a fraction of the fat, sugar, and calories of store-bought cereal, this tasty recipe can be made in a big batch and stored for up to a month. It makes a great snack, too.

Ingredients:

3 cups rolled whole oats (not instant)

¼ cup flax seeds

1 cup frozen blueberries, thawed

½ cup walnuts, crushed

½ teaspoon cinnamon

2 teaspoons honey

2 tablespoons pure olive oil

Instructions:

Preheat oven to 275 degrees. Combine all ingredients in a bowl and mix well. Bake on a cookie sheet for 45 minutes to 1 hour, or until blueberries are dried and oats are crispy.

Tips and Notes:

Try other fruit in this recipe, like frozen raspberries or strawberries. Add other types of nuts or seeds such as pepitas (pumpkin seeds), sesame seeds, shelled sunflower seeds, or even shredded coconut.

Nutrition Facts:

Serving Size 68g, Calories 239, Total Fat 12g, Sat. Fat 1g, Cholesterol 0mg, Sodium 4mg, Carbs 26g, Fiber 6g, Sugars 6g, Protein 6g

Satisfying Cinnamon Almond Pancakes with Blueberry Sauce

Serves: 4–6

Total Time: 20 minutes

You won't miss the maple syrup with these fluffy, whole grain pancakes. The cinnamon and almonds are oh so yummy—and the fresh blueberry sauce (rich and decadent) will have you licking the plate when no one is looking.

Ingredients:

½ cup brown rice flour

½ cup oat flour

¾ cup rice bran

1 teaspoon cinnamon

1 teaspoon baking powder

½ teaspoon baking soda

1 ¼ cups Greek yogurt

1 teaspoon honey

2 omega-3 eggs, beaten

½ teaspoon almond extract

Coconut oil cooking spray

For the Topping:

1 cup fresh blueberries

Juice of 1 orange

Garnish: 2 tablespoons toasted almonds, slivered

Instructions:

Combine the flours, bran, cinnamon, baking powder, and baking soda in a large bowl. Combine the yogurt, honey, almond extract and eggs and stir into the flour mixture until smooth—add a little milk if batter is very thick. For the sauce, puree the blueberries in a blender with the juice. Lightly spray a griddle or large cast iron pan with the cooking spray and ladle ¼ cup of batter for each pancake. Cook for 2–3 minutes or until underside is brown and top is bubbly. Flip and cook for 2–3 minutes more.

Repeat with all the batter. Serve with the sauce over the top and the almonds sprinkled over.

Tips and Notes:

Different berry sauces are amazing on so many things. Try strawberries with yogurt in an oat flour crepe or raspberries and ginger over homemade granola. You can also substitute other nuts like walnuts or pecans.

Nutrition Facts:

Serving Size 149g, Calories 198, Total Fat 6g, Sat. Fat 1g, Cholesterol 1mg, Sodium 158mg, Carbs 37g, Fiber 6g, Sugars 11g, Protein 11g

Mini Caprese Quiche with Fresh Mozzarella, Tomato and Basil

Serves: 4

Total Time: 35–45 minutes

These blood pressure-friendly, single-serving quiches are elegant and tasty but also a cinch to make. No need for refined flour to get a crispy-crusted, deliciously fluffy breakfast that is perfect for a weekend brunch or even as a light lunch with a mixed green salad

Ingredients:

6 omega-3 eggs, beaten

½ cup milk

1 medium tomato, diced

½ cup fresh mini mozzarella balls or larger ball diced

¼ cup fresh basil, chopped

2 quinoa or other gluten-free tortillas, cut in half

Instructions:

Preheat the oven to 375 degrees. Combine the eggs and milk and whisk. Lightly oil four large ramekins and press the tortillas down into them to make a cup form. The tortilla does not have to cover all sides but should stick up above the rim on at least one side. Pour the egg mixture into the cups. Sprinkle the cheese, tomatoes and basil into the eggs. Bake for 20–25 minutes or until custard is set. Serve immediately with extra basil as garnish.

Tips and Notes:

This is a great way to use leftover steamed vegetables from the night before. Add broccoli, zucchini or peppers to give extra crunch and nutrition.

Nutrition Facts:

Serving Size 154g, Calories 196, Total Fat 4g, Sat. Fat 1g, Cholesterol 1mg, Sodium 160mg, Carbs 37g, Fiber 6g, Sugars 12g, Protein 9g

High-Fiber Pear Mango Pecan Breakfast Bars

Serves: 16 bars

Total Time: 1 hour

Scrumptious, wholesome bars don't cost an arm and a leg and are full of healthful nuts, whole grains, and yogurt. This grab-and-go breakfast is full of fiber and protein to keep you satisfied all morning.

Ingredients:

1¾ cup oat flour

¼ cup honey

½ cup unsweetened dried mango, chopped

¼ cup oat bran

1 teaspoon baking powder

½ teaspoon salt

2 tablespoons unsweetened coconut, shredded

¼ teaspoon baking soda

½ cup pecans, chopped

1 pear, grated

¾ cup plain Greek yogurt

¼ cup pure olive oil

2 omega-3 eggs

Instructions:

Preheat oven to 350 degrees. In a large bowl, mix flour, honey, mango, bran, baking powder, salt, coconut, baking soda, nuts, and pear. Whisk together yogurt, oil, and eggs. Stir into dry ingredients just until combined. Spread in a lightly oiled casserole dish. Bake for 35-40 minutes or until toothpick inserted in center comes out clean. Let cool, then cut into 16 bars.

Tips and Notes:

Make these the evening before. Bars can be stored in an airtight container for up to three days, or individually wrapped and frozen for up to one month.

Nutrition Facts:

Serving Size 62g, Calories 154, Total Fat 9g, Sat. Fat 2g, Cholesterol 19mg, Sodium 74mg, Carbs 21g, Fiber 5g, Sugars 7g, Protein 5g

Poached Eggs with Creamy Herb Sauce, Turkey Sausage, and Spinach

Serves: 4

Total Time: 20 minutes

This is a perfect Sunday brunch dish that won't have you slaving away in the kitchen all morning. Sit down, relax with the newspaper, and still impress your family and friends with this unique, diabetes-friendly take on Eggs Benedict. Forgo the traditional hollandaise for this flavorful herb sauce over your perfectly poached eggs. Nutrient-rich spinach is a perfect complement to low-fat turkey sausage.

Ingredients:

4 omega-3 eggs

4 slices oat or other gluten-free bread

2 cups spinach, chopped

6 oz ground organic turkey sausage

Sauce:

½ cup plain Greek yogurt

Juice of ½ lemon

1 teaspoon honey

2 tablespoons fresh herbs (tarragon, basil, oregano, parsley, thyme), minced

Instructions:

Combine the ingredients for the sauce in a bowl and mix well. Set aside.

Cook the sausage in a small sauté pan for 5–7 minutes or until cooked through. Add the spinach and cook 2–3 minutes more or until spinach is wilted. In a sauté pan bring about 2 inches of water to a light simmer. Add a splash of white vinegar to keep the eggs together or use ring molds. Poach the eggs for 3–4 minutes or until desired doneness is reached.

Toast the bread and layer the spinach-sausage mixture on top. Place the eggs over the spinach and spread the sauce around the edges of the plate.

Tips and Notes:

Try this sauce with different proteins like grilled chicken or fish. For an on-the-go breakfast scramble the eggs instead and make a sandwich wrapped in aluminum foil.

Nutrition Facts:

Serving Size 165g, Calories 218, Total Fat 10g, Sat. Fat 2g, Cholesterol 211mg, Sodium 457mg, Carbs 16g, Fiber 3g, Sugars 6g, Protein 21g

Antioxidant-Rich Raspberry Papaya Smoothie

Serves: 4

Total Time: 5 minutes

The deep red color of raspberry invites me to savor this delicious breakfast drink. The unique combination of papaya and raspberry are enhanced by a dash of coriander and a splash of pomegranate juice. It takes just minutes to make and the high-protein yogurt will satisfy your hunger all morning.

Ingredients:

1 papaya, peeled, seeded, and chopped

1 cup plain Greek yogurt

½ cup fresh or frozen raspberries

1-2 tablespoons pomegranate juice

1 cup ice cubes

1 teaspoon honey

1 tablespoon wheat bran

1 tablespoon flax meal

¼ teaspoon ground coriander

Instructions:

Combine all ingredients in blender or food processor and blend until smooth. Pour into chilled glasses and sprinkle with extra coriander. Serve immediately.

Tips and Notes:

Freeze any leftover in a shallow baking dish and serve as a yummy frozen dessert topped with fresh raspberries or even a sprinkling of dark chocolate chips.

Nutrition Facts:

Serving Size 173g, Calories 121, Total Fat 2g, Sat. Fat 0g, Cholesterol 1mg, Sodium 51mg, Carbs 20g, Fiber 4g, Sugars 15g, Protein 7g

Fiber-Full Sour Cream Corn Muffins with Turkey Bacon and Jalapeño

Serves: 1 dozen muffins

Total Time: 30 minutes

If you like a wake-me-up kick in the morning, this is the way to get it! Grab one of these spicy, smoky muffins and you're out the door, feeling ready to tackle the world. Fiber-rich whole grains are seen in a whole new light when paired with protein-rich low-fat turkey bacon and sour cream.

Ingredients:

1 cup oat flour

¾ cup cornmeal

2 teaspoons baking powder

½ teaspoon baking soda

1 omega-3 egg, beaten

½ cup sour cream

1 cup milk

4 slices all-natural turkey bacon, diced

1 large jalapeño, seeded and diced

Instructions:

Preheat the oven to 400 degrees. In a small sauté pan, cook the bacon on medium heat until crispy. Drain on paper towels. Combine the flour, cornmeal, baking powder and baking soda and mix. Add the egg, milk, and sour cream and stir just to combine. Fold in the bacon and jalapeño. Fill 12 lightly oiled muffin cups ¾ of the way full and bake for 18-20 minutes.

Tips and Notes:

Garnish these with a sprinkle of cheddar cheese or even a small spread of salsa or guacamole.

Nutrition Facts:

Serving Size 106g, Calories 172, Total Fat 4g, Sat. Fat 1g, Cholesterol 37mg, Sodium 216mg, Carbs 33g, Fiber 4g, Sugars 3g, Protein 9g

Vanilla French Toast Sticks with Banana Cashew Butter

Serves: 4–6

Total Time: 20 minutes

Try not to eat breakfast on the run, but if you have to cook-n-carry, this breakfast is both portable and blood pressure-friendly. Whole grain French toast in a stick is the right portion size as well as slow-digesting for sustained energy all morning. The cashew butter is a nutrient-rich delectable topping instead of sugary jam.

Ingredients:

French Toast:

3 omega-3 eggs, beaten

3 tablespoons milk

½ teaspoon vanilla extract

4 slices oat or other gluten-free bread, cut into 4 sticks each

2 tablespoons unsalted butter

Cashew Butter:

½ cup freshly ground cashew butter

1 ripe banana

¼ cup milk

1 teaspoon honey

Instructions:

In a blender puree the ingredients for the cashew butter until smooth. If the topping is too thick, add a few tablespoons of water until desired consistency is reached. Whisk together the eggs, milk, and vanilla, until combined. Heat half the butter in a large sauté pan or griddle on medium heat. Dip each piece of bread in the egg mix and cook for 2-3 minutes on each side or until golden. Repeat with the remaining butter and the rest of the bread. Serve the French toast sticks with the cashew butter on the side to dip or pour over the top.

Tips and Notes:

Dense flavorful gluten-free breads are great for this recipe because they don't get soggy when cooked. Try almond butter or all natural peanut butter as well. For garnish use extra slices of banana or some chopped up cashews for crunch.

Nutrition Facts:

Serving Size 89g, Calories 222, Total Fat 13g, Sat. Fat 4g, Cholesterol 103mg, Sodium 110mg, Carbs 20g, Fiber 3g, Sugars 7g, Protein 9g

Wild Mushroom Frittata with Sage and Blue Cheese

Serves: 4

Total Time: 30 minutes

No need for an omelet pan or any fancy flipping skills with this easy delicious frittata. Simply add veggies and protein-packed eggs to a pan and pop it in the oven. You'll have a savory herbal meal with the earthiness of mushroom and the tang of blue cheese. Serve this as breakfast, nibble a slice as a midmorning snack, or have it with a salad for a light lunch or dinner.

Ingredients:

2 cups mushrooms (shitake, crimini, oyster, Portobello), sliced

1 tablespoon pure olive oil

1 tablespoon unsalted butter

6 omega-3 eggs, beaten

2 tablespoons milk

½ small onion, diced

¼ cup gorgonzola, crumbled

2 tablespoons fresh sage, minced

Instructions:

Preheat the oven to 375 degrees. Heat the oil in a large sauté pan and cook the mushrooms on medium high heat for 5–7 minutes or until they start to wilt and caramelize. Add the onion and cook for 3 minutes more, stirring often. Add the butter and let melt. Stir together the milk, eggs and sage and add the mixture to the pan. Stir quickly to mix in the mushrooms and onions. When the edges start to set up, sprinkle the cheese over the top and transfer to the oven for 7–10 minutes or until center is set.

Tips and Notes:

Try this with feta cheese and oregano, instead, for a Greek-flavored frittata or add cooked turkey sausage for extra protein.

Nutrition Facts:

Serving Size 134g, Calories 198, Total Fat 17g, Sat. Fat 6g, Cholesterol 293mg, Sodium 217mg, Carbs 4g, Fiber 1g, Sugars 2g, Protein 12g

APPENDIX G

BEST BLOOD PRESSURE–HEALING SNACK CHOICES

It may come as a surprise, but snacking is good for you, especially if you are concerned about your blood pressure. Between-meal eating keeps your energy high and—believe it or not—helps control your weight by minimizing your hunger. When you go for a long time between meals, your blood sugar and your energy level starts to drop until you feel so hungry that you will reach for the first thing available—which usually is a sugary, bready, salty, or greasy snack food that is devoid of nutrients and is no good for your weight and blood pressure.

A blood pressure-healing snack made with healthy fats, protein, and high-fiber fruits or vegetables can make all the difference between a midday blood-sugar bomb and a healing helper that keeps your energy levels and blood pressure stable.

You can safely assume that virtually every snack food stocked in a vending machine, convenience store, or snack-food aisle at the grocery store has high-fructose corn syrup (HFCS) or other added sweeteners—plus trans fats, polyunsaturated vegetable oils like soybean or canola, refined white flour, excessive salt, and a myriad of chemicals used as preservatives, stabilizers, dough conditioners, artificial colors, and artificial flavors. And don't forget the high calorie count. All of these are bad for your blood pressure.

THE PERFECT SNACK

Unfortunately, when it comes to healthful snack options in our daily environment, there are few-to-none. Your best strategy is to pack your snacks from home, and keep them close at hand at work and when you're traveling. There is a science to healthy snacking, especially for the person with high blood pressure. Your perfect snack should contain between 100 and 150 calories, should include a slow-carb food coupled with either fat or protein, and should be relatively high in fiber content.

Your basic recipe of fresh vegetables or fruit plus cheese equals great snacking. Try sliced apples with a pinky-sized piece of sharp cheddar, berries with cottage cheese, pears and bleu cheese, and even raw broccoli with goat cheese. These fiber-plus-fat combos are endless and so are the nutritional benefits. Vegetables are the ultimate slow-carb foods because they break down slowly into blood sugar—thanks to all that fiber. The result is you receive a steady and sustained supply of energy. And, because the protein and good fats digest even more slowly, you feel full sooner and your appetite is quickly appeased. In addition, a protein snack will perk up your brain and mental functions.

Other high-protein snack options to enjoy with vegetables include hummus and yogurt-based dips. Hummus brings together several blood pressure-healing foods: Chickpeas (also known as garbanzo beans), olive oil, and the sesame-seed butter called *tahini,* along with lemon juice and garlic. Or add herbs, a dash of hot sauce, and some curry powder (all of which are beneficial for blood pressure and healthy blood sugar) to some plain yogurt. Another satisfying dip can be made by seeding and dicing cucumbers and stirring them into yogurt with fresh chopped mint and cracked pepper. These dips are perfect with raw carrot sticks, bell peppers, celery and/or radishes (called *crudités* in gourmet circles).

Don't forget high-quality dark chocolate (containing at least 75% to 85% cocoa solids) in small amounts (about 150 calories). Italian researchers gave a group of healthy people a daily dose of either white or dark chocolate and measured their blood sugar. Insulin resistance (a condition in which the body's cells don't use insulin properly) was significantly lower after subjects ate dark chocolate than after they ate white chocolate, thanks to the flavanols in dark chocolate (white chocolate doesn't contain flavanols).[361]   Remember, the higher your insulin levels, the higher your blood pressure will rise.

Nuts and nut butters are great for snacking, too. Eat them out of hand, spread nut butter on whole grain, gluten-free bread or celery sticks, or chop and add them to yogurt. No matter how you enjoy them, nuts are a quick, nutritious snack that's rich in healthful monounsaturated fats, antioxidants, vitamins, and minerals that reduce the risk of high blood pressure and keep it under control. Nuts are also high in protein (ounce for ounce, nearly as much as lean meat!) and have a low glycemic index (GI), so they won't spike your blood sugar and insulin.

Almonds are especially good at keeping blood sugar levels under control. A study published in the medical journal *Metabolism* reported that almonds not only have a low GI, but also actually help lower the GI of the entire meal. [362] They are also rich in the antioxidant vitamin E. Try natural almond butter on celery sticks. Whole grain, gluten-free bread or sliced apples are delectable snacks when spread with a little almond butter.

Walnuts are a great snack choice as well, because they are exceptionally high in omega-3 essential fatty acids—and have the lowest ratio of omega-6 to omega-3 of any nut (4.2 to 1). Numerous studies show that a diet rich in omega-3s helps prevent the blood clotting and plaque build-up that can lead to atherosclerosis. And omega-3s also improve the ratio of HDL cholesterol to LDL cholesterol, while reducing inflammation. Walnuts and apples are a classic combo eaten by hand or mixed into yogurt with a generous sprinkle of cinnamon, making it a fantastically healthful snack.

Let us not forget our old favorite, the peanut, which contains oleic acid, the same healthy fat found in olive oil. Peanuts—and peanut butter—are high in vitamin E and a great source of antioxidants. Peanuts are also high in resveratrol, a heart-healthy antioxidant. According to a study[363] published in the *Journal of Agricultural and Food Chemistry*, resveratrol improves blood flow to the brain by as much as 30%, significantly reducing the risk of stroke.

SOME NUTTY ADVICE

It is best to buy organically grown raw nuts. If you want, you can lightly toast them in a dry frying pan over very low heat (or in your oven). Keep nuts in a tightly sealed glass jar in the refrigerator, to prevent their natural oils from going rancid. Do not buy roasted nuts because they lose their potency when subjected to high heat and often have added salt and oils. And remember to keep nut snacking to a small handful, or no more than two tablespoons of nut butter daily.

Make sure you purchase peanut and other nut butters without anything else added (you should be a well-practiced food label reader by now)—and avoid added sugar, oils, and excessive salt in packaged nuts.

Also avoid packaged trail mix that includes added candy or dried fruit. Limit yourself to one or two dried apricots or dates, sliced and mixed into yogurt, or a spoonful of raisins or dried cranberries (and make sure the dried fruit has no added sweeteners).

OTHER HEALING SNACK OPTIONS

Popcorn. This is a bonafide whole grain that's loaded with fiber—if you pop your own. Forget microwave popcorn and movie theatre popcorn (toxic chemicals, artificial flavors, excess salt). Buy your own (organic is best) and pop it in an inexpensive air popper or on the stove. Two tablespoons of melted butter or extra virgin olive oil on a large bowl of popcorn is a sufficient snack for two to four people; or you can divide it, pack it up in a sealed container, and take it to work for a midday snack. Sprinkle it with parmesan cheese, chili powder, garlic powder, dry mustard, cinnamon, or herbs such as basil or oregano.

Turkey. A piece of thinly sliced turkey rolled up around a slim stalk of cheese or fruit makes a fine protein boost mid-afternoon.

A **few canned sardines** in olive oil (or a forkful or two of canned salmon) with a smear of cream cheese (after Day 12, you can eat these on whole grain crackers).

- **Hard-boiled egg**.

- **Half a cup of plain Greek yogurt**.

- **Cottage cheese** with cinnamon.

- **Warmed vegetarian refried beans** from a can as a dip for raw veggies.

Let your imagination run wild!

THE TOP 10 BLOOD PRESSURE-FRIENDLY
SNACK SUBSTITUTIONS

Instead of	**Choose**
Chips	Air-popped popcorn (with a little olive oil or butter and grated parmesan cheese).
Soda pop	Sparkling water flavored with 100% pomegranate juice.
Cookies	Apple slices and five walnut halves.
Candy bar	Four prunes and four almonds.
Ice cream	Plain Greek yogurt with berries, chopped nuts, and cinnamon.
Granola bar	Tablespoon peanut butter + raisins on whole grain toast pieces.
Nachos	Baked potato skins with spinach or broccoli slices, onion and a bit of cheese.
Milkshake	Smoothie with plain yogurt, berries, and flaxseed.
Popsicle	10 tart fresh cherries.

APPENDIX H

BLOOD PRESSURE-HEALING LUNCHES

If you think you can do yourself a favor by skipping lunch and eating a bag of chips or pretzels and a soda from the vending machine, think again. You already know how little energy such a nutritionally empty "lunch" is going to provide for your afternoon's work. Snack-food and fast-food lunches can lead to increased snacking (and more calories) later in the afternoon, as well as a lack of energy and ability to concentrate. Without a substantial meal, your blood sugar levels plunge, only to spike when you eat a high-carb snack in search of energy. It's a deadly cycle.

But what if you could have an inexpensive lunch that filled you up, was low in calories, high in fiber, and actually helped balance your blood sugar and lower your blood pressure? The good news is that you can! But you won't find it at some newly opened restaurant. Instead, it's going to come from the same place all your other Blood Pressure-Healing Superfoods come from: Your own pantry and fridge.

As lunch is not always easy to plan and fit into our hectic schedules, we have placed special importance on that meal in this section. Note, however, that all of the blood pressure-healing lunch recipes can be enjoyed equally for dinner.

THE BLOOD PRESSURE-HEALING "BROWN BAG LUNCH"

If you are serious about healing your blood pressure with every bite of food you eat, then you are going to want to pack a healthful lunch with you to take to work, or to know your options when you go out. You might also want to re-think the entire concept of lunch. Lunch should not be a sandwich and a salty, fatty side dish like chips or fries. Or a full entrée complete with breadbasket and sugary drink. Or a cluster of unidentifiable leftovers, rescued with a sugary coffee drink topped with whipped cream.

Your healing brown bag lunch might be a number of small containers offering a wide variety of tastes and textures. It might have some fruit, some vegetables, and a one-bowl meal of brown rice, vegetables and a bit of last night's grass-fed steak, grilled salmon, or chicken breast. You might have a jar of mixed nuts, an apple, and some slices of cheese, or a salad with cold chicken and sliced almonds.

Fresh vegetables, prepared raw or lightly steamed, are loaded with phytonutrients like antioxidants, vitamins, and minerals. They also are a centerpiece of the Blood Pressure Healing Diet—and are easy to take to work. You can even buy carrots and other vegetables already peeled and sliced in small packages, for those mornings when prep time is limited. Sliced carrots, sweet bell peppers (red, yellow, and green), and cucumbers are easy to prepare; just rinse, toss in a container, and go. Try a light sprinkle of salt on peeled cucumber; add peanut butter or cream cheese to your celery sticks for a nutritious treat.

Chopped broccoli and cauliflower are abundant sources of antioxidants and the anti-inflammatory chemical sulforaphane. Rinse and chop, then lightly stem. Add a pat of butter or a drizzle of olive oil to help you absorb the fat-soluble nutrients in the vegetables. Add to a container of cooked brown rice.

You know that wild Alaskan salmon is one of your best sources of omega-3 essential fatty acid, an important anti-inflammatory. But, you might not know that most canned salmon is wild Alaskan salmon, making it a convenient choice for a healthful lunch. Canned salmon can be made into a number of delicious dishes, including salmon patties, salmon salad, or salmon loaf, all of which work perfectly well as lunchtime alternatives.

9 BLOOD PRESSURE-HEALING LUNCH TIPS

1. Avoid plastic containers. The most important decision you can make about your lunch away from home is to avoid using any plastic containers, especially in the microwave (and that includes containers labeled "microwave-safe," a term that is unregulated and therefore meaningless). Plastic containers and beverage bottles are often made with bisphenol A (BPA); the National Institute of Health reports that BPA may lodge in tissue and affect the prostate, brain, and development of fetuses, infants, and children. Microwaved plastic also can release dioxins, which are known carcinogens, into your food from the high heat.

You'll want to have a stash of small glass containers on hand for your lunches, and don't use the plastic lids or plastic wrap in the microwave (a piece of wax paper or a paper napkin on top of the food is sufficient). While microwaving makes brown-bagging more convenient, keeping a toaster-oven in the office lunchroom can go a long way toward reducing your risk while still allowing you to enjoy a hot meal in minutes.

2. Skip the "brown bag." Instead, purchase a re-useable tote bag in which to carry your lunch to work. This signals your commitment to making your own Blood Pressure-Healing meals. Lunch bags today have a wide array of features, including insulated pouches, pockets for different sizes of containers and matching Thermoses (make sure the Thermos is stainless steel or glass on the inside rather than plastic). In addition to the kids' lunch box aisle, you can also try an outdoor supply shop for larger, more rugged lunch containers. Or if you want to recycle, small gift bags are the perfect size to take a light lunch to work in and are usually pretty, too.

3. Be prepared. Planning takes the guesswork and the frantic last-minute frenzy out of your morning routine. Slice or chop vegetables the night before. Put dinner leftovers in containers you can take for lunch. Put all your lunch components in one place in the fridge so you can find them easily in the morning, or pack your whole lunch and leave your lunch bag in the fridge overnight.

4. Use leftovers. Before making dinner, assess its lunch potential. If you are making a casserole or large meal for dinner, make an extra serving or two for tomorrow's lunch. Remember that almost anything you've had for dinner—grilled salmon, steamed broccoli, brown rice—can be mixed together for a one-bowl meal the next day. Grate some cheese on top, or sprinkle in some lightly roasted almonds for a new twist to yesterday's meal.

5. Soup is "super." Add a small Thermos of soup to your brown bag lunch. Eat it before the rest of your meal, because studies show that when you have soup as a first course, it will fill you up and you'll actually eat 20% fewer calories. Beans are a superior blood pressure-healing food, and make for a hearty soup, along with plenty of vegetables. Soup can be made at night or on the weekend and divided into several containers for easy lunches later in the week. Freeze homemade soup in small BPA-free containers, as well, so you have a back-up supply.

6. Find some allies. Dine with co-workers who are committed to eating healthful lunches, too. Not only will you have support for bucking the fast-food trend, you'll have someone with whom to share meal ideas. Research shows that lifestyle choices like exercise and weight loss, as well as obesity and smoking, are all influenced by the people you interact with the most. You might even make some new friends at the office.

7. Break your routine. If you always eat at your desk, go outside to a local park and have a picnic on a bench, or take a brisk walk after you eat. If you have access to a bookstore or museum, hop inside for 15 minutes and nourish yourself with new ideas. You'll face your afternoon refreshed and energized in mind and body. The downside to eating at your desk is that you tend to eat without thinking—thus eating more and gaining weight. You also end up spending more sedentary time, which is bad for your circulation and your metabolism, and leads to a host of medical conditions from arthritis to heart disease. Physical activity is a necessity for healing your blood pressure, so take every chance you can to get out and walk around for a while.

8. Get help in the kitchen. If you have a houseful of family members all getting ready in the morning, put everyone to work, so that making a healthful breakfast and lunch is easy. Your kids can assemble an appropriate lunch with just a few directions to make sure nothing gets missed. Teaching them responsibility early on not only prepares them for a life of healthier eating, it gives parents a big break in the caretaking department.

9. Make lunch simple. It's just lunch, after all. A jar of mixed nuts, an apple, and a slice of cheese or some leftover chicken and rice make a satisfying meal that can be thrown together in minutes. Don't stress—it's bad for your heart! Enjoy the many ways that the Blood Pressure Healing Superfoods can be mixed and matched to provide a super-healthful brown bag lunch.

BLOOD PRESSURE-HEALING LUNCH RECIPES

Black Bean and Roasted Corn Quesadilla with Green Chile Grapefruit Dip

Serves: 4

Prep Time: 30 minutes

Craving a taste of Mexico? Here is a super easy meal that you can snack on anytime of the day. It will provide you with the nutrients and flavor that keep you going strong while healing your blood pressure and making your coworkers jealous.

Ingredients:

Quesadilla:

4 quinoa or other gluten-free tortillas

1 cup organic cheddar, shredded

3 cloves garlic, minced

2 green onions, sliced

1 small red bell pepper, diced

1 cup frozen corn, thawed

1 tablespoon pure olive oil

1 cup cooked black beans, drained and rinsed

Green Chile Grapefruit Dip:

Juice of 1 grapefruit

¾ cup plain Greek yogurt

¼ cup green chile

1 teaspoon honey

Instructions:

Combine all ingredients for the dip in a small bowl and mix gently. Preheat the oven to 350 degrees. Roast the corn in a little coconut oil for 5–7 minutes or until it starts to caramelize. In a large sauté pan, heat the olive oil on medium. Sauté the onion, garlic and bell pepper for 3–4 minutes. Add the beans and heat through. Smash lightly with a fork and stir in the corn. Layer the tortillas with the cheese and bean mixture and fold in half. Bake on a cookie sheet for 5–7 minute, or until cheese is melted. Serve with the dip on the side.

Tips and Notes:

Add chicken or shrimp. Try another citrus juice in the dip like lime juice. For an exotic twist dice up a mango and add it to the bean mixture.

Nutrition Facts:

Serving Size 260g, Calories 260, Total Fat 8g, Sat. Fat 2g, Cholesterol 7mg, Sodium 346mg, Carbs 37g, Fiber 5g, Sugars 8g, Protein 11g

Broccoli Soup with BLT Rolls

Serves: 4–6

Prep. Time: 30 minutes

Broccoli and bacon is a pair made in heaven. And bacon, lettuce, and tomato sandwiches are a classic never to be forgotten. Here we combine all four in a blood pressure-friendly and easy-to-make lunch. Dip the rolls in the soup or eat them side by side for a hearty meal that will have you reminiscing for your childhood without your blood sugar going through the roof.

Ingredients:

BLT Rolls:

4–6 slices turkey bacon

1 large tomato, cut in half and sliced

4 romaine lettuce leaves, spine removed

2–3 tablespoons olive oil mayonnaise

Broccoli Soup:

1 small carrot, sliced

1 celery stalk, sliced

1 small onion, chopped

2 cloves garlic, minced

½ teaspoon cayenne peeper

½ cup low-sodium chicken stock

2 cups milk

2 cups broccoli florets, chopped

½ cup plain Greek yogurt

Instructions:

Combine the carrot, onion, garlic, celery, and stock in a saucepan and bring to a simmer. Cook for 5-7 minutes. Add the milk and broccoli and cook for 3-5 minutes more or until broccoli is just tender. Cook the bacon until crisp. Drain on paper towels. Puree the soup with an immersion blender or in batches in a food processor or blender until smooth. Return to the stove and reheat if necessary. Stir in the yogurt. Roll the bacon and tomato in the lettuce like an eggroll. Serve the mayonnaise on the side to spread on at lunch or to dip.

Tips and Notes:

For an even healthier lunch, substitute plain yogurt for the mayonnaise. Add extra vegetables like bell peppers, carrot, or avocado.

Nutrition Facts:

Serving Size 237g, Calories 117, Total Fat 5g, Sat. Fat 1g, Cholesterol 16mg, Sodium 304mg, Carbs 13g, Fiber 2g, Sugars 8g, Protein 10g

Creamy Mushroom Soup with Roasted Pepper Salad

Serves: 6–8

Prep Time: 30 minutes

Soup and salad is a classic healing lunch—and in this version you get blood pressure-healing onion, garlic, yogurt, romaine, and olive oil, all together in a delicious melody of smoky, sweet, crispy, and creamy. A thermos of earthy mushroom soup will have you dreaming of noon all morning; and the fresh, sweet salad will keep you energized all afternoon.

Ingredients:

Soup:

1 cup dried shitake mushrooms, soaked in 2 cups boiling water

4 cups mushrooms (button, crimini, shitake, portobello), sliced

1 medium onion, chopped

1 tablespoon pure olive oil

4 cups low-sodium vegetable stock

1 cup milk

¼ cup plain Greek yogurt

2 tablespoons balsamic vinegar

Salad:

1 large red bell pepper

1 large yellow bell pepper

½ small red onion, sliced

1 small head romaine, chopped

¼ cup red wine vinegar

1 tablespoons extra virgin olive oil

1 teaspoon honey

2 teaspoons Dijon mustard

Instructions:

Preheat the oven to 400 degrees. Roast the peppers in the oven for 15–20 minutes or until charred and soft. Place in a paper bag and let sit for 10 minutes to cool and loosen skins. For the soup, heat the olive oil in a Dutch oven or stock pot on medium heat. Sauté the onion and fresh mushrooms for 7–10 minutes. Drain the dried mushrooms and slice, reserving the liquid. Add the dried mushrooms, reserved liquid and stock to the pot and bring to a boil. Cook for 30–35 minutes. Puree the soup with an immersion blender or in batches in a blender or food processor. Garnish with a drizzle of balsamic vinegar.

Combine the red wine vinegar, olive oil, honey and mustard and whisk. Take the stems and seeds out of the peppers and slice thin. Serve the romaine with the sliced onions, peppers and dressing drizzled over the top.

Tips and Notes:

To make this an even quicker lunch, use jarred roasted peppers instead (just read ingredient labels to be sure there are no added sweeteners). Try adding other vegetables to the salad like cucumber, carrot or red cabbage. For a crispier salad, keep the dressing separate until you are about to eat.

Nutrition Facts:

Serving Size 363g, Calories 158, Total Fat 5g, Sat. Fat 1g, Cholesterol 1mg, Sodium 325mg, Carbs 27g, Fiber 5g, Sugars 6g, Protein 5g

Eggplant Mushroom Melt with Marinara and Mozzarella

Serves: 4

Prep Time: 45 minutes

This may not be the neatest sandwich to eat at your desk, but the flavor combinations will let you fly away to Italy for at least a half hour. Bring a knife and fork and gobble up this succulent blood pressure-friendly lunch that will have you licking your fingers and slurping up every drop of sauce.

Ingredients:

Marinara:

2 cups canned (labeled BPA-free) crushed tomatoes

3 cloves garlic, minced

1 teaspoon red chili flakes

¼ cup fresh basil, chopped

Sandwich:

1 tablespoon pure olive oil

1 small eggplant, peeled and diced

2 cups button mushrooms, sliced

½ small onion, chopped

¾ cup low-fat mozzarella, shredded

1 cup spinach

4 oat or other gluten-free sandwich rolls

Instructions:

In a small saucepan, combine the tomato, garlic, and red chili flakes. Bring to a simmer and cook for 15–20 minutes or until slightly thickened. Stir in the basil.

In a sauté pan, heat the olive oil on medium heat and sauté the eggplant and mushrooms for 7–10 minutes or until soft. Add the onion and cook 3–5 minutes more. Add the marinara to the vegetables and stir to combine. Using a slotted spoon, ladle the vegetable mixture onto a toasted bun, draining off most of the sauce. Top with the mozzarella and broil for 3–4 minutes or until cheese is melted. Top with the spinach and the other half of the bun. Serve the remaining marinara on the side to dip.

Tips and Notes:

This is a great dish to make the night before. Serve it over quinoa, millet, or gluten-free pasta. You can also just make a big batch of the super simple marinara and freeze it in individual portions. This way you can bring it for your lunch with any kind of sandwich or make it into an easy dinner or weekend lunch.

Nutrition Facts:

Serving Size 317g, Calories 219, Total Fat 5g, Sat. Fat 1g, Cholesterol 4mg, Sodium 4mg, Carbs 34g, Fiber 11g, Sugars 7g, Protein 15g

Lamb and Sun Dried Tomato Tabouli

Serves: 4–6

Total Time: 30 minutes

Here is a dish with the refreshing tastes of the Middle East where you can heal your blood pressure, get your fill of delicious protein-filled lamb and have a lunch that will be the envy of everyone. Citrusy lemon, fiber-rich tabouli, and crisp vegetables combine to make this a refreshing and hearty lunch.

Ingredients:

12 oz ground lamb

2 cups bulgur wheat, cooked

1 small onion, diced

½ cup fresh mint, chopped

½ cup fresh parsley, chopped

1 medium cucumber, seeded and diced

½ cup sun dried tomatoes, diced

Juice of 3 lemons

2 tablespoons extra virgin olive oil

Instructions:

Preheat the oven to 400 degrees. Place the pita triangles on a baking sheet and brush with the olive oil. Sprinkle with the garlic powder and bake for 5–7 minutes or until crispy. Sauté the lamb in a pan on medium heat until cooked through. Cool. Combine all ingredients for the salad and mix gently.

Tips and Notes:

To make this even tangier, serve with a small bowl of plain yogurt to serve on the crackers as well.

Nutrition Facts:

Serving Size 195g, Calories 237, Total Fat 9g, Sat. Fat 4g, Cholesterol 21mg, Sodium 179mg, Carbs 18g, Fiber 4g, Sugars 3g, Protein 9g

Muffaletta Tuna Salad in Red Cabbage Pockets

Serves: 4

Prep Time: 15 minutes

A taste of New Orleans without all the regrets. You'll be able to tell everyone about this experience as you help your blood pressure and bounce around the office. These crispy, tasty wraps take no time to make in the morning and will stay fresh and delicious until you gobble them up at lunchtime.

Ingredients:

6 pitted black olives, drained and chopped

6 pitted green olives, drained and chopped

½ small red onion, chopped

2 tablespoons red wine vinegar

Juice of 1 lemon

2 tablespoons extra virgin olive oil

1 teaspoon honey

2 cloves garlic, minced

1 teaspoon dried oregano

1 teaspoon dried basil

¾ teaspoon black pepper

½ cup artichoke hearts, chopped

1 small tomato, seeded and diced

¼ cup turkey salami, diced

8 oz tuna, canned in water and drained

8 small red cabbage leaves, spine removed

4–6 tablespoons Dijon mustard

Instructions:

Combine all ingredients for the salad and mix gently. Spread each cabbage leaf with a spoonful of mustard and fill with about ¼ cup of filling. Roll into an eggroll shape.

Tips and Notes:

Try this salad with canned salmon or diced chicken instead. You can also use lettuce leaves or gluten-free tortillas instead of the cabbage.

Nutrition Facts:

Serving Size 219g, Calories 212, Total Fat 10g, Sat. Fat 2g, Cholesterol 27mg, Sodium 421mg, Carbs 14g, Fiber 4g, Sugars 6g, Protein 18g

Pad Thai Salad with Peanuts and Romaine

Serves: 6

Prep Time: 30 minutes

Traditional Pad Thai is already a blood pressure-friendly Thai classic, and here we serve it over romaine lettuce. This easy salad gives a taste of the East that just gets better as it waits for you to munch it up at lunchtime.

Ingredients:

8 oz brown rice noodles

1 tablespoon pure olive oil

6 oz chicken breast, boneless and skinless, cut into 1-inch cubes

12 medium shrimp, shelled and deveined

½ cup chicken stock

1 tablespoon fish sauce

2 tablespoons gluten-free soy sauce

1 teaspoon honey

1 tablespoon lime juice

1–2 teaspoons red chili paste

1 cup bean sprouts

1 medium carrot, shredded

½ small onion, sliced

3 garlic cloves, minced

1 egg, beaten

3 cups romaine, chopped

1 green onion, sliced

2 limes, cut into wedges

2 tablespoons roasted peanuts, finely chopped

Instructions:

Cook the rice noodles in boiling water for 10–15 minutes or until al dente. Heat the olive oil on medium heat and sauté the chicken for 3–5 minutes. Add the shrimp and onions and cook for 3–5 minutes more. Push the mixture to one side and stir in the egg. Scramble for 2–3 minutes and mix with the meat and onions.

Add the chicken stock, fish sauce, soy sauce, honey, lime juice, garlic and chili paste and bring to a simmer. Add the carrots and half the bean sprouts and simmer for 2–3 minutes. Turn off the heat and stir in the noodles. Cool. Serve the Pad Thai over the romaine garnished with the remaining bean sprouts, peanuts, and lime wedges.

Tips and Notes:

Make a big batch and serve this hot the night before. Use leftovers for your lunch. Try it with tofu, salmon fillet, or scallops.

Nutrition Facts:

Serving Size 259g, Calories 217, Total Fat 7g, Sat. Fat 1g, Cholesterol 65mg, Sodium 426mg, Carbs 25g, Fiber 4g, Sugars 5g, Protein 14g

Roast Buffalo Sandwich with Cucumber Slaw and Horseradish Cream

Serves: 4 serves

Prep Time: 15 minutes

This is the perfect application for leftover roast. No need to get store-bought sandwich meats when you can use leftovers for a lunch that is 10 times better than any ham and cheese from the vending machine. Easy slaw and horseradish cream elevate this blood pressure-healing meal to the level of royalty.

Ingredients:

Cucumber Slaw:

1 large cucumber sliced thin

1 small carrot, shredded

½ small red onion, sliced thin

1 medium red bell pepper

Juice of 1 lemon

1 tablespoon extra virgin olive oil

2 teaspoons Dijon mustard

Horseradish Cream:

¼ cup plain yogurt

2 tablespoons sour cream

2–4 tablespoons prepared horseradish

Juice of ½ lemon

Sandwiches:

12 oz cooked roast bison, sliced thin on a bias

1 medium tomato, sliced

4 thin oat rolls

Instructions:

Combine all the ingredients for the slaw and mix gently. Combine the ingredients for the horseradish cream and mix well. Toast the bread and layer the meat on the bottom, then the cream, then the slaw. Keep any remaining cream to dip.

Tips and Notes:

Layer the sandwich like this so the meat and cheese protect the bread from getting soggy. If you prefer an even crispier sandwich, eat the slaw on the side.

Nutrition Facts:

Serving Size 327g, Calories 322, Total Fat 11g, Sat. Fat 3g, Cholesterol 75mg, Sodium 279mg, Carbs 28g, Fiber 5g, Sugars 9g, Protein 29g

Roasted Black Pepper Turkey Sandwich with Brie and Apples

Makes: 4

Total Time: 15 minutes

Everyone in your office will be begging to trade you their lunch for this gourmet sandwich that fits in your hand, but has the flavors of a fabulous summer picnic. The homemade turkey breast is easy to make the night before and you'll know exactly how many calories it has...or doesn't have. No preservatives, no added salt—this sandwich will fight your high blood pressure and fill you up.

Ingredients:

12-oz turkey breast, boneless and skinless

1 tablespoon pure olive oil

2 teaspoons coarsely ground black pepper

1 medium green apple, cored, sliced

4 oz brie, sliced

1 cup mixed greens

¼ cup almonds, slivered

3 tablespoons yellow mustard

2 tablespoons plain Greek yogurt

1 teaspoon honey

2 thin oat rolls

Instructions:

Preheat the oven to 350 degrees. Butterfly the turkey breast and coat with the oil and pepper on both sides. Bake for 25–30 minutes or until cooked through. Slice the turkey breast into thin slices and cool. Combine the mustard, yogurt, and honey, and mix well. Spread the rolls with the honey mustard and layer with the turkey, apple, brie, and greens.

Tips and Notes:

Heat the rolls or try pita bread (gluten-free) in the oven with the turkey and cheese for 5 minutes to make a yummy hot melt. Add the apples and greens at the end so they don't get soggy. To keep the apples from turning brown by lunchtime, soak them in a bowl of cold water with a squeeze of lemon or orange juice before putting them in the sandwich. For some extra crunch, sprinkle the sandwiches with a few tablespoons of slivered almonds.

Nutrition Facts:

Serving Size 275g, Calories 349, Total Fat 13g, Sat. Fat 6g, Cholesterol 1mg, Sodium 432mg, Carbs 23g, Fiber 3g, Sugars 12g, Protein 35g

Tomato Herb Soup with Cheese Avocado Wrap

Makes: 4–6 servings

Total Time: 30 minutes

You'll feel like a kid again with this classic lunchtime meal. The soup is easy yet sophisticated and the wrap is a perfect combination of fresh and sharp flavors. Dip the sandwich in the soup and slurp it all up for an afternoon of energy.

Ingredients:

Soup:

1 tablespoon pure olive oil

2 cloves garlic, minced

½ medium onion, diced

2 cups low-sodium vegetable stock

2 cups milk

2 cups canned diced tomatoes with juice

1 teaspoon dried basil

1 teaspoon dried marjoram

½ teaspoon dried oregano

½ teaspoon dried thyme

1 bay leaf

Wrap:

4 brown rice tortillas

4–6 slices extra sharp cheddar cheese

½ avocado, sliced

½ cup sprouts

4 tablespoons Dijon mustard

Instructions:

In a large saucepan, heat the olive oil on medium heat. Sauté the onions for 3–5 minutes. Add the garlic and sauté for 1 minute more. Add the stock, tomatoes, milk and spices and bring to a simmer. Cook for 15–17 minutes and remove the bay leaf. Puree the soup with an immersion blender or in batches in a blender or food processor. Spread the mustard on the tortillas and layer with the avocado, sprouts, and cheese.

Tips and Notes:

Keep the soup warm in a thermos or bring it in a covered glass bowl to microwave at lunch. Wrap the wrap in foil to keep it fresh and intact.

Nutrition Facts:

Serving Size 313g, Calories 187, Total Fat 7g, Sat. Fat 2g,

Cholesterol 7mg, Sodium 380mg, Carbs 21g, Fiber 4g, Sugars 10g, Protein 11

ENDNOTES

Chapter 1

1 http://todaysseniorsnetwork.com/Blood_Pressure_Study.htm

2 http://www.medpagetoday.com/Cardiology/Hypertension/34552

3 http://www.everydayhealth.com/hypertension/understanding/what-is-hypertension.aspx

4 http://www.sciencedaily.com/releases/2004/10/041027113516.htm

5 http://health.usnews.com/health-news/family-health/heart/articles/2011/05/25/study-finds-almost-1-in-5-young-adults-has-high-blood-pressure

6 http://www.mayoclinic.com/health/high-blood-pressure/HI00062

7 Metabolic Syndrome published by Web M.D. at http://www.webmd.com/heart-disease/guide/metabolic-syndrome

8 Metabolic Syndrome published by Web M.D. at http://www.webmd.com/heart-disease/guide/metabolic-syndrome—also see: http://www.medicinenet.com/metabolic_syndrome/page3.htm

9 http://en.wikipedia.org/wiki/Metabolic_syndrome

10 http://www.pritikin.com/eperspective/0509/hypertension.shtml

11 http://www.everydayhealth.com/hypertension/understanding/what-is-hypertension.aspx

Chapter 2

12 http://www.heart.org/HEARTORG/Conditions/HighBloodPressure/AboutHighBloodPressure/Understanding-Blood-Pressure-Readings_UCM_301764_Article.jsp

13 http://www.baptistjax.com/health-library/health-news/ninety-percent-stroke-risk-due-to-ten-risk-factors

14 http://www.msnbc.msn.com/id/35063248/ns/health-aging/t/high-blood-pressure-linked-dementia/

15 http://www.mayoclinic.com/health/pulmonary-hypertension/DS00430

16 http://ndt.oxfordjournals.org/content/16/6/1095.full

17 Ibid.

18 http://www.sciencedaily.com/releases/2012/02/120210111250.htm

Chapter 3

19 http://www.cdc.gov/mmwr/preview/mmwrhtml/mm6004a4.htm?s_cid=mm6004

20 Furberg, MD, Curt D., "Treatment of Hypertension: A Failing Report Card" Oxford Jounals, *American Journal of Hypertension* (2009); 22, 1, 1–2

21 http://www.theheart.org/article/1434701.do

22 http://www.medpagetoday.com/Cardiology/Hypertension/34225?utm

23 http://www.drlam.com/articles/2001-No2-Hypertension.asp

24 "ß-Blocker Use and Clinical Outcomes in Stable Outpatients With and Without Coronary Artery Disease." *JAMA* October 03, 2012, Vol 308, No. 13

25 *Eur Heart J.* 2007 Sep;28 (18):2249-55. Epub 2007 July 19

[26] http://www.sciencedaily.com/releases/2010/08/100819112222.htm

[27] http://www.anh-usa.org/high-blood-pressure-just-burn-away-overactive-nerves/

[28] http://www.mayoclinic.com/health/high-blood-pressure/DS00100/DSECTION=treatments-and-drugs

[29] Each of the anti-hypertensive drug classes mentioned in this interview has numerous brand names for each medication. Only two are given as examples.

[30] http://medicalconsumers.org/2003/08/01/prehypertension%E2%80%94how-real-is-this-new-"disease"

[31] http://medicalconsumers.org/2009/09/10/no-benefit-to-reducing-blood-pressure-below-14090/

[32] Christopher I. Li, MD, PhD, et al., Use of Antihypertensive Medications and Breast Cancer Risk Among Women Aged 55 to 74 Years; *JAMA Internal Medicine*—September 23, 2013; Vol. 173, No. 17

[33] Channel Blocker BP Meds Tied to Breast Cancer Risk published online at WebMD—Aug. 5, 2013; *http://www.webmd.com/breast-cancer/news/20130805/channel-blockers-for-blood-pressure-linked-to-breast-cancer-risk-study-finds*

Chapter 4

[34] http://www.theheart.org/article/982461.do

[35] http://hyper.ahajournals.org/cgi/content/abstract/57/5/898

[36] Magid DJ, et al "A Pharmacist-led, American Heart Association Heart360 Web-Enabled Home Blood Pressure Monitoring Program" *Cicr Cardiov Qual Outc* 2013; DOI: 10.1161/CIRCOUTCOMES.112.968172; http://www.medpagetoday.com/Cardiology/Hypertension/37694

[37] Lisa Nainggolan. Large between-arm BP Differences Don't Bode Well. theheart.org. [Clinical Conditions > Hypertension > Hypertension]; June 23, 2011. Accessed at http://www.theheart.org/article/1243889.do on June 26, 2013

Chapter 5

[38] http://www.webmd.com/hypertension-high-blood-pressure/guide/new-low-for-high-blood-pressure?page=3

[39] http://www.nhlbi.nih.gov/guidelines/hypertension/index.htm

[40] http://www.webmd.com/hypertension-high-blood-pressure/guide/new-low-for-high-blood-pressure?page=3

[41] http://www.nhlbi.nih.gov/guidelines/hypertension/index.htm.

[42] Pre-Hypertension—How Real Is This New "Disease" published by the Center for Medical Consumers on August 1, 2003—available online at http://medicalconsumers.org/2003/08/01/prehypertension%E2%80%94how-real-is-this-new-%E2%80%9Cdisease%E2%80%9D/

[43] http://medicalconsumers.org/2003/08/01/prehypertension%E2%80%94how-real-is-this-new-"disease"

[44] http://summaries.cochrane.org/CD004349/aiming-for-blood-pressure-targets-lower-than-14090-mmhg-is-not-beneficial

[45] Taubes, Gary, *Why We Get Fat*; Knopf, 2011, p. 183

[46] http://www.medscape.com/viewarticle/471536_2

[47] http://www.npr.org/templates/story/story.php?storyId=121609815

[48] Just the opposite occurs in indigenous culture where the Western diet has yet to penetrate. We'll see why this is in Chapter Nine.

[49] http://www.westonaprice.org/ask-the-doctor/205-high-blood-pressure

[50] http://www.webmd.com/hypertension-high-blood-pressure/guide/new-low-for-high-blood-pressure?page=3

[51] Ibid.

Chapter 6

52 http://www.webmd.com/hypertension-high-blood-pressure/hypertension-in-african-americans

53 http://www.mayoclinic.org/atherosclerosis/

54 Article Source: http://EzineArticles.com/3647643

55 http://kidney.niddk.nih.gov/kudiseases/pubs/highblood/#how

56 http://www.3fatchicks.com/how-weight-gain-can-cause-hypertension-2/

57 High Blood Pressure May Be Due To Excess Weight in Half of Overweight Adults; *ScienceDaily* (Oct. 3, 2007) http://www.sciencedaily.com/releases/2007/09/070928180348.htm

58 http://articles.mercola.com/sites/articles/archive/2012/11/14/waist-size-matters.aspx

59 http://www.3fatchicks.com/how-weight-gain-can-cause-hypertension-2/

60 http://www.health.state.ny.us/diseases/chronic/cvd.htm

61 http://www.deerfieldsclinic.com/declining-fitness-over-a-decade-doubles-risks-of-ami-death

62 http://www.mayoclinic.com/health/high-blood-pressure/HI00027

63 http://www.mayoclinic.com/health/blood-pressure/AN00318

64 https://www.ttuhsc.edu/som/internalmedicine/general/education/ambulatory/documents/isolated_systolic_htn_elderly.pdf

65 http://www.uptodate.com/contents/smoking-and-hypertension

66 http://www.nhlbi.nih.gov/hbp/prevent/factors/smoke.htm

67 http://www.uptodate.com/contents/smoking-and-hypertension

68 http://www.webmd.com/hypertension-high-blood-pressure/guide/kicking-habit

69 Ibid.

70 *The Merck Manual of Health and Aging* by Mark H. Beers and Thomas V. Jones; p. 556

71 http://highbloodpressure.about.com/od/highbloodpressure101/a/diabetes-hbp.htm

72 http://jcem.endojournals.org/content/95/7_Supplement_1/s1.long

73 Nash, P., Magder, L., Lustberg, M., et al., "Blood Lead, Blood Pressure, and Hypertension in Perimenopausal and Postmenopausal Women," *Journal of the AMA*, 2003, 289 (12): 1523-32.

74 http://www.sonasimc.com/2011/03/silent-killer-in-the-us/

Chapter 7

75 http://www8.nationalacademies.org/onpinews/newsitem.aspx?RecordID=18311

76 http://medicalconsumers.org/2003/08/01/prehypertension%E2%80%94how-real-is-this-new-"disease"/

77 http://www.fitnessmagazine.com/recipes/healthy-eating/nutrition/with-a-grain-of-salt/

78 http://www.age-well.org/hyponatraemia.html

79 Source: *The Cochrane Library*, Cochrane Database of Systematic Reviews, doi: 10.1002/14651858.CD009217 *"Reduced dietary salt for the prevention of cardiovascular Disease"*, Authors: R.S. Taylor, K.E. Ashton, T. Moxham, L. Hooper, S. Ebrahim

80 http://www.foodnavigator.com/Science-Nutrition/Lancet-paper-blasts-Cochrane-salt-study

[81] http://douglassreport.com/2011/08/03/low-salt/

[82] http://jama.jamanetwork.com/issue.aspx?journalid=67&issueid=20327&direction=P

[83] http://www.ncbi.nlm.nih.gov/pubmed/18465175

[84] http://medicalconsumers.org/Search for "Prehypertension How-Real-Is-This-New-Disease"

[85] Ibid.

[86] http://www.nature.com/ki/journal/v78/n8/full/ki2010280a.html

[87] http://www.foodnavigator-usa.com/Science/Cochrane-review-doesn-t-change-our-advice-on-salt-reduction-AHA

[88] http://www.stat.berkeley.edu/users/rice/Stat2/salt.html

[89] Ibid.

[90] Taubes, Gary, *Good Calories, Bad Calories*, Knopf, 2007; p. 146, 147

[91] http://www.foodnavigator.com/Science-Nutrition/Lancet-paper-blasts-Cochrane-salt-study

[92] http://www.theheart.org/article/1262843.do

[93] van Mierlo LAJ, Greyling A, Zock PL, et al. Suboptimal potassium intake and potential impact on population BP. *Arch Intern Med* 2010; 170:1501-1502

[94] Yang Q, Liu T, Kuklina EV, et al. Sodium and potassium intake and mortality among U.S. adults. Prospective data from the Third National Health and Nutrition Examination Survey. *Arch Intern Med* 2011; 171:1183-1191.

[95] Silver LD and Farley TA. "Sodium and potassium intake. Mortality effects and policy implications," *Arch Intern Med* 2011; 171:1191-1192.

[96] http://www.nytimes.com/2012/06/03/opinion/sunday/we-only-think-we-know-the-truth-about-salt.html?_r=1&pagewanted=all&pagewanted=print

[97] It's Time to End the War on Salt by Melinda Wenner Moyer; *The Scientific American*—July 8, 2011

[98] Ibid.

Chapter 8

[99] http://www.livestrong.com/article/323499-why-have-a-low-fat-diet-in-hypertension/#ixzz1Rje0h7pZ

[100] Taubes, Gary, *Why We Get Fat,* Knopf, 2011; p. 187

[101] Ibid. pp.187–188

[102] Ibid. p. 190

[103] Ibid. pp. 190–191

[104] Ibid. p. 192

[105] A Reversal On Carbs by Marni Jameson: *Los Angeles Times*—December 20, 2010; http://articles.latimes.com/2010/dec/20/health/la-he-carbs-20101220

[106] Ibid.

[107] Ibid.

[108] In 1998, Dr. Heilbron published the first study named on the beneficial effects of a low-carb diet, which later became The South Beach Diet. This was landmark at the time. (http://www.jaccjournaloftheacc.com/article/S0735-1097(98)81029-2)

109 The Skinny On Fats by Mary G. Enig, PhD, and Sally Fallon @ http://www.westonaprice.org/know-your-fats/the-skinny-on-fats

110 http://en.wikipedia.org/wiki/Monounsaturated_fat

111 The Skinny On Fats by Mary G. Enig, PhD, and Sally Fallon @ http://www.westonaprice.org/know-your-fats/the-skinny-on-fats

112 http://www.healthyeatingontherun.com/good-fat.html

113 The Skinny On Fats by Mary G. Enig, PhD, and Sally Fallon @ http://www.westonaprice.org/know-your-fats/the-skinny-on-fats

114 http://www.healthyeatingontherun.com/good-fat.html

115 The Skinny On Fats by Mary G. Enig, PhD, and Sally Fallon @ http://www.westonaprice.org/know-your-fats/the-skinny-on-fats

116 http://www.willardswater.com/newsletters/July09WebVersion.pdf

117 Ibid.

118 http://www.hsph.harvard.edu/nutritionsource/nutrition-news/transfats/

119 The Skinny On Fats by Mary G. Enig, PhD and Sally Fallon @ http://www.westonaprice.org/know-your-fats/the-skinny-on-fats

120 Ibid.

121 http://www.menshealth.com/health/saturated-fat

122 *Good Calories, Bad Calories* by Gary Taubes; p. 27, (Anchor, 2008)

123 *Why We Get Fat* by Gary Taubes; p. 182

124 http://www.menshealth.com/health/saturated-fat/page/3

125 Ibid

126 http://www.nytimes.com/2002/07/07/magazine/what-if-it-s-all-been-a-big-fat-lie.html

127 According to Dr. Mary Enig: "The best evidence indicates that our intake of PUFAs should not be more than approximately four percent of total calories as compared to native populations in temperate and tropical regions whose intake of polyunsaturated oils comes from the small amounts found in legumes, grains, nuts, green vegetables, fish, olive oil and animal fats but not from commercial vegetable oils." From The Skinny On Fats by Mary G. Enig, PhD, and Sally Fallon @ http://www.westonaprice.org/know-your-fats/skinny-on-fats

128 Ibid.

129 http://www.gfo.ca/Community/ConsumerResourcesforCorn.aspx

130 http://www.ninds.nih.gov/disorders/stroke/detail_stroke.htm

131 Study Raises Questions about Dietary Fats and Heart Disease Guidance; *Science Daily*—February 5, 2013

132 Hibbeln JR. Hong Lin Y, Alvheim AR. A century of change in linoleic acid: Endocannabinoids, obesity and addiction. National Institute on Alcohol Abuse and Alcoholism, U.S.A.

133 *Nutrition Week* 3/22/91 21:12; http://www.westonaprice.org/basics/myths-a-truths-about-nutrition

134 Felton, CV, et al.,"Dietary polyunsaturated fatty acids and composition of human aortic plaques." Lancet 1994 Oct 29; 344:1195

135 http://www.pbs.org/wgbh/pages/frontline/shows/diet/interviews/willett.html#ixzz1UblW4fu4

[136] Ripich, Stefan and Jim Healthy, *The 30-Day Diabetes Cure* Jim Healthy Publications, NM 2010; p. 97

[137] Ibid.

[138] Ibid.

[139] Ibid. p. 124

[140] Boughton, Barbara,"Processed meat linked to increased stroke risk"; adapted from Medscape Medical News—a professional news service of WebMD—August 19, 2011

[141] Ripich, Stefan and Jim Healthy, *The 30-Day Diabetes Cure* Jim Healthy Publications, NM 2010; p. 125

[142] http://www.cholesterol-and-health.com/Vitamin-D.html

[143] Does Supplementation of Diet with Fish Oil Reduce Blood Pressure? A Meta-Analysis of Controlled Clinical Trials; published by *JAMA Internal Medicine* (formerly: *Archives of Internal Medicine*) June 28, 1993, Vol. 153, No. 12—published online at http://archinte.jamanetwork.com/article.aspx?articleid=617401

Chapter 9

[144] Taubes, *Why We get Fat*; pp. 180–181

[145] Ibid. p. 181

[146] Ibid.

[147] *Good Calories, Bad Calories* by Gary Taubes; pp. 148–149

[148] Ibid.

[149] Ibid.

[150] Ibid. p. 150

[151] Ibid. p. 151

[152] Ibid. p. 145

[153] Ibid. p. 145

[154] Ibid. pp. 145–146

[155] "Fructose Consumption Increases Risk Factors for Heart Disease: Study Suggests US Dietary Guideline for Upper Limit of Sugar Consumption Is Too High," *ScienceDaily* (July 28, 2011).

[156] Ibid.

[157] Broadcast on Feb. 4, 2010

[158] http://articles.mercola.com/sites/articles/archive/2010/07/22/high-fructose-diet-contributes-to-high-blood-pressure.aspx

[159] http://articles.mercola.com/sites/articles/archive/2010/03/13/richard-johnson-interview.aspx

[160] Ibid.

[161] Ibid

[162] Insulin Resistance Can Predict Hypertension Development, Wake Forest Researchers Report; *ScienceDaily* (Nov. 17, 2000)

[163] *The 30-Day Diabetes Cure*; pp. 89–91

[164] Ibid.

[165] Ibid.

[166] *Why We Get Fat;* p. 177

[167] Ibid. pp. 177–178

[168] http://www.proteinpower.com/drmike/ketones-and-ketosis/metabolism-and-ketosis/

[169] *Why We Get Fat*; p. 78

[170] Individual Treatment Goals in Type 2 Diabetes by Jill Shuman published in MedPage Today online at http://www.medpagetoday.com/resource-center/diabetes/Making-Personal-Individual-Treatment-Goals-Type-2-Diabetes/a/31637 and Rethinking "Normal" Blood Sugar Levels by Beth Levine published in Baseline of Health Foundation's *Daily Health Tips* Newsletter; October 10, 2012, online at http://world-food-cooking.blogspot.com/2012/10/rethinking-normal-blood-sugar-levels.html

[171] http://emedicine.medscape.com/article/127943-overview

[172] *Why We Get Fat*; p. 187

[173] http://health.usnews.com/health-news/diet-fitness/heart/articles/2010/04/21/should-the-food-industry-ban-added-salt-and-sugar

[174] *Why We Get Fat*; pp. 193–194, 187

[175] http://www.guyleechfitness.com/Latest/the-metabolic-syndrome-more-evidence-of-the-dangers.html

[176] http://www.uthct.edu/newsinfo/release.asp?id=540

[177] Glucose tolerance and mortality: comparison of WHO and American Diabetes Association diagnostic criteria. The DECODE study group. European Diabetes Epidemiology Group. Diabetes Epidemiology: Collaborative analysis Of Diagnostic criteria in Europe. http://www.ncbi.nlm.nih.gov/pubmed/10466661

[178] Khaw KT, et al. Association of hemoglobin A1c with cardiovascular disease acute mortality in adults: the European prospective investigation into cancer in Norfolk. *Ann Intern Med.* 2004 Sep 21;141(6):413-20. pp. 395

[179] McGlothin, P, Averill M. Glucose Control: The Sweet Spot in Longevity. *The CR Way: Using the Secrets of Calorie Restriction for a Longer, Healthier Life.* NY: HarperCollins; 2008:57-78.

[180] Bjornholt JV, Erikssen G, Aaser E, et al. Fasting blood glucose: an underestimated risk factor for cardiovascular death. Results from a 22-year follow-up of healthy nondiabetic men. Diabetes Care. 1999 Jan;22(1):45-9.

[181] "The Lie That's Killing Us: Pre-Diabetes" by Riva Greenberg; Huffington Post—Posted: 05/29/2013

[182] AACE: CAD Risk for Pre-Diabetes Similar to Diabetes—http://www.diabetesincontrol.com/index.php?option=com_content&view=article&id=14598&catid=1&Itemid=17

[183] Jessani S, et al. Should oral glucose tolerance testing be mandatory following acute myocardial infarction? *Int J Clin Pract.* 2007 Apr;61(4):680-83. pp. 395

[184] Khaw KT, et al. "Association of hemoglobin A1c with cardiovascular disease acute mortality in adults: the European prospective investigation into cancer in Norfolk." *Annals of Internal Medicine*—2004 Sep 21;141(6):413-20. pp. 395

Chapter 10

[185] http://beyondhealth.com/CustomPages/articles/TheCholesterolMyth.pdf

[186] Inflammation and oxidation are interrelated processes. Inflammation is the body's normal response to injury, irritation, or infection. Chronic inflammation is an unhealthy condition that generates a constant supply of free radicals that overwhelm the body's antioxidant reserves and allow inflammation to run rampant everywhere.

[187] Low-Total-Fat Diet Did Not Reduce the Risk of Cardiovascular Events; Michael Pignone, MD, MPH—American Diabetes Assn. online at: http://clinical.diabetesjournals.org/content/24/3/143.full and "A low-fat dietary pattern intervention did not reduce breast cancer, colorectal cancer, or CVD in postmenopausal women" from *Evidence-Based Nursing* (Volume 9, Issue 4) online at http://ebn.bmj.com/content/9/4/112.extract

[188] http://beyondhealth.com/CustomPages/articles/TheCholesterolMyth.pdf

[189] http://www.pbs.org/wgbh/pages/frontline/shows/diet/interviews/willett.html#ixzz1TuKMGkan

[190] Renaud S, de Lorgeril M, Delaye J, Guidollet J, Jacquard F, Mamelle N, Martin JL, Monjaud I, Salen P, Toubol P: Cretan Mediterranean diet for prevention of coronary heart disease. *American Journal of Clinical Nutrition* (1995) Jun; 61(6 Suppl):1360S-1367S. http://www.ncbi.nlm.nih.gov/pubmed/7754988

[191] de Lorgeril M, Salen, P, Martin JL, Monjaud I, Delaye J, Mamelle N. Mediterranean Diet, Traditional Risk Factors, and the Rate of Cardiovascular Complications after Myocardial Infarction: Final Report of the Lyon Diet Heart Study. *Circulation* (1999) 99(6):779-785. http://www.ncbi.nlm.nih.gov/pubmed/9989963

[192] Read more from the Mayo Clinic: http://www.mayoclinic.com/health/mediterranean-diet/CL00011

Chapter 11

[193] *What to Eat*, Marion Nestle; p 17 (North Point Press, 2007)

[194] "Plant-animal subsistence ratios and macronutrient energy estimations in worldwide hunter-gatherer diets," L Cordain, et al., *American Journal of Clinical Nutrition* March, 2000; Vol. 71, No.3.

[195] http://www.naturalnews.com/aspartame.html

[196] Chen, Jennifer, MD, et al.,"Fitness, fatness and systolic blood pressure," *Amer. Heart Journal,* Vol. 160, Issue 1, pp. 166-170, July 2010.

[197] http://news.bioscholar.com/2011/05/exercise-protects-heart-from-injury-through-nitric-oxide.html

[198] http://health.nytimes.com/health/guides/specialtopic/physical-activity/exercise's-effects-on-the-heart.html

[199] http://next-level-nutrition.com/?p=5000

Chapter 12

[200] http://www.johnshopkinshealthalerts.com/alerts/hypertension_stroke/JohnsHopkinsHealthAlertsHypertensionStroke_541-1.html

[201] http://dx.doi.org/10.1016/j.jff.2012.08.010

[202] http://nutritionistic.blogspot.com/2012/12/banana-nutrition-health-benefits.html

[203] http://www.msnbc.msn.com/id/41139434/ns/health-heart_health/t/blueberries-lower-chance-high-blood-pressure/

[204] http://articles.mercola.com/sites/articles/archive/2012/09/23/broccoli-health-benefits.aspx?e_cid=20120923_SNL_Art_1

[205] http://www.umm.edu/altmed/articles/celery-seed-000231.htm

[206] Sinatra, S. and Healthy, J., *The Healing Kitchen*, p. 209 (Bottom Line Books, 2012)

[207] Ibid.

[208] http://www.health-care-tips.org/herbal-medicines/parsley.htm

[209] http://www.cbsnews.com/8301-504763_162-57494718-10391704/flavonol-rich-dark-chocolate-may-help-reduce-blood-pressure/

[210] http://www.ehow.com/how_2071293_normalize-blood-pressure-apple-cider.html#ixzz2NAP4lRVZ

[211] http://www.livestrong.com/article/308115-how-use-apple-cider-vinegar-to-lower-high-blood-pressure/

[212] http://ireport.cnn.com/docs/DOC-708294

[213] http://www.medpagetoday.com/Cardiology/Hypertension/34859

[214] http://www.redorbit.com/news/health/1112697824/yogurt-blood-pressure-092012/

[215] *The Healing Kitchen*; p. 206

[216] http://www.whfoods.com/genpage.php?tname=foodspice&dbid=60

[217] http://umm.edu/health/medical/altmed/herb/garlic

[218] http://www.nlm.nih.gov/medlineplus/druginfo/natural/961.html

[219] *The Healing Kitchen*; p. 210

[220] Ibid.

[221] Ibid.

[222] http://jn.nutrition.org/content/136/12/2987.abstract?sid=3e9f0f71-b173-422f-b13f-8cfe98f23701

[223] http://www.whfoods.com/genpage.php?pfriendly=1&tname=disease&dbid=3

[224] http://www.nutraingredients.com/Research/Resveratrol-could-protect-against-stroke-says-lab-study

[225] *The Healing Kitchen*; p. 206

[226] http://www.livestrong.com/article/322686-olive-oil-and-high-blood-pressure/

[227] *The Healing Kitchen;* p. 206

[228] http://www.naturalnews.com/022987.html

[229] http://www.nutraingredients-usa.com/Research/Orange-juice-flavanone-may-benefit-heart-health-Study?utm_source=RSS_text_news

[230] http://www.livestrong.com/article/368733-can-papaya-lower-blood-pressure/

[231] *The Healing Kitchen;* pp. 206–207

[232] http://www.organicfacts.net/health-benefits/vegetable/health-benefits-of-potato.html

[233] *The Healing Kitchen*; p. 209

[234] *The Healing Kitchen*; p. 206

[235] www.bcerc.org/.../BCERC.FactSheet_Phytoestrogen_Genistein.pdf

[236] http://www.thehealthierlife.co.uk/natural-health-articles/high-blood-pressure/b-vitamin-lower-risk-hypertension-00732.html

[237] *The Healing Kitchen*; p. 210

[238] http://pubs.acs.org/doi/abs/10.1021/jf026186y

[239] http://www.bastyrcenter.org/content/view/984/

[240] Whitaker, MD, Julian, *Reversing Hypertension*; Warner Books, 2000; p.144

[241] http://www.medscape.com/viewarticle/570051

[242] *The Healing Kitchen*; p. 210

[243] http://www.foods-healing-power.com/green-tea-blood-pressure.html

[244] *The Healing Kitchen*; p. 215

[245] http://naturalmedicinejournal.com/article_content.asp?article=215

[246] Ibid.

[247] http://www.thereadystore.com/katadyn-combi-water-filter

[248] http://healthss.wordpress.com/2011/06/01/himalayan-crystal-salt/

Chapter 13

[249] http://www.stroke.org/site/PageServer?pagename=STROKE

[250] http://www.nature.com/jhh/journal/v27/n8/full/jhh20136a.html

[251] http://www.nutritionalreviews.org/alphalipoic_acid.htm

[252] http://www.bastyrcenter.org/content/view/1029/

[253] http://www.theheart.org/article/1509041.do

[254] Ibid.

[255] http://www.naturalnews.com/030039_high_blood_pressure_prevention.html

[256] http://www.ncbi.nlm.nih.gov/pubmed/23169470

[257] http://altmedicine.about.com/od/completeazindex/a/grapeseed.htm

[258] http://www.umm.edu/altmed/articles/grape-seed-000254.htm

[259] http://nccam.nih.gov/health/grapeseed/ataglance.htm

[260] http://www.umm.edu/altmed/articles/hawthorn-000256.htm

[261] http://www.smart-publications.com/articles/hawthorn-the-safe-heart-tonic-that-improves-blood-supply-to-the-heart

[262] http://www.webmd.com/vitamins-supplements/ingredientmono-875-L-ARGININE.aspx?activeIngredientId=875&activeIngredientName=L-ARGININE

[263] http://www.mayoclinic.com/health/fish-oil/NS_patient-fishoil

[264] http://www.umm.edu/altmed/articles/omega-3-000316.htm

[265] http://www.health.harvard.edu/fhg/updates/update0705c.shtml

[266] http://www.ext.colostate.edu/pubs/foodnut/09355.html

[267] http://ezinearticles.com/?Naturally-Lower-High-Blood-Pressure-HBP-With-Vitamin-B&id=785840

[268] http://www.sciencedaily.com/releases/1999/12/991221080724.htm

Chapter 14

[269] http://www.psychologytoday.com/articles/200602/make-gratitude-adjustment

[270] http://heartdisease.about.com/od/hypertension/a/acupunctureBP.htm

[271] http://nccam.nih.gov/health/taichi/introduction.htm

[272] http://www.ncbi.nlm.nih.gov/pubmed/12943180

[273] http://nccam.nih.gov/health/yoga/introduction.htm

[274] http://www.mayoclinic.com/health/high-blood-pressure/HI00016

Chapter 15

[275] http://www.epa.gov/oia/toxics/pop.htm

[276] Ibid.

[277] Sources of Hormone-Disrupting Chemicals in San Francisco Bay; Environmental Working Group—July 12, 2007, online at: http://www.ewg.org/research/down-drain

[278] Sources of Hormone-Disrupting Chemicals in San Francisco Bay; Environmental Working Group—July 12, 2007 online at: http://www.ewg.org/research/down-drain

[279] Comments for Public Meeting on "International Cooperation on Cosmetics Regulations (ICCR) Preparations"—Environmental Working Group; Thursday, June 19, 2008, online at: http://www.ewg.org/news/testimony-official-correspondence/comments-public-meeting-international-cooperation-cosmetics

[280] Hooper, Rowan, "Top 11 compounds in US drinking water" *New Scientist*, 12 January 2009

[281] http://chicagoist.com/2010/04/18/trib_tackles_gender_bending_chemica.php

[282] http://www.treehugger.com/files/2009/08/todays-toxin-atrazine.php

[283] http://www.webmd.com/balance/natural-liver-detox-diets-liver-cleansing?page=2

[284] http://www.ehow.com/way_5840323_chiropractic-liver-detox.html

[285] http://www.healthyhealing.com/herbs-articles-safety/bid/175715/Self-Tests

[286] http://www.wholehealthchicago.com/knowledge-base/m/milk-thistle/

[287] http://aje.oxfordjournals.org/cgi/content/short/164/9/898

[288] http://www.renegadeneurologist.com/turmeric-and-brain-health/

[289] http://www.thereadystore.com/katadyn-combi-water-filter

[290] http://www.consumerreports.org/cro/magazine-archive/december-2009/food/bpa/overview/bisphenol-a-ov.htm

[291] http://www.telegraph.co.uk/news/uknews/1555173/Body-absorbs-5lb-of-make-up-chemicals-a-year.html

[292] http://www.nhregister.com/articles/2008/11/26/opinion/doc492d4214d2c89772087215.txt

[293] http://www.ncbi.nlm.nih.gov/pmc/articles/PMC3018511/

Part 2, Day One

[294] http://www.bmj.com/content/344/bmj.e1327

[295] http://www.mayoclinic.com/health/high-blood-pressure/HI00016

Day Two

[296] http://www.dukehealth.org/health_library/news/5687

Day Three

[297] http://www.webmd.com/diet/news/20050613/drink-more-diet-soda-gain-more-weight

[298] http://shine.yahoo.com/healthy-living/sweet-sodas-soft-drinks-may-raise-risk-depression-183000091.html

[299] http://aspartame.mercola.com/

[300] http://www.nytimes.com/2012/06/06/opinion/evolutions-sweet-tooth.html

Day Four

[301] Hypertension 2008; DOI: 10.1161/HYPERTENSIONAHA.107.103523. Available at: http://hyper.ahajournals.org.

[302] http://www.medpagetoday.com/Cardiology/Hypertension/38465

[303] http://articles.mercola.com/sites/articles/archive/2012/09/23/broccoli-health-benefits.aspx?e_cid=20120923_SNL_Art_1

[304] http://www.nlm.nih.gov/medlineplus/druginfo/natural/961.html

[305] http://www.livestrong.com/article/483532-parsley-blood-pressure/

[306] *The Healing Kitchen* by Sinatra and Healthy; Bottom Line Books, 2012; p. 210

Day Seven

[307] New Evidence That Egg White Protein May Help High Blood Pressure; ScienceDaily—April 9, 2013. http://www.sciencedaily.com/releases/2013/04/130409155814.htm

Day Eight

[308] Brooks, Megan "Fiber-rich diet may protect against stroke" April 9, 2013. http://www.theheart.org/article/1526195.do

Day Ten

[309] http://www.holisticmed.com/aspartame/abuse/methanol.html and http://www.holisticmed.com/aspartame/abuse/

[310] http://ajpregu.physiology.org/content/295/5/R1370

[311] http://www.iatp.org/documents/table-a-total-mercury-detected-in-55-brand-name-foods-and-beverages-high-in-hfcs

[312] http://www.washingtonpost.com/wp-dyn/content/article/2009/01/26/AR2009012601831.html

Day 12

[313] http://www.whfoods.com/genpage.php?tname=foodspice&dbid=98

[314] http://www.sciencedirect.com/science?_ob=ArticleURL&_udi=B6T6R-4CWBKYV-2&_user=10&_coverDate=05%2F31%2F2005&_rdoc=1&_fmt=high&_orig=search&_sort=d&_docanchor=&view=c&_searchStrId=1331517642&_rerunOrigin=google&_acct=C000050221&_version=1&_urlVersion=0&_userid=10&md5=ebbd6626cbee00d825c94ef44c6cdf92

[315] http://jn.nutrition.org/cgi/content/abstract/138/9/1671

Day 13

[316] http://www.medicalnewstoday.com/articles/260247.php

Day 14

[317] http://www.ncbi.nlm.nih.gov/pubmed?orig_cmd=Search&term=%22The+American+journal+of+medicine%22%5BJour%5D+AND+77%5Bvolume%5D+AND+785%5Bpage%5D+AND+1984%5Bpdat%5D

[318] http://shared.web.emory.edu/whsc/news/releases/2011/05/exercise-protects-the-heart-via-nitric-oxide.html

Day 15

[319] http://www.uea.ac.uk/mac/comm/media/press/2011/january/berries

Day 18

[320] http://www.cnn.com/2011/HEALTH/06/24/sitting.shorten.life/

Day 20

[321] http://www.npr.org/blogs/health/2013/04/25/178407883/gut-bacterias-belch-may-play-a-role-in-heart-disease

Day 21

[322] http://www.journalsleep.org/ViewAbstract.aspx?pid=27857

[323] http://www.psychologytoday.com/articles/200602/make-gratitude-adjustment

Day 22

[324] http://www.nytimes.com/health/guides/symptoms/depression/print.html

[325] http://www.webmd.com/healthy-aging/omega-3-fatty-acids-fact-sheet?page=2

[326] Sandyk, Reuven, MD. (1992) *International Journal of Neuroscience*, Volume 67

[327] http://umm.edu/health/medical/altmed/supplement/5hydroxytryptophan-5htp

Day 24

[328] http://www.epa.gov/oia/toxics/pop.htm

[329] http://www.epa.gov/oia/toxics/pop.html

[330] http://www.epa.gov/oia/toxics/pop.htm#table

[331] http://www.ncbi.nlm.nih.gov/pmc/articles/PMC1247187/

[332] http://www.ncbi.nlm.nih.gov/pmc/articles/PMC1332699/

[333] Reprinted (updated and excerpted) with permission from *Vitality Magazine*, www.vitalitymagazine.com

[334] http://www.epa.gov/osw/hazard/wastemin/minimize/factshts/dioxfura.pdf

[335] http://www.ewg.org/skindeep/myths-on-cosmetics-safety/

[336] www.perfumerbook.com/Dark%20Side%20of%20Fragrance's.pdf

[337] http://www.womensconference.org/7-healthy-lifestyle-tips-on

[338] http://greencentury.com/wp-content/uploads/2013/05/bpareport2010.pdf

[339] http://www.telegraph.co.uk/news/uknews/1555173/Body-absorbs-5lb-of-make-up-chemicals-a-year.html

[340] http://ajrccm.atsjournals.org/cgi/content/full/176/8/735

[341] Hooper, Rowman, "Top 11 compounds in US drinking water," *New Scientist*, 12 January 2009.

[342] http://www.unc.edu/courses/2009fall/envr/442/001/Pesticide%20Toxicity%2005nov2009.pdf

Day 25

[343] http://www.nutraingredients.com/Research/Magnesium-may-benefit-blood-pressure-in-hypertensives

[344] http://www.livestrong.com/article/464027-what-is-l-arginine-hcl/

[345] http://www.webmd.com/vitamins-supplements/ingredientmono-875-L-ARGININE.aspx?activeIngredientId=875&activeIngredientName=L-ARGININE

[346] http://lpi.oregonstate.edu/infocenter/othernuts/coq10/

[347] http://www.mayoclinic.com/health/coenzyme-q10/NS_patient-coenzymeq10/DSECTION=evidence

[348] http://lpi.oregonstate.edu/infocenter/othernuts/coq10/

[349] Duffy, Stephen J., et al. Treatment of hypertension with ascorbic acid. The Lancet, Vol. 354, December 11, 1999, pp. 2048-49 (research letter)

Day 26

[350] http://www.upi.com/Health_News/2012/09/13/Anger-management-lower-blood-pressure/UPI-66821347515289/#ixzz2LH4cXlqg

Day 27

[351] http://benpercent-musingaloud.blogspot.com/2010/08/note-on-cocao-vs-cocoa.html

[352] "Key to Changing Habits Is in Environment, Not Willpower, Duke Expert Says," DukeToday, Dec. 17, 2007; http://news.duke.edu/2007/12/habit.html

Day 28

[353] http://www.health.harvard.edu/special_health_reports/simple-changes-big-rewards-a-practical-easy-guide-for-healthy-happy-living

[354] http://www.health.harvard.edu/special_health_reports/simple-changes-big-rewards-a-practical-easy-guide-for-healthy-happy-living

Appendix A

[355] http://www.medicalnewstoday.com/releases/70445.php

[356] http://www.livestrong.com/article/244400-side-effects-of-renin-inhibitors/

Appendix E

[357] http://www.johnshopkinshealthalerts.com/alerts/hypertension_stroke/JohnsHopkinsHealthAlertsHypertensionStroke_1458-1.html

[358] http://www.ncbi.nlm.nih.gov/pubmed/20537171##

[359] http://www.nejm.org/doi/full/10.1056/NEJMoa1200303?query=featured_home&

[360] http://www.ucsf.edu/news/2010/05/5986/type-2-diabetes-cholesterol-heart-disease-kidney-risks-paleolithic-diet

Appendix G

[361] http://ajcn.nutrition.org/content/81/3/541.full

[362] http://www.ncbi.nlm.nih.gov/pubmed/17292730

[363] http://www.nutraingredients.com/Research/Resveratrol-could-protect-against-stroke-says-lab-study

INDEX

ACKNOWLEDGMENTS

From Dr. Heilbron:

- To my wife, Angelique Hart, MD, I love you.

- To my children — Onima, Karina and Roy III, you guys are awesome.

- To my parents, Roy and Celia, thanks for having me and for your amazing support all these years.

- To my brother, Karl, you rock.

- To Jim, thank you for your patience and letting me fulfill my destiny to finally get this thing going. We are going to change the world of medicine and teach people how to move "keep getting better."

- To my friends Jorge, Yaffa, Pete, Bill, Paco, Kevin, Rachel, Orlando, Eduardo, Robyn, Little Grandmother — thanks for your friendship.

- To my departed spiritual friend, Mahavatar Babaji, for showing me how to be in this world.

- To my patients in Miami Beach and Santa Fe, thank you for teaching me and allowing me to share in your lives.

- To Arthur Agatston, MD, for allowing me to help in the creation of what became The South Beach Diet and for showing me what is possible.

- To Adhemar Hart, MD, for showing us how to do chelation and opening the world of holistic/integrative/alternative medicine to us.

- To Dr. Norman Shealy MD, for your pioneering efforts in holistic and energy medicine, and for your ongoing contributions to the advancement of medicine.

From Jim Healthy:

- To Carlos Mendivil and Miguel Yi-Sandino for layout and cover design, and Suzanne Herzstam for her eagle-eye proofreading.

- To Michael Cawdrey for his excellent scientific research and feedback.

- To Tony (Gervasio) Lamas MD, my mentor, who trained me, later becoming a friend, for your dedication to completing this monumental task (TACT) and for letting me be a part of it; and

- To the seven billion people on Earth: Let's conquer today's "lifestyle diseases" so we can get on with other important things, like cooperating to make this planet a healthier place for our children and yours.

ABOUT THE AUTHORS

Roy Heilbron, MD, is board-certified in cardiology (2009), internal medicine (1993), and nuclear cardiology (1998). He is a Diplomat in Cardiovascular Disease of the American Board of Internal Medicine, a Diplomat of the American Board of Holistic Medicine, a certified chelation therapist, former Clinical Assistant Professor, University of Miami School of Medicine, and current Clinical Assistant Professor of Medicine, University of New Mexico School of Medicine. One of the original National Institutes of Health researchers for the TACT (Trial to Assess Chelation Therapy) study, he is the co-author of *Healing Heart Disease with Chelation Therapy* (2012) and is the subject of a documentary film on chelation therapy entitled "Unleaded."

Dr. Heilbron is also a co-developer and original researcher of The South Beach Diet, in collaboration with Arthur Agatston, MD. He is also the winner of numerous awards and citations, including the Genentech Research Award and the Paul Furlong Clinical Medicine Award, awarded to the outstanding physician of Mount Sinai Medical Center, Miami Beach, Florida.

He is currently in private practice in Santa Fe, New Mexico.

Jim Healthy™ is a health coach and activist, medical reporter, publisher, and author. He is the founder and editor of JimHealthy.com and MyHealingKitchen.com, where he coaches and instructs readers on how to improve their personal health through wiser diet and lifestyle choices.

Jim is the co-author of *The Healthy Body Book* (Penguin, 1991), *Arthritis Interrupted* with Stephen Sinatra, MD (Jim Healthy Publications, 2009), *The 30-Day Diabetes Cure* (co-authored with Stefan Ripich, ND, CNP, 2010), *The Diabetes Healing Cookbook* (Jim Healthy Publications, 2010), and *Healing Heart Disease with Chelation Therapy* (co-authored with Roy Heilbron, MD, 2012).